Study Guide
Linton

Introduction to Medical-Surgical Nursing

Fifth Edition

Nancy K. Maebius, PhD, RN
Consultant
Galen College of Nursing
San Antonio, Texas

Reviewers

Michele Cislo, MA, RN
Associate Professor,
Union County College
Plainfield, NJ

Dolores Cotton, MSN, RN
Practical Nursing Coordinator
Meridian Technology Center
Stillwater, Oklahoma

ELSEVIER
SAUNDERS

ELSEVIER
SAUNDERS

3251 Riverport Lane
St. Louis, Missouri 63043

Study Guide
Introduction to Medical-Surgical Nursing, 5th Edition   ISBN: 978-1-4377-2214-7

Copyright © 2012, 2007, 2003, 2000, 1995 by Saunders, an imprint of Elsevier Inc.

Notices

Knowledge and best practice in this field are constantly changing. As new research and experience broaden our understanding, changes in research methods, professional practices, or medical treatment may become necessary.

Practitioners and researchers must always rely on their own experience and knowledge in evaluating and using any information, methods, compounds, or experiments described herein. In using such information or methods they should be mindful of their own safety and the safety of others, including parties for whom they have a professional responsibility.

With respect to any drug or pharmaceutical products identified, readers are advised to check the most current information provided (i) on procedures featured or (ii) by the manufacturer of each product to be administered, to verify the recommended dose or formula, the method and duration of administration, and contraindications. It is the responsibility of practitioners, relying on their own experience and knowledge of their patients, to make diagnoses, to determine dosages and the best treatment for each individual patient, and to take all appropriate safety precautions.

To the fullest extent of the law, neither the Publisher nor the authors, contributors, or editors, assume any liability for any injury and/or damage to persons or property as a matter of products liability, negligence or otherwise, or from any use or operation of any methods, products, instructions, or ideas contained in the material herein.

Executive Editor: Teri Hines Burnham
Associate Developmental Editor: Jennifer Shropshire
Publishing Services Manager: Deborah Vogel
Project Manager: John Gabbert
Designer: Margaret Reid

Printed in the United States of America
Last digit is the print number: 9 8 7 6 5 4 3 2 1

To my family:

My husband, Jed

My children, Stephen, Maria, Elizabeth, Tom, Brian, Justine, Andrew and Clayton

My grandchildren, Allison, Sarah, Jessica, Erica, George, Ella, Henry, Anna, Emma, Colter, Hudson, Stormy, and Mary John

To my vocational nursing students:

From you I have learned so much about thinking, learning, dedication, and commitment to nursing.

Preface

TO THE STUDENT

Welcome to the fifth edition of the Study Guide for *Introduction to Medical-Surgical Nursing*. This Study Guide is a companion to the textbook *Introduction to Medical-Surgical Nursing* by Adrianne Dill Linton, and is designed to help reinforce the material studied in the textbook and learned in class. It utilizes medical terminology and key chapter objectives originally introduced in the textbook. Each chapter in the Study Guide corresponds to a chapter in the textbook and contains questions and activities related to the chapter content. Some questions are easy and require simple recall; other exercises are more difficult and are designed to help you apply, analyze, and synthesize basic concepts. This requires you to view previously learned content and encourages you to integrate it with new content. Some of the questions encourage you to think critically and integrate a variety of concepts. By answering many different types of questions, you will establish a solid base of knowledge in medical-surgical nursing.

It is recommended that you work through all the exercises in every chapter. For some of you, working in groups may be valuable and make the learning process more enjoyable. Student-to-student interaction often encourages active learning.

This new edition brings a greater focus on preparation for the NCLEX-PN examination. Many new alternate format practice questions were added. The practice questions are reflective of the framework and the content identified in the current NCLEX-PN test plan. The beginning of each chapter lists the related NCLEX categories that are covered in that chapter. There are questions in every chapter related to the NCLEX client needs categories and subcategories.

A complete Answer Key has been provided for your instructor which includes the rationales for Part III, Challenge Yourself! Getting Ready for the NCLEX. Your Evolve site (http://evolve.elsevier.com/Linton/medsurg/) also has many helpful resources, including additional activities, a pharmacology tutorial, and NCLEX questions (see the inside cover of this Study Guide for a complete list of assets).

ORGANIZATION

The Study Guide chapters are divided into three parts: Part I, Mastering the Basics; Part II, Putting It All Together; and Part III, Challenge Yourself! Getting Ready for NCLEX.

Part I, Mastering the Basics, contains matching, multiple-response, labeling, diagram reading, and fill-in-the-blank questions related to major content areas in the corresponding textbook chapter. These exercises help you learn medical-surgical nursing knowledge. The questions in Part I are at the basic knowledge and comprehension levels.

Part II, Putting It All Together, contains multiple-choice and multiple-response questions that integrate the chapter content. Most of the questions in Part II are at the comprehension and application levels, and are related to basic pathophysiology and basic nursing content.

Part III, Challenge Yourself! Getting Ready for NCLEX contains multiple-choice, multiple-response, case studies, fill-in-the-blank calculations, ordering, and prioritizing questions that are related to the NCLEX client needs and integrated processes content. Because the practice of practical/vocational nursing involves application of knowledge, skills, and abilities, the majority of questions in Part III are written at the application or analysis levels of cognitive ability and are related to nursing application content.

Acknowledgments

Sincere thanks and appreciation go to the many individuals who have contributed to the publication of this Study Guide.

I thank my helpers at Elsevier: Executive Editor Teri Hines Burnham and Associate Developmental Editor Jennifer Shropshire for their continuous support and expert professional guidance. I also thank Jenn for keeping me on schedule with manuscript submission, and for her accessibility and encouragement. In addition, thank you to Lisa Hernandez, who was always one step ahead of me in producing the pages, and to Heather Rippetoe, Associate Developmental Editor, who helped me coordinate the Study Guide with the textbook.

I especially want to thank my family: Jed, Stephen, Elizabeth, Brian, and Andrew, and all of my 13 grandchildren, who provide unconditional support and humorous moments. My dog, Puff, and my cat, Rita, sat by my side as I have written all of the Study Guide editions, and I value their company.

Lastly, very special thanks go to my nursing students. I want to thank all of my nursing students at Galen College of Nursing, who have come to me since 1991 asking for extra help with practice questions in order to prepare for the NCLEX examination. Their questions, enthusiasm, commitment, and energy have helped me become a better teacher. I thank these students for sharing their ideas and thoughts with me. I am grateful for their dedication to nursing and providing nursing care.

Contents

The Health Care System

 Go to http://evolve.elsevier.com/Linton/medsurg/ for additional activities and exercises.

NCLEX CATEGORIES:

Safe and Effective Care Environment:
Coordinated Care, Safety and Infection Control

OBJECTIVES

1. Describe the organization of the health care system in the United States.
2. Describe the focus of public health services.
3. Discuss financing of health care in the United States, including Medicare and Medicaid programs.
4. Describe the components of the health care system that provide both outpatient and inpatient care and the types of service each system provides.
5. Describe the impact of cost-containment measures on the delivery of care.
6. Discuss the contribution nurses can make to cost containment.
7. Describe the six aims of health care.
8. Define the QSEN quality and safety competencies for nurses.
9. Explain the potential benefits of a national health information infrastructure.

PART I: MASTERING THE BASICS

A. Key Terms.
Match the definition in the numbered column with the most appropriate term in the lettered column.

1. _____ Provision of comprehensive health care at a reasonable cost through enrollment in HMO or PPO with incentives to reduce costs

2. _____ System of reimbursement standards for hospitals for care based on a fixed fee for a diagnostic category, regardless of cost

3. _____ Steps taken to prevent disease recurrence or complications of diagnosed disease or injury

4. _____ Project focused on patient-centered care, evidence-based practice, and informatics

5. _____ Fees for services at prenegotiated rates with health care providers in return for the number of patients brought into the health care system

6. _____ Steps taken to improve health and prevent disease and injury

7. _____ Program that provides health care services for needy, low-income, and disabled individuals with funds distributed at the state level

8. _____ Health insurance program administered by the federal government funded by Social Security payments

9. _____ Steps taken that focus on early detection and treatment of disease

A. Diagnosis-related group (DRG)
B. Medicaid
C. Medicare
D. Managed health care
E. Preferred provider group (PPO)
F. Quality and safety education for nurses (QSEN)
G. Primary prevention
H. Secondary prevention
I. Tertiary prevention

B. Prevention.

1. Which of the following are examples of primary prevention? Select all that apply.
   1. Providing Pap smears at reduced cost
   2. Educating people to wear seat belts
   3. Teaching a person with diabetes proper diet and foot care
   4. Educational programs to prevent people from smoking
   5. Use of physical therapy to prevent contractures in a stroke patient

PART II: PUTTING IT ALL TOGETHER

C. Multiple Choice/Multiple Response.

Choose the most appropriate answer or select all that apply.

1. Which age group of Americans is least likely to be covered by health insurance?
   1. Children
   2. Young adults
   3. Middle-aged adults
   4. Older adults

2. Which is the largest component of health care costs?
   1. Hospital care
   2. Prescription drugs
   3. Professional services
   4. Outpatient centers

3. Which statements refer to Medicare? Select all that apply.
   1. Funded by monthly premium from paycheck; funds matched by federal government
   2. Funded by federal, state, and local taxes
   3. Needy, low-income, disabled persons under age 65 and their dependent children
   4. All people 65 years and older and those younger than 65 who are disabled or have permanent kidney damage
   5. Administered by federal government
   6. Administered by both federal and state governments

4. Which of the following correctly describes skilled nursing facilities?
   1. A licensed nursing staff provides skilled care, including rehabilitative care
   2. Provide care for those who need observation during acute or unstable phase of illness
   3. Permit a high degree of independence with limited access to nursing care
   4. Residents' units have kitchen, but group meals are usually provided
   5. Purpose is to care for and provide palliative care to dying people
   6. Extended care for people who have the potential to regain function

5. A patient admitted to a skilled nursing facility asks who will be the main type of health care worker. Who provides the most patient care to residents in skilled nursing facilities?
   1. RNs
   2. LPNs
   3. Physical therapists
   4. Nursing assistants

6. Which of the following do health insurance companies, HMOs, and PPOs have in common?
   1. Health care service delivery for low-income people
   2. Delivery of health care services at a reasonable cost
   3. Establishment of ambulatory care centers
   4. Diagnosis-related groups (DRGs)

7. In which setting is the number of patients decreasing?
   1. Ambulatory care
   2. Home health
   3. Clinics
   4. Hospitals

8. A stroke patient who is aphasic will need the services of a(n):
   1. occupational therapist.
   2. physical therapist.
   3. speech therapist.
   4. social worker.

9. The focus of hospice care is to:
   1. extend life of the terminally ill.
   2. provide a better quality of life for dying patients and their families.
   3. provide assistance to families trying to manage chronic illness in the home.
   4. provide emergency care to dying patients at home.

10. Nursing care used by hospice nurses is centered around:
    1. palliative care.
    2. treatment of disease.
    3. preservation of life.
    4. infection control.

11. In public health, the focus of attention is on:
    1. emphasizing patients' rights.
    2. improving health of aggregates.
    3. increasing cost-sharing.
    4. decreasing home health care.

12. Since the beginning of cost-effective health care methods starting with DRGs, what method of health care delivery today is aimed at cost-effectiveness?
    1. Ambulatory care
    2. Long-term care
    3. Managed health care
    4. Extended care

13. Which of the following are outpatient settings? Select all that apply.
    1. Physicians' offices
    2. Ambulatory surgery centers
    3. Emergency departments
    4. Rehabilitation centers
    5. Long-term care facilities
    6. Mammography centers

14. One aim of primary prevention is to:
    1. promote health.
    2. detect disease early.
    3. treat disease to improve patient outcomes.
    4. prevent complications of disease.

PART III: CHALLENGE YOURSELF!

D. Getting Ready for NCLEX.

Choose the most appropriate answer or select all that apply.

1. Which statements relate to QSEN? Select all that apply.
   1. Minimize risk of harm to patients and providers
   2. Use technology to mitigate error and support decision-making
   3. Integrate best current evidence when providing nursing care
   4. Reduce waits and harmful delays for patients and providers
   5. Avoid waste of equipment, supplies, and energy
   6. Provide care that is equitable

2. Which type of health care treatment receives the most attention today?
   1. Health promotion
   2. Disease prevention
   3. Treatment of illness
   4. Home health care

3. What factors contribute to the nurse's role in cost-containment? Select all that apply.
   1. Nurses experience firsthand the organizational decisions made to control spending.
   2. Nurses emphasize safe and effective nursing care.
   3. Nurses participate in patient-centered care.
   4. Nurses provide private nursing care when needed.
   5. Nurses have direct, comprehensive, and ongoing contact with patients.
   6. Nurses identify strategies to streamline care and provide quality care with limited resources.

4. Which of the following describes a characteristic of managed care?
   1. Incentives to save costs
   2. Increased treatment of acute diseases
   3. Increased hospital care
   4. Decreased cost-sharing

5. Which conditions are included in the five most frequent reasons for hospitalization? Select all that apply.
   1. Surgery for fractures
   2. Cardiovascular disease
   3. Trauma from accidents
   4. Osteoporosis
   5. Depression
   6. Pneumonia

6. Why does the demand for professional home health care services continue to increase for all age categories? Select all that apply.
   1. Ambulatory surgery center services are decreasing.
   2. Health care costs are decreasing.
   3. Managed health care is focused on acute care.
   4. Hospitals are reducing the length of hospital stays.
   5. Increased need for prescription drugs.
   6. Early discharge with needs for special care.

7. The effects of managed care include:
   1. increase in fee-for-service.
   2. decrease in home health care.
   3. decreased focus on wellness.
   4. increased focus on prevention.

8. An older patient's son is considering taking his father with dementia to an adult day care center. He asks the nurse what the benefits would be. Which of the following are advantages of adult day care centers? Select all that apply.
   1. Provides a respite from constant caregiving.
   2. Provides primary skilled nursing services.
   3. Patients can continue to live at home and have supervision during the day.
   4. Current illnesses in patients are diagnosed and treated.
   5. Provides health promotion programs and nutritional meals.

9. Which type of medical insurance is appropriate to use for a 70-year-old patient recovering from a broken wrist?
   1. Medicare
   2. Medicaid
   3. Private insurance
   4. Social Security

10. The priority type of care for a 68-year-old patient who is on a rehabilitation unit following a stroke is:
    1. palliative care.
    2. acute care.
    3. assisted living care.
    4. skilled nursing care.

11. Which patient is entitled to receive Medicare insurance?
    1. 25-year-old patient with asthma
    2. 72-year-old patient with hypertension
    3. 60-year-old patient with pneumonia
    4. 55-year-old patient with brain injury

12. Which low-income patient is most likely to be eligible for Medicaid funding?
    1. 35-year-old patient with multiple sclerosis
    2. 65-year-old patient with a stroke
    3. 70-year-old patient with acute myocardial infarction
    4. 40-year-old patient with chronic allergies

13. A patient with a brain tumor is admitted to hospice care. Which are requirements for admission to hospice care? Select all that apply.
    1. A diagnosis of a terminal illness
    2. A prognosis of less than 12 months to live
    3. Treatment including chemotherapy
    4. IV infusions for antibiotics
    5. Informed consent by the physician to elect hospice care
    6. Placement of nasogastric tube for feedings

14. The purpose of hospice is to:
    1. provide home health care services to terminally ill patients.
    2. provide observation during acute or unstable phases of illness.
    3. enable patients to receive IVs and tube feedings at home.
    4. enable terminally ill patients to live as full a life as possible.

15. Which are Institute of Medicine (IOM) recommendations to reduce medication errors? Select all that apply.
    1. Better patient education
    2. Use of information technologies
    3. Better drug labeling and information sheets
    4. Increased use of informed consent
    5. Double-check of opioid administration

16. What accounts for the majority of preventable medical errors? Select all that apply.
    1. Individual carelessness
    2. System problems
    3. Health care process problems
    4. Lack of concentration

17. Which characteristics of a national health information infrastructure would prevent errors and allow nurses to learn from errors when they do occur? Select all that apply.
    1. Maintenance of complete patient database
    2. Use of electronic health records
    3. Rapid dissemination of best practices information
    4. Increased patient-centered care
    5. Use of teamwork
    6. Reduced wait times for patients

18. Which are aims for the 21st Century Health Care System? (Cited in the IOM's *Crossing the Quality Chasm*)? Select all that apply.
    1. Safe
    2. Effective
    3. Efficient
    4. Comprehensive
    5. Patient-centered
    6. Cost-contained

19. Which are included in the QSEN quality and safety competencies? Select all that apply.
    1. Primary nursing care
    2. Evidence-based practice
    3. Quality improvement
    4. Teamwork and collaboration
    5. Informatics
    6. Cost-containment

20. Using data to monitor the outcomes of care processes is an example of which QSEN competency?
    1. Teamwork
    2. Quality improvement
    3. Safety
    4. Informatics

21. A 66-year-old patient is admitted to the rehabilitation unit of a hospital following surgery for a fractured hip. Which type of preventive care is provided?
    1. Primary
    2. Secondary
    3. Tertiary
    4. Comprehensive

Patient Care Settings

Go to http://evolve.elsevier.com/Linton/medsurg/ for additional activities and exercises.

NCLEX CATEGORIES:

Safe and Effective Care Environment:
Coordinated Care, Safety and Infection Control

Psychosocial Integrity

Physiological Integrity: Basic Care and Comfort, Physiological Adaptation

OBJECTIVES

1. Describe the role of the nurse in community and home health, rehabilitation, and long-term care settings.
2. Differentiate community health and community-based nursing.
3. Describe the types of specialty care that nurses may provide in home health care.
4. Describe the principles of rehabilitation.
5. List the four levels of disability.
6. Discuss legislation passed to protect the rights of disabled persons.
7. Identify the goals of rehabilitation.
8. Name the members of the rehabilitation team.
9. List the types of long-term care facilities.
10. Discuss the effects of institutionalization on the elderly person.
11. Describe the principles of nursing home care in long-term residential facilities.

PART I: MASTERING THE BASICS

A. Key Terms.
Match the definition in the numbered column with the most appropriate term in the lettered column.

1. _____ Measurable loss of function, usually delineated to indicate a diminished capacity for work

2. _____ Physical or psychological disturbance in functioning

3. _____ Inability to perform one or more normal daily activities because of mental or physical disability

   A. Impairment
   B. Handicap
   C. Disability

B. Disability Terms.
Match the definition in the numbered column with the most appropriate term in the lettered column.

1. _____ Severe limitations in one or more activities of daily living (ADLs); unable to work

2. _____ Slight limitation in one or more ADLs; usually able to work

3. _____ Total disability characterized by near complete dependence on others for assistance with ADLs; unable to work

4. _____ Moderate limitation in one or more ADLs; able to work but workplace may need modifications

   A. Level I
   B. Level II
   C. Level III
   D. Level IV

PART II: PUTTING IT ALL TOGETHER

C.   Multiple Choice/Multiple Response.

Choose the most appropriate answer or select all that apply.

1. Which of the following basic criteria for home health care must be met to receive Medicare reimbursement? Select all that apply.
   1. Care must be continuous for 24 hours per day.
   2. Care must be skilled.
   3. Care must be reasonable and necessary.
   4. The patient must be homebound.
   5. The physician must authorize a plan of care.
   6. The patient must be bedridden.

2. Which are the five most common intravenous therapies that can be given in a home health setting? Select five that apply.
   1. Hydration
   2. Chemotherapy
   3. Blood transfusion
   4. Total parenteral nutrition (TPN)
   5. Antibiotics
   6. Platelet infusion
   7. Pain control

3. Which are examples of long-term care facilities? Select all that apply.
   1. Personal care homes
   2. Board and care homes
   3. Hospitals
   4. Nursing homes
   5. Assisted-living facilities
   6. Acute care facilities

4. Care delivered in a long-term care residential facility is based upon what three principles? Select three that apply.
   1. Maintenance of autonomy
   2. Prevention of illness
   3. Maintenance of function
   4. Treatment of disease
   5. Promotion of independence

5. Which are four levels of modern long-term residential care? Select four that apply.
   1. Domiciliary care
   2. Ambulatory care
   3. Sheltered housing
   4. Primary care
   5. Intermediate care
   6. Skilled care

6. What are positive responses to institutionalization of residents in long-term care facilities? Select all that apply.
   1. Increased depersonalization
   2. Improved nutrition
   3. Management of medical problems
   4. Surgical treatment of fractures
   5. Improved socialization
   6. Social withdrawal

7. By providing clear documentation of functional losses and goals for care, the nurse is meeting the Medicare criterion of:
   1. skilled care.
   2. reasonable and necessary care.
   3. homebound patient care.
   4. intermittent care.

PART III: CHALLENGE YOURSELF!

D.   Getting Ready for NCLEX.

Choose the most appropriate answer or select all that apply.

1. The focus in rehabilitation is to:
   1. restore maximal possible functioning.
   2. function independently.
   3. assist with ADLs.
   4. eliminate impairment.

2. People born without arms can perform ADLs by using their feet and assistive devices. These people are said to have:
   1. a disability.
   2. a handicap.
   3. paralysis.
   4. impairment.

3. An individual with an injured back who has a diminished capacity for work is classified as:
   1. handicapped.
   2. impaired.
   3. disabled.
   4. dependent.

4. Which actions play a role in preventing a secondary disability for a post-stroke patient at risk for falls? Select all that apply.
   1. Use of walker
   2. Passive range of motion exercises
   3. Exercise three times a day for 30 minutes
   4. Modifications of the environment
   5. Teach patient about use of call bell
   6. Keep the side rails up

5. A patient was hospitalized with a stroke and is being transferred to a rehabilitation facility. Which of the following are goals of rehabilitation? Select all that apply.
   1. Improve health status of communities or groups of people through public education
   2. Return disabled individuals to maximum state of functioning
   3. Prevent further disabilities in patients
   4. Provide specialty home care services
   5. Perform skilled nursing procedures in the home
   6. Respond promptly to patient requests for assistance with care

6. Which requires the LVN to call the RN case manager? Select all that apply.
   1. Changes in vital signs
   2. Changes in weight
   3. Wound parameter changes
   4. Signs of patient abuse or neglect

7. Which is an example of safety measures a nurse provides to prevent a secondary disability?
   1. Perform dressing changes for a postoperative patient
   2. Provide walker for post-stroke patient
   3. Teach patient with diabetes how to draw up insulin in a syringe
   4. Remove small rugs for patient who has had a hip replacement

8. Which nursing interventions are examples of the long-term residential care principle of maintenance of autonomy? Select all that apply.
   1. Place a urinal near the bed for immobile, incontinent patients.
   2. Allow nursing home residents to assist in establishing care goals.
   3. Give long-term care residents choices in activities.
   4. Explore factors that may be responsible for the patient's incontinence.
   5. Set specific goals for each resident that encourage independence.

9. A health care team with one RN, one LVN, and a nursing assistant are working together in a clinic. Which of the following can be performed by an LVN that cannot be performed by a nursing assistant? Select all that apply.
   1. Development of a teaching plan
   2. Comprehensive patient assessment
   3. Administration of chemotherapy
   4. Sterile wound dressing change
   5. Insertion of Foley catheter
   6. Focused patient assessment

10. Which examples of secondary disabilities in a patient with a stroke is the nurse planning to prevent? Select all that apply.
    1. Eye infection
    2. Pneumonia
    3. Paralysis
    4. Pressure ulcers
    5. Limb contractures
    6. Urinary incontinence

11. Which are considered to be skilled nursing procedures? Select all that apply.
    1. Unsterile dressing changes
    2. Teaching a patient to draw up insulin
    3. Foley catheter insertion
    4. Enema administration
    5. Venipuncture
    6. Injecting insulin

12. A patient rings the call bell. What is the first action the nurse should take to prevent the patient feeling indignity?
    1. Knock on the patient's door before entering.
    2. Talk with the patient about events inside and outside the long-term care facility.
    3. Simplify language and activities for the patient and avoid baby talk.
    4. Give the patient some flexibility and measure of control in the daily activities.

13. A patient in a long-term care facility exhibits new behaviors that include staying in bed most of the day, expressing difficulty with walking, and losing conversational skills. Which effect of institutionalization is this patient exhibiting?
    1. Social withdrawal
    2. Indignity
    3. Regression
    4. Depersonalization

14. A 72-year-old patient who has had a recent stroke has been transferred to a rehabilitation facility. The nurse notices an unused walker in the corner of the room. What referral needs to be made to improve his mobility?
    1. Physical therapist may need to increase strengthening exercises and gait training
    2. Social worker to address fears of the patient
    3. Speech therapist to improve communication
    4. Occupational therapist to help patient improve fine motor skills

15. What can the nurse do to maintain autonomy in the patient in long-term care? Select all that apply.
    1. Set up flexible routine with the patient.
    2. Allow the patient to decide the time of his bath.
    3. Select specific goals for the patient.
    4. Plan with the patient hours to watch television.

Legal and Ethical Considerations

chapter

3

e Go to http://evolve.elsevier.com/Linton/medsurg/ for additional activities and exercises.

NCLEX CATEGORIES:

Safe and Effective Care Environment:
Coordinated Care, Safety and Infection Control

OBJECTIVES

1. Define ethics, bioethics, values, morality, moral uncertainty, moral distress, moral outrage, and moral or ethical dilemma.
2. Explain the principles of ethics: autonomy, justice, fidelity, beneficence, and nonmaleficence.
3. Explain how values are formed.
4. Explain how values clarification is useful in nursing practice.
5. Discuss the relationship between culture and values.
6. Describe the following philosophical bases for ethics: deontology, utilitarianism, feminist ethics, and ethics of care.
7. Describe the steps in processing ethical dilemmas.
8. Describe the role of institutional ethics committees.
9. Explain the role of the licensed vocational nurse/licensed practical nurse (LVN/LPN) in relation to informed consent.

PART I: MASTERING THE BASICS

A. Key Terms.
Match the definition in the numbered column with the most appropriate term in the lettered column.

1. _____ Principles or standards shared by members of a society that determine what is desirable or worthwhile

2. _____ Shared ideas of what is right and good

3. _____ Ethical questions related to health care

4. _____ Belief that one's own culture is superior to others

A. Ethnocentrism
B. Values
C. Bioethics
D. Morality

B. Ethics Key Terms.
Match the basic concept of ethics in the numbered column with the proper label in the lettered column.

1. _____ Do no harm
2. _____ Obligation to do good
3. _____ Obligation to be fair to everyone
4. _____ Right to make one's own decisions
5. _____ Obligation to be faithful to agreements
6. _____ Telling the truth

A. Veracity
B. Beneficence
C. Justice
D. Nonmaleficence
E. Fidelity
F. Autonomy

C. Legal Terms.
Match the definition in the numbered column with the most appropriate term in the lettered column.

1. _____ Civil or criminal law
2. _____ Result of judicial decisions made when individual cases are decided in the courts
3. _____ Rules created by administrative bodies such as state boards of nursing
4. _____ Civil wrong against a person or property
5. _____ Conduct falling below the standard of care
6. _____ Condition when injury was caused by the nurse's failure to carry out the duty
7. _____ Spoken false information that could damage a person's reputation
8. _____ Written false information that could damage a person's reputation

A. Common law
B. Malpractice
C. Negligence
D. Regulatory law
F. Tort
G. Slander
H. Libel

D. Negligence.
Which of the following are common negligence errors? Select all that apply.
1. Failure to give complete report to oncoming shifts.
2. Restraining a patient against his wishes.
3. Failure to use aseptic technique when required.
4. Improper release of medical information.
5. Medicating a patient to keep him quiet.
6. Falls resulting in injury to a patient.

E. Autonomy.
Which of the following are related to the recognition of autonomy? Select all that apply.
1. Reporting a coworker who is impaired
2. Advance directives
3. Patient's right to refuse treatment
4. Patient's right to expect that staff will not abandon him or her
5. Policies for fair distribution of scarce resources
6. Informed consent

F. Ethical Dilemmas.
The nurse is faced with an ethical dilemma. List the seven steps for processing ethical dilemmas in sequential order. (Letter A is the first step and letter G is the last step.)

A. _____ Gather all of the information relevant to this case.
B. _____ Verbalize the problem.
C. _____ Negotiate the outcome.
D. _____ Evaluate the action.
E. _____ Determine if this is an ethical dilemma.
F. _____ Consider possible courses of action.
G. _____ Examine and determine your own values on this issue.

PART II: PUTTING IT ALL TOGETHER

G. Multiple-Response Questions.
Choose the most appropriate answer.

1. When the nurse takes the right action that produces the greatest good for the greatest number of people, the nurse is demonstrating:
   1. feminist ethics.
   2. ethics of care.
   3. utilitarianism.
   4. deontology.

2. When the nurse feels powerless because moral beliefs cannot be followed due to institutional barriers, she is experiencing moral:
   1. outrage.
   2. uncertainty.
   3. confusion.
   4. distress.

3. What is the initial task when the nurse encounters an ethical dilemma?
   1. State the ethical problem clearly so that everyone can agree on the problem.
   2. Decide whether the situation constitutes an ethical problem.
   3. Consider own values in relation to the problem.
   4. Outline possible courses of action and consequences.

4. Where are the legal boundaries of nursing practice in a given state defined?
   1. Hospital policy and procedures books
   2. Professional nursing organizations
   3. State legislatures
   4. Nurse practice acts

5. What group creates regulatory laws that address the conduct of nurses?
   1. Professional organizations
   2. State legislatures
   3. State boards of nursing
   4. State supreme courts

6. A threat of some contact without the patient's consent is called:
   1. assault.
   2. battery.
   3. libel.
   4. slander.

7. The nurse's professional duty to help others is an example of:
   1. veracity.
   2. beneficence.
   3. fidelity
   4. autonomy.

8. A system or code of behavior related to what is right is known as:
   1. ethics.
   2. empathy.
   3. caring.
   4. empowerment.

9. Which ethical concept is applied when the nurse provides quality care to patients regardless of their socioeconomic status?
   1. Justice
   2. Veracity
   3. Autonomy
   4. Fidelity

10. When the nurse reports substandard nursing practice, she is utilizing:
    1. beneficence.
    2. veracity.
    3. fidelity.
    4. nonmaleficence.

11. Which patient cannot give informed consent?
    1. Patient having an appendectomy
    2. Patient receiving chemotherapy following a mastectomy
    3. Patient who just received a preoperative sedative
    4. Patient having cataract surgery as day surgery

12. The nurse's best protection against negligence and malpractice is to follow:
    1. hospital policies.
    2. scope of practice rules.
    3. standards of care.
    4. state nurse practice acts.

13. Which right do all patients have regarding informed consent?
    1. Explanation of rehabilitation
    2. Have all questions answered
    3. The patient will not be abandoned
    4. Recommendations will be made indicating the best treatment

14. Who is responsible for obtaining informed consent?
    1. Hospital
    2. Nurse supervisor
    3. Staff nurse
    4. Physician

15. The release of medical information or publication of patient photographs without the patient's consent constitutes:
    1. defamation of character.
    2. slander.
    3. invasion of privacy.
    4. malpractice.

16. The nurse is obtaining informed consent for a surgical procedure. What action should the nurse take if the patient states that he does not understand the surgical procedure for which he is scheduled?
    1. Explain the procedure to the patient.
    2. Ask the patient if he has any questions
    3. Inform the patient that he may want to discuss this with his family members.
    4. Contact the physician.

PART III: CHALLENGE YOURSELF!

H. Getting Ready for NCLEX.

Choose the most appropriate answer or select all that apply.

1. Which topics must be discussed with patients to constitute sufficient information for the patient to give informed consent? Select all that apply.
   1. Recommended treatment
   2. Risks
   3. Benefits
   4. Alternatives
   5. Consequences of refusing treatment
   6. Research data about treatment

2. What conditions must be met to be found liable for malpractice? Select all that apply.
   1. The nurse owed a duty to the patient.
   2. The nurse communicated with other members of the health care team.
   3. The patient was injured.
   4. The nurse refused to work overtime.
   5. The nurse did not carry out the duty to the patient.
   6. Injury was caused by the nurse's failure to carry out the duty.

3. Which of the following are essential elements of informed consent? Select all that apply.
   1. Mandatory agreement
   2. Patient decision-making capability
   3. Sufficient information
   4. Physician present when patient signs consent

4. Which of the following constitutes assault? Select all that apply.
   1. Nurse touches the patient in offensive manner.
   2. Nurse threatens to restrain a patient against his wishes.
   3. Nurse gives false information that damages the patient's reputation.
   4. Nurse improperly releases information about the patient to a relative.
   5. Nurse threatens to medicate a patient against his wishes.

5. According to the NAPNES Standards of LPN/LVN Responsibilities for Nursing Practice Implementation, which responsibilities does the LPN/LVN have? Select all that apply.
   1. Conducts a focused nursing assessment
   2. Identifies patient needs, forming nursing diagnoses
   3. Contributes to the evaluation of patient care
   4. Implements treatments and procedures
   5. Documents care provided
   6. Completes the admission assessment on new patients

6. According to the NAPNES Standards of LPN/LVN as Member of Interdisciplinary Health Care Team, which responsibilities does the LPN/LVN have? Select all that apply.
   1. Functions as a member of the health care team
   2. Develops an integrated health care plan
   3. Respects the property of others
   4. Protects confidential information of the patient

7. When the LVN posts information about the patient she is caring for on Facebook, which standard of practice is she violating?
   1. Communicate relevant, accurate, and complete information.
   2. Document assessments and interventions.
   3. Maintain organizational and patient confidentiality.
   4. Utilize information technology to communicate the provision of patient care.

8. Which of the following are caring interventions as described in the NAPNES Standards of Care? Select all that apply.
   1. Utilize knowledge of normal values to identify deviation in health status to plan care.
   2. Assess data related to the patient's health status.
   3. Modify patient care as indicated by the evaluation of stated outcomes.
   4. Provide and promote the patient's dignity.
   5. Identify and honor the emotional and spiritual influences on the patient's health.
   6. Assist the patient to cope with and adapt to stressful events and changes in health status.

9. Which are common negligence errors? Select all that apply.
   1. Copying or removing a part of a patient's record
   2. Medication injuries that result in injury to patients
   3. Falls relating to injury to patients
   4. Failure to carry out physician's orders
   5. Failure to give report to an oncoming shift
   6. Failure to notify a physician of a significant change in a patient's status

10. What constitutes a breach in confidentiality? Select all that apply.
    1. Discussing a patient's medical treatment with colleagues at lunch
    2. Avoiding public discussion of patient information
    3. Providing family members with results of diagnostic tests
    4. Turning in care plans for nursing school assignments that include a patient's name

11. According to NAPNES Standards of Practice, which of the following competencies indicate that the outcome of professional behavior has been met? Select all that apply.
    1. Communicate relevant, accurate, and complete information.
    2. Utilize knowledge of normal values to identify deviation in health status to plan care.
    3. Identify own LPN/LVN strengths and limitations for the purpose of improving nursing performance.
    4. Demonstrate accountability for nursing care provided by self and/or directed to others.
    5. Function as an advocate for the health care consumer, maintaining confidentiality as required.
    6. Provide and promote the patient's dignity.

The Leadership Role of the Licensed Practical Nurse

Go to http://evolve.elsevier.com/Linton/medsurg/ for additional activities and exercises.

NCLEX CATEGORIES:

Safe and Effective Care Environment:
Coordinated Care, Safety and Infection Control

Psychosocial Integrity

OBJECTIVES

1. Differentiate leadership from management.
2. Describe leadership styles.
3. Discuss management theories.
4. Discuss management theories.
5. List tips for effective management.
6. Describe the role of the licensed vocational nurse as a team leader.
7. Discuss the processes involved in managing care.

PART I: MASTERING THE BASICS

A. Leadership Styles and Management Theories.

Match the definition in the numbered column with the most appropriate term in the lettered column.

1. _____ Authoritarian, directive, or bureaucratic types of leadership

2. _____ Mixture of autocratic and democratic leadership; feedback from group members is used by the leader to make a final decision

3. _____ Achievement of goals through participation by all group members

4. _____ Nondirective type of leadership

5. _____ Management by autocratic rule with little participation in decision-making by workers

6. _____ Democratic style of management with some participation in decision-making by workers

7. _____ Management with full participation in decision-making by workers

8. _____ All group members may assume leadership and follower roles in various circumstances based upon their unique skills and talents

A. Autocratic leadership
B. Theory X
C. Laissez-faire leadership
D. Democratic leadership
E. Participative leadership
F. Transformational leadership
G. Theory Y
H. Theory Z

B. Key Terms.

Match the definition in the numbered column with the most appropriate term in the lettered column.

1. _____ Turning over part of one person's responsibility to another person with that person's consent

2. _____ Identification and delegation of specific tasks to a specific person who is hired and paid to perform these tasks

3. _____ Guidance, or showing the way to others

4. _____ Effective use of selected methods to achieve desired outcomes

A. Leadership
B. Management
C. Assignment
D. Delegation

C. Management Theory.
Choose the most appropriate answer.

1. Which of the following characteristics of people in their work environments refer to Theory X management style? Select all that apply.
   1. Work together for the good of the company
   2. Care about what they are doing
   3. Find no pleasure in work
   4. Do not want to think for themselves
   5. Work only because they fear being fired
   6. Constantly striving to grow

2. Which of the following characteristics of people in their work environment refer to Theory Y management style? Select all that apply.
   1. Mature and responsible
   2. Self-directed
   3. Child-like and prefer being told what to do
   4. Not capable of making decisions for themselves
   5. Work for rewards other than money
   6. Active and enjoy setting their own goals

3. Which of the following characteristics of people in their work environment refer to Theory Z management style? Select all that apply.
   1. Dislike responsibility
   2. Accept responsibility
   3. Dynamic, flexible, and adaptive
   4. Based on mutual trust and loyalty
   5. Complete knowledge of organizational objectives
   6. Involved in every phase of operation of the company

4. Which stage of conflict occurs when each party formulates a view of the basis of conflict?
   1. Frustration
   2. Conceptualization
   3. Action
   4. Outcomes

5. Which characteristics are related to autocratic leadership style? Select all that apply.
   1. Leader turns group over to the group to manage.
   2. Leader leads by suggestion rather than domination.
   3. Leader is authoritarian and directive.
   4. Leader analyzes feedback from the group and then makes decisions.
   5. Leader presents personal views to group members who provide critique and comment.
   6. Leader believes that leader should not be questioned by group.

6. Which are factors contributing to the evolution in leadership of LPNs as they move from a focus on tasks to a focus on facilitating the care process? Select all that apply.
   1. Health care delivery system is predictable
   2. One generally accepted "right way to do things"
   3. Rapid change in information and technology
   4. Cost control measures
   5. Consumers of care expect high-quality care
   6. Expansion of managed health care

D. Conflict Resolution.
Match the positive outcomes and uses of conflict resolution modes in the numbered column with the related mode of conflict in the lettered column.

1. _____ Generates commitment to work together
2. _____ Produces mutually acceptable solutions
3. _____ Agreement is reached
4. _____ Reflects strong stance to defend principles
5. _____ Temporarily defuses highly charged emotional disagreement

A. Accommodation
B. Collaboration
C. Compromise
D. Avoidance
E. Competition

E. Management Tips.

Choose the most appropriate answer.

1. Which of the following are tips for effective management? Select all that apply.
    1. _____ Produce mutually acceptable solutions
    2. _____ Defuse highly charged emotional disagreement
    3. _____ Seek help and support from a variety of sources
    4. _____ Take active approach to planning
    5. _____ Have a clear vision
    6. _____ Generate commitment to work together

PART II: PUTTING IT ALL TOGETHER

F. Multiple Choice/Multiple Response.

Choose the most appropriate answer or select all that apply.

1. Which of the following methods does the democratic leader use to make decisions?
    1. Participation of all group members and group consensus
    2. Nondirective style, letting group members decide
    3. Makes decisions independently from group
    4. Presents personal views to group members for comments before making final decision

2. Individuals who achieve their goals by setting objectives and having them carried out without input or suggestions from others display what style of leadership?
    1. Democratic
    2. Autocratic
    3. Laissez-faire
    4. Cooperative

3. Which style do leaders who use Theory Y of management usually have?
    1. Autocratic
    2. Democratic
    3. Bureaucratic
    4. Laissez-faire

4. The benefit of taking an active approach to planning is that the nurse is likely to:
    1. emphasize the importance of documentation.
    2. avoid conflict before it occurs.
    3. make employees accountable for their actions.
    4. treat other employees with respect.

5. Which leadership style provides the quickest response?
    1. Laissez-faire
    2. Democratic
    3. Participative
    4. Autocratic

6. In making assignments, an attempt should be made to match the skills of the assigned personnel with:
    1. patient personalities.
    2. nursing needs.
    3. patient needs.
    4. institutional needs.

7. When making assignments for patient care, which approach encourages cooperation and tends to get more work done?
    1. Directly ordering that a task be done
    2. Requesting that a task be done
    3. Delegating tasks to more than one person
    4. Asking to see the staffing plan

8. Which should *not* be delegated to unlicensed assistive personnel?
    1. Making a bed
    2. Weighing a patient
    3. Writing a nursing care plan
    4. Feeding a patient

9. Continuous quality improvement (CQI) is a term frequently used in relation to:
    1. organization.
    2. direction.
    3. coordination.
    4. control.

10. Which of the following is likely to occur when an autocratic leader hires an autocratic manager?
    1. Group concerns
    2. Problem-solving
    3. Power struggle
    4. Confusion

11. Which type of leadership style requires a highly motivated, focused group to work well?
    1. Democratic
    2. Laissez-faire
    3. Autocratic
    4. Participative

12. When delegating a task or making an assignment to unlicensed assistive personnel, the nurse has the duty to maintain:
    1. patient safety.
    2. caring relationships.
    3. patient autonomy.
    4. autocratic leadership.

13. Involving others and brainstorming are used in the decision-making process as part of:
    1. identifying the problem.
    2. exploring possible solutions.
    3. choosing the most desirable action.
    4. planning evaluation.

14. The purpose of state nurse practice acts is to _____. Select all that apply.
    1. Protect the public.
    2. Address scope of practice
    3. Set standards of care
    4. Describe policies and procedures
    5. State organizational chart
    6. Promote the nursing profession

15. Which are characteristics of effective leaders and managers? Select all that apply.
    1. Must be competent
    2. Have respect of people who work with them
    3. Be able to communicate with others
    4. Control behavior of others
    5. Set realistic goals
    6. Be able to motivate others

16. Which are ways that leaders and managers motivate others? Select all that apply.
    1. Organizational benefits
    2. Merit pay raises
    3. Personal values
    4. Clear vision

17. According to Theory X, people who do not want to think for themselves want to:
    1. have a democratic manager.
    2. be a team member.
    3. be directed and controlled.
    4. have a laissez-faire leader.

18. According to Maslow's human need for security, what takes precedence for nurses in difficult economic times?
    1. Belonging to a harmonious work group
    2. Striving for self-actualization
    3. Job security
    4. Praise and recognition

19. Which steps are necessary when directing people to carry out their assignments? Select all that apply.
    1. Skills of assigned personnel must match patient needs.
    2. More personnel are assigned to tasks that take a long time.
    3. The patient must understand the assignment.
    4. Directions are given in a clear, logical order.
    5. All team members are responsible for making assignments.
    6. All assigned activities must fall within the state's nurse practice act.

20. Which of the following are structure standards related to quality improvement? Select all that apply.
    1. Care delivery standards
    2. Health care–associated infection rates
    3. Patient satisfaction surveys
    4. Job descriptions
    5. Policies and procedures
    6. Documentation expectations

21. The purpose of quality assurance committees is to:
    1. evaluate compliance for set standards of care.
    2. measure the number of medical errors.
    3. promote patient safety.
    4. develop policies and procedures.

PART III: CHALLENGE YOURSELF!

G. Getting Ready for NCLEX.

Choose the most appropriate answer or select all that apply.

1. Which of the following are specific quality indicators for nursing care that have been identified for monitoring and focused continuous quality improvement? Select all that apply.
   1. Health care–associated infections
   2. Patient satisfaction
   3. Pressure ulcers
   4. Number of patients with strokes
   5. Nurse staffing
   6. Patient falls

2. Under the supervision of an RN, the LPN can help the RN team leader carry out which of the following responsibilities? Select all that apply.
   1. Carry out and document medical orders and plans
   2. Initiate discharge planning
   3. Identify referral needs
   4. Facilitate patient education
   5. Keep care plans current
   6. Develop organizational structure charts

3. On which of the following are assignments made by LPNs based? Select all that apply.
   1. Educational background of the nursing assistants
   2. Patient needs
   3. Scope of practice for LPNs
   4. Available staff
   5. Job descriptions

4. When the LPN is delegating a task, the LPN always has the duty to maintain patient:
   1. confidentiality.
   2. autonomy.
   3. safety.
   4. satisfaction.

5. Which characteristics describe the authoritarian leadership style? Select all that apply.
   1. Little freedom
   2. No control
   3. Decision-making by the leader
   4. Shared responsibility
   5. High quantity output of the group
   6. Minimal leader activity

6. Which of the following are major leadership theories? Select all that apply.
   1. Multicratic
   2. Trait
   3. Attitudinal
   4. Situational
   5. Laissez-faire

7. Which are characteristics of leaders and managers? Select all that apply.
   1. Sets realistic goals
   2. Is easily self-satisfied
   3. Makes decisions not involving risks
   4. Answers questions of co-workers

8. List in sequential order the steps in the decision-making process.
   A. _____ Implement action
   B. _____ Identify the problem
   C. _____ Plan evaluation
   D. _____ Choose the most desirable action
   E. _____ Explore possible solutions

9. List in sequential order the steps in the management process.
   A. _____ Coordinating
   B. _____ Controlling
   C. _____ Planning
   D. _____ Organizing
   E. _____ Directing

The Nurse-Patient Relationship

chapter

5

 Go to http://evolve.elsevier.com/Linton/medsurg/ for additional activities and exercises.

NCLEX CATEGORIES:

Psychosocial Integrity

OBJECTIVES

1. Define holistic view of nursing.
2. Define the concept of *self*.
3. Discuss the use of self in the practice of nursing.
4. Compare the meaning of the terms *patient* and *client*.
5. List commonly held expectations of patients and families.
6. Describe the meaning of the American Hospital Association Patient Care Partnership document.
7. Describe guidelines for nurse-patient relationships.
8. Describe basic components of communication.

PART I: MASTERING THE BASICS

A. Helper Roles.

What characteristics must a nurse must have to assume the helper role in a nurse-patient relationship? Select all that apply.

1. Sense of responsibility to the patient
2. Ability to express feelings and attitudes with the patient
3. Ability to form a long-term relationship
4. Nonjudgmental attitude
5. Ability to keep secrets
6. Ability to form friendship or support relationships

B. Nonverbal Communication.

Which are examples of nonverbal communication? Select all that apply.

1. Laughing
2. Facial expression
3. Explanation of patient care
4. Patient is a partner in care
5. Assertive communication
6. Body position
7. Making gestures

C. Helper Roles.

1. Which are characteristics of the nurse in a professional helping person role? Select all that apply.
   1. Shares personal information
   2. Responsible to patient
   3. Sexual overtones or a sexual relationship may develop
   4. Both individuals express feelings, attitudes, and opinions
   5. Attitude is nonjudgmental
   6. Relationship is goal-directed
   7. Individuals meet each other's needs
   8. Relationship is time-limited

2. Which are characteristics of the nurse, acting in the role of friend, that can interfere with the therapeutic process? Select all that apply.
   1. Objective of relationship is to meet patient's needs
   2. Relationship may continue
   3. No plan involved
   4. Discourages any sexual overtones in relationship
   5. Each tries to influence the other in discussing issues
   6. Does not keep secrets
   7. Attempts to influence patient to his or her way of thinking

D. Communication.

Match the example of communication technique in the numbered column with the proper label in the lettered column.

1. _____ Resisting the urge to fill quiet periods with conversation.

2. _____ "Tell me your reactions to your new treatment."

3. _____ "You say you're feeling better since your brother has returned?"

4. _____ "So you have decided to have surgery, but delay it until after Christmas."

5. _____ "I hear you're concerned about your son."

6. _____ "Do you mean 'sad' when you say 'upset'?"

A. Reflecting
B. Clarifying
C. Silence
D. Restating
E. Summarizing
F. Open-ended statement

E. Communication.

Which of the following are examples of nontherapeutic communication techniques? Select all that apply.
   1. "You shouldn't worry about the new treatment."
   2. "Try to think positively."
   3. "Tell me more about what you are feeling about your surgery."
   4. "The first thing you need to do is to make your teenagers help you more."
   5. "It sounds like you would like to learn more about losing weight."
   6. "You must quit smoking immediately."
   7. "It's incredible that your doctor did not tell you when to take this medication."

PART II: PUTTING IT ALL TOGETHER

F. Multiple-Response Questions.

Choose the most appropriate answer.

1. The ability to be open and honest about one's feelings is characteristic of:
   1. self-image.
   2. self-esteem.
   3. self-disclosure.
   4. self-trust.

2. What is the first step in developing a therapeutic relationship?
   1. See the patient's experiences from his or her perspective.
   2. Accept the patient's values.
   3. Build up trust.
   4. Encourage the patient to share thoughts freely.

3. Understanding another's feelings and becoming immersed in the situation is:
   1. empathy.
   2. helping.
   3. sympathy.
   4. apathy.

4. The main difference between a therapeutic relationship and a social relationship is that the therapeutic helping person:
   1. has a spontaneous approach.
   2. discusses own beliefs.
   3. shares feelings and opinions.
   4. is responsible to the patient.

5. A goal-directed focus on one patient is a description of:
   1. self-disclosure.
   2. self-awareness.
   3. therapeutic relationship.
   4. reflection.

6. The ability to be honest and open about one's feelings relates to:
   1. reflection.
   2. clarification.
   3. self-disclosure.
   4. nonjudgmental attitude.

7. According to the AHA Patient Care Partnership, which of the following can patients expect during their hospital stay?
   1. Complete medical care regardless of the ability to pay
   2. Choice of the best method of health care delivery
   3. Understanding of the patient's health care goals and values
   4. Determination of treatment for medical care by a physician

PART III: CHALLENGE YOURSELF!

G. Getting Ready for NCLEX.

Choose the most appropriate answer or select all that apply.

1. Which of the following are patient rights described in the AHA Patient Care Partnership? Select all that apply.
   1. Discussion of the treatment plan
   2. Promotion of self-image
   3. Understanding of health goals
   4. Therapeutic communication
   5. Protection of privacy

2. Which are physical needs of a surgical patient? Select all that apply.
   1. Fear about surgery
   2. Fluid replacement
   3. Wound healing
   4. Worry about returning to work
   5. Pain management

3. What are the best ways to make patients feel respected? Select all that apply.
   1. Introduce them by name.
   2. Explain your own values and beliefs to the patient.
   3. Provide a backrub before sleep.
   4. Express sympathy for the patient's condition.
   5. Introduce the patient by name to other health care providers.
   6. Provide interpreters, if needed, to explain treatment.

Cultural Aspects of Nursing Care

Go to http://evolve.elsevier.com/Linton/medsurg/ for additional activities and exercises.

NCLEX CATEGORIES:

Psychosocial Integrity

OBJECTIVES

1. Describe cultural concepts related to nursing and health care.
2. Identify traditional health habits and beliefs of major ethnic groups in the United States.
3. Explain cultural influences on the interactions of patients and families with the health care system.
4. Discuss cultural considerations in providing culturally sensitive nursing care.
5. Discuss ways in which planning and implementation of nursing interventions can be adapted to a patient's ethnicity.

PART I: MASTERING THE BASICS

A. Key Terms.
Match the definition in the numbered column with the most appropriate term in the lettered column. Answers may be used more than once.

1. _____ A group of individuals within a culture whose members share different beliefs, values, and attitudes from those of the dominant culture

2. _____ Replacing values and beliefs with those of another culture

3. _____ The existence of many cultures in a society

4. _____ Learned values, beliefs, and practices that are characteristic of a society and that guide individual behavior

5. _____ Integration of cultural considerations into all aspects of nursing care

6. _____ Group of individuals with a unique identity based on shared traditions and customs

7. _____ The process of learning to be part of a culture

A. Cultural diversity
B. Enculturation
C. Subculture
D. Culture
E. Assimilation
F. Ethnic group

B. Culture.
What are the three basic characteristics of all cultures? Select the three that apply.

1. Culture is based on symbols.
2. Culture is based on ethnic background.
3. Culture is shared.
4. Culture is learned.
5. Culture is based on religious background.
6. Culture is based on health literacy.

C. Ethnic Groups.

Match the healers in the numbered column with the ethnic group that may be likely to use them in the lettered column. Answers may be used more than once.

1. _____ Spiritualists
2. _____ Curanderos
3. _____ Root doctors
4. _____ Medicine men
5. _____ Herbalists
6. _____ Acupuncturists

A. Asian
B. Native American
C. Latino
D. African-American

D. Culture Shock.

List in the proper sequence the three phases of culture shock associated with hospitalization.

A. _____ Patient becomes disenchanted with the whole situation, frustrated, and withdraws.

B. _____ Patient begins to adapt to new environment and is able to maintain a sense of humor.

C. _____ Patient asks questions regarding the hospital routine and the hospital's expectations of the patient.

PART II: PUTTING IT ALL TOGETHER

E. Multiple-Response Questions.

Choose the most appropriate answer.

1. Which cultural group member is likely to become oversedated when diazepam (Valium) is given to him?
   1. Chinese descent
   2. German descent
   3. Italian descent
   4. French descent

2. The integration of cultural considerations into all aspects of nursing care is called:
   1. cultural diversity.
   2. transcultural nursing.
   3. enculturation.
   4. subcultural nursing.

3. Which ethnic group values self-respect, respect for elders, and pride?
   1. Whites
   2. African-Americans
   3. Latinos
   4. Asians

4. Which religious group believes that the body should not be left alone until buried?
   1. Judaism
   2. Protestant
   3. Eastern Orthodox
   4. Mormon

5. Which religious group believes in reincarnation and calls in a priest at the time of death, who ties a thread around the neck of the dead person as a blessing?
   1. Mormon
   2. Hinduism
   3. Eastern Orthodox
   4. Judaism

6. Which religious group believes that the body should be washed, prepared, and placed in a position facing Mecca following death?
   1. Judaism
   2. Eastern Orthodox
   3. Catholic
   4. Muslim

7. Which ethnic group responds better to diuretics for treatment of hypertension than the other groups?
   1. African-Americans
   2. Latinos
   3. Native Americans
   4. Whites

8. Utilizing interpersonal skills to adapt nursing care to the cultural differences of patients is called:
   1. holistic care.
   2. complementary care.
   3. cultural competence.
   4. cultural diversity.

PART III: CHALLENGE YOURSELF!

F. Getting Ready for NCLEX.

Choose the most appropriate answer or select all that apply.

1. A patient claims that his illness is a result of punishment for a sin that he has committed. This patient believes in:
   1. divine punishment.
   2. corporal punishment.
   3. legal punishment.
   4. ethnic punishment.

2. The nurse is caring for a patient who believes that her stomachaches are caused by phlegm and black bile. This patient's belief system about illness is called:
   1. divine punishment theory.
   2. balance with nature theory.
   3. sacred healing theory.
   4. hot-and-cold theory.

3. What are the three stages of culture shock associated with hospitalization? Select three that apply.
   1. Asking questions
   2. Denial
   3. Adaptation
   4. Bargaining
   5. Being disenchanted
   6. Generalization

4. Which religious group believes in Kosher dietary laws which state that there is no mixing of milk and meat at a meal?
   1. Seventh-Day Adventist
   2. Eastern Orthodox
   3. Judaism
   4. Protestant

5. A 24-year-old woman has been given an antidepressant for depression. Which ethnic group will respond better to a lower dose of antidepressants?
   1. Whites
   2. African-Americans
   3. Europeans
   4. Asians

6. Why are antihypertensive drugs less effective in Japanese patients?
   1. They metabolize the drug more quickly.
   2. They eat Kosher foods.
   3. Their diet is high in salt.
   4. They are at greater risk for drug toxicity.

7. A 62-year-old patient in the hospital states that he does not like to take baths routinely and is very modest about disrobing in front of strangers. Which are appropriate responses of the nurse? Select all that apply.
   1. Explain to the patient that baths will be taken every morning before noon.
   2. Knock before entering the room.
   3. Ask permission before touching the patient.
   4. Reassure the patient that it is all right to disrobe in the hospital, as you will pull the curtain to provide privacy.
   5. Ask permission from the patient to assist with personal hygiene.
   6. Explain the importance of personal hygiene for all patients in the hospital.

8. Which are characteristics of patients who have the highest health literacy level? Select three that apply.
   1. Male
   2. Female
   3. African-American adult
   4. White adult
   5. 50-year-old adult
   6. 70-year-old adult

9. A 45-year-old Muslim male is on bedrest in the hospital. What action should the nurse take to facilitate his personal devotion time?
   1. Place the Koran in his bed beneath his prayer book.
   2. Assist the patient with washing required before prayer time.
   3. Encourage a prayer practitioner to come pray with him.
   4. Prepare the patient for foot washing as a part of holy communion.

10. A Chinese-American patient has been admitted to the hospital. Which are traditional dietary practices that the nurse will work to accommodate while the patient is hospitalized? Select all that apply.
    1. High amounts of poultry and fish
    2. High amounts of rice or noodles
    3. Stir-fried food
    4. High amounts of corn and dried beans
    5. Most calories from legumes and vegetables
    6. Low dairy products

The Nurse and the Family

chapter

7

 Go to http://evolve.elsevier.com/Linton/medsurg/ for additional activities and exercises.

NCLEX CATEGORIES:

Health Promotion and Maintenance

Psychosocial Integrity

OBJECTIVES

1. Describe the concept of *family* and its relationship to society.
2. Compare various family structures or lifestyles that characterize modern American families.
3. Discuss the family from a developmental perspective.
4. Describe roles and communication patterns within families.
5. Describe adaptive and maladaptive mechanisms used by families to cope with various stressors.
6. Describe the role of the nurse in dealing with families experiencing various stresses.
7. Identify community resources that may help to meet the family's needs.

PART I: MASTERING THE BASICS

A. Family Types.
Match the description in the numbered column with the most appropriate type of family in the lettered column.

1. _____ Cohabiting couples
2. _____ Blended family
3. _____ Relatives of either spouse who live with the nuclear family
4. _____ Biologic or adoptive mother and father and their children
5. _____ One widowed head of household

A. Nuclear family
B Extended family
C. Step-parent
D. Single-parent
E. Nontraditional

B. Developmental Tasks.
Match the developmental task in the numbered column with the correct stage of the family life cycle in the lettered column.

1. _____ Establish mutually satisfying marriage; make decisions about parenthood
2. _____ Set up young family as a stable unit; socialize children
3. _____ Balance freedom with responsibility for children; communicate openly between parents and children
4. _____ Expand family circle to include new family members acquired by marriage; assist aging and ill parents of husband or wife
5. _____ Maintain a satisfying living arrangement; adjust to loss of spouse; maintain intergenerational family ties

A. Launching children and moving on
B. Families with adolescents
C. Families with young children
D. Families in later life
E. Beginning families

C. Family Roles.

Which family roles are considered to be informal roles within the family? Select all that apply.
1. Harmonizer
2. Family caretaker
3. Wife-mother
4. Family scapegoat
5. Son-brother

D. Family Communication.

Which are examples of functional family communication? Select all that apply.
1. Dynamic, two-way process
2. Acceptance of individual differences
3. Unclear transmission of a message
4. Verbal messages of caring
5. Inability to focus on one issue
6. Forbidden subjects for discussion
7. Mutual respect for each other's feelings

PART II: PUTTING IT ALL TOGETHER

E. Multiple Choice/Multiple Response.

Choose the most appropriate answer or select all that apply.

1. Which is a negative strategy for adapting to family stress?
   1. Problem-solving
   2. Mastery
   3. Coping behavior
   4. Defense mechanism

2. Which is an external family coping strategy?
   1. Joint family problem-solving
   2. Seeking information to maintain control of situation
   3. Maintaining as normal a life as possible
   4. Relieving anxiety and tension with humor

3. Maintaining ties between aging parents and growing children is a developmental task of:
   1. beginning families.
   2. families with young children.
   3. launching children and moving on.
   4. families in later life.

4. Which are internal family coping strategies? Select all that apply.
   1. Family group reliance
   2. Role flexibility and changing roles
   3. Using support groups
   4. Obtaining spiritual support

PART III: CHALLENGE YOURSELF!

F. Getting Ready for NCLEX.

Choose the most appropriate answer or select all that apply.

1. What is the most consistent family developmental task that must be met throughout the family life cycle?
   1. Defining the roles of the family members
   2. Continuing education
   3. Maintaining the marital relationship
   4. Maintaining individual independence

2. Which of the following is the most important influence on family interaction?
   1. Self-esteem of each member
   2. Family income
   3. Family size
   4. Type of family configuration

3. Which are ways for the nurse to collect data about families and their coping strategies? Select all that apply.
   1. Determine stressors being experienced.
   2. Assess family communication patterns.
   3. Find out what kinds of coping strategies are used.
   4. Explore each family member's political views.

4. What is the most important strategy for assisting families to cope?
   1. Encourage all family members to be involved in the process.
   2. Work with the most influential member of the family.
   3. Support new coping strategies instead of using old coping strategies that have worked in the past.
   4. Reinforce coping styles that have been helpful in the past.

5. When taking care of a patient in the hospital, how can the nurse best assist the patient and the family?
   1. Keep the family members out of the room.
   2. Focus care on the patient and have the family members wait in the family room.
   3. Determine whether the family members are supportive or detrimental in the patient's recovery process.
   4. Provide information only to the patient because of confidentiality.

6. The nurse is caring for a family that is suddenly homeless due to an earthquake. The family is working on finding temporary living quarters. Which kind of coping strategy does this represent?
   1. Attaching meaning to the experience
   2. Providing comfort to each other
   3. Dealing directly with the cause of the problem
   4. Sharing feelings and thoughts to maintain a cohesive unit

7. A coping strategy used by one family is to participate in clubs or community organizations to serve family members' needs. What type of coping strategy is this?
   1. Internal family coping strategy
   2. External family coping strategy
   3. Defense mechanism strategy
   4. Role switching strategy

Health and Illness

 Go to http://evolve.elsevier.com/Linton/medsurg/ for additional activities and exercises.

NCLEX CATEGORIES:

Health Promotion and Maintenance

Psychosocial Integrity

OBJECTIVES

1. Describe the health-illness continuum.
2. Discuss traditional and current views of health and illness.
3. List Maslow's five basic human needs, explaining why they constitute a hierarchy.
4. Explain the four levels of adaptability to stress.
5. Discuss concepts related to health promotion, disease prevention, and health maintenance.
6. Define acute and chronic illness.
7. Discuss illness behavior and the impact of illness on the family.
8. Describe nursing measures for health promotion, health maintenance, and illness.
9. Describe complementary and alternative therapies and the nurse's role in relation to both.

PART I: MASTERING THE BASICS

A. Maslow's Hierarchy.

List the five levels of human needs in order of priority from Maslow's hierarchy.

⑤

④

③

② Physical safety | Psychological safety

① Oxygen | Fluids | Nutrition | Body temperature | Elimination | Shelter | Sex

1. _____

2. _____

3. _____

4. _____

5. _____

B. Maslow's Hierarchy.

Match the need in the numbered column with the correct level in the lettered column.

1. _____ Oxygen, fluid, nutrition, temperature, elimination, shelter, rest, and sex

2. _____ Security, protection from harm, freedom from anxiety and fear

3. _____ Feeling loved by family and friends, and accepted by peers and community

4. _____ Feeling good about oneself and feeling that others hold one in high regard

5. _____ Self-fulfillment; able to problem-solve, accept criticism from others, and eager to acquire new knowledge; self-confidence; maturity

A. Self-esteem
B. Safety and security
C. Physiologic
D. Self-actualization
E. Love and belonging

C. Adaptation.

Which are stages of the general adaptation syndrome? Select all that apply.

1. Anxiety
2. Resistance
3. Exhaustion
4. Tachycardia
5. Fear
6. Alarm

D. Maslow's Hierarchy.

Which components of nursing care are related to physiologic needs of Maslow's hierarchy of human needs? Select all that apply.

1. Breathe normally.
2. Work so that there is a sense of accomplishment.
3. Worship according to one's faith.
4. Eat and drink adequately.
5. Eliminate body wastes.
6. Avoid dangers in the environment.

E. Views of Health.

Which descriptions represent current views of health, as compared to traditional views of health? Select all that apply.

1. Emphasis is on maintenance of health and prevention of disease.
2. Health and illness are separate entities.
3. Focus is on curing disease or injury.
4. Health and illness are relative and ever-changing.

F. Herbal-Drug Interactions.

Which of the following herb-drug interactions increase the risk of bleeding in patients? Select all that apply.

1. Echinacea and immunosuppressants
2. Garlic and anticoagulants
3. Ephedra and antihypertensives
4. Kava-kava and CNS depressants
5. Ginseng and aspirin
6. Hawthorne and cardiac glycosides

G. Complementary Therapies.

Which of the following complementary therapies are commonly used herbal medicines? Select all that apply.

1. *Ginkgo biloba*
2. Antioxidants
3. Echinacea
4. High-dose vitamin therapy
5. St. John's wort

H. Maslow's Hierarchy.

Which of the following findings indicate safety and security needs of the patient? Select all that apply.

The patient is a 45-year-old male who has been admitted to the hospital with pneumonia. As the nurse is conducting the admission interview, she finds out the following:

1. He has recently separated from his wife and three children.
2. He is afraid to jog due to crime in his neighborhood.
3. He states that he feels like he will never amount to anything.
4. His parents live 300 miles away; he has few close friends in town.
5. He states he fears he will lose his job if he is in the hospital too long.
6. He states he feels alone a lot.

PART II: PUTTING IT ALL TOGETHER

I. Multiple Choice/Multiple Response.

Choose the most appropriate answer or select all that apply.

1. Which of the following are internal stressors? Select all that apply.
    1. Loss of relationship
    2. Boredom
    3. Economic inadequacies
    4. Sensory deprivation
    5. Feelings of powerlessness

2. What is the type of stress that occurs when a person feels angry, while fearing the consequences of expressing it?
    1. Physical overexertion
    2. Psychological perceived threat
    3. Interpersonal relations, loss of relationship
    4. Socioeconomic sensory deprivation

3. A patient's refusal of treatment is an example of which coping strategy?
    1. Confrontation
    2. Denial
    3. Problem-solving
    4. Event review

4. Wound healing and inflammation are examples of:
    1. general adaptation syndrome.
    2. local adaptation syndrome.
    3. negative feedback response.
    4. countercurrent response.

5. A physiologic response of the body to stress is:
    1. bronchoconstriction.
    2. increased heart rate.
    3. decreased respirations.
    4. decreased blood pressure.

6. Slowed speech, inability to concentrate, and hesitant speech may be signs of:
    1. stress.
    2. adaptation.
    3. depression.
    4. alarm.

7. Activities directed toward maintaining or enhancing well-being as a protection against illness are related to:
    1. health adaptation.
    2. health promotion.
    3. prevention of illness.
    4. homeostasis measures.

8. Which is an example of a psychological internal stressor?
    1. Unemployment
    2. Sensory deprivation
    3. Feeling of powerlessness
    4. Ethnic difference

9. Which are examples of complementary and alternative therapies? Select all that apply.
    1. Acupuncture
    2. Surgery
    3. Guided imagery
    4. Antioxidants
    5. Generic drugs
    6. Biofeedback

10. Which are focus areas of the *Healthy People 2020* document? Select all that apply.
    1. Cancer
    2. Thyroid disorders
    3. Diabetes
    4. HIV
    5. Autoimmune disorders
    6. Access to quality health services

11. Which are leading health indicators of *Healthy People 2020*? Select all that apply.
    1. Substance abuse
    2. Occupational health
    3. Mental health
    4. Physical activity
    5. Environmental quality

12. Following a fight-or-flight alarm reaction to stress, the body stabilizes. This adaptation to the stressor is called:
    1. initial stress stage.
    2. resistance stage.
    3. exhaustion stage.
    4. physiologic stage.

13. Which are examples of self-actualization, according to Maslow? Select all that apply.
    1. Ability to solve problems
    2. Willingness to accept criticism from others
    3. Desire for new experiences and knowledge
    4. Maturity
    5. Feeling loved by one's family
    6. Feeling confident about oneself

PART III: CHALLENGE YOURSELF!

J. Getting Ready for NCLEX.

Choose the most appropriate answer or select all that apply.

1. Nursing interventions to increase adaptability in older adults should be geared toward helping older patients to:
   1. use past successful coping mechanisms to deal with new stressors.
   2. assess their strengths and weaknesses in dealing with new stressors.
   3. develop new coping mechanisms to deal with new stressors.
   4. learn new methods of dealing with stressors.

2. Tasks for chronically ill individuals include:
   1. ignoring disease.
   2. preventing and managing crises.
   3. curing disease.
   4. promoting social isolation.

3. The nurse assists with the admission to the hospital of a 42-year-old patient who has the following signs and symptoms. Which of the following are signs and symptoms of stress? Select all that apply.
   1. Slowed speech
   2. Cold hands and feet
   3. Excessive sweating
   4. Nervous movements
   5. Decreased body movement
   6. Withdrawal

4. A patient is newly admitted to the hospital for the first time, stating he feels "very stressed." Which are characteristics of the alarm reaction to stress? Select all that apply.
   1. Decreased heart rate
   2. Increased cardiac output
   3. Increased respiratory rate
   4. Decreased mental energy
   5. Pinpoint pupils
   6. Increased oxygen intake

5. Which question will the nurse ask the patient to help determine what the external coping strategies of the patient are?
   1. "What is your worst possible stressor, and how does this present stress compare with the worst?"
   2. "What ways have you coped with stress in the past that have been successful for you?"
   3. "What kinds of things do you do when you are stressed? Do you eat more or less?"
   4. "Whom do you turn to when you are feeling stressed?"

Nutrition

 Go to http://evolve.elsevier.com/Linton/medsurg/ for additional activities and exercises.

NCLEX CATEGORIES:

Health Promotion and Maintenance

Psychosocial Integrity

Physiological Integrity: Basic Care and Comfort, Physiological Adaptation

OBJECTIVES

1. Explain the role of the gastrointestinal system in the digestion of food.
2. Describe how food is digested and absorbed.
3. List the functions of each of the six classes of essential nutrients.
4. Define macronutrient and micronutrient.
5. Identify the food sources of proteins, carbohydrates, and fats.
6. Identify the food sources of dietary fiber.
7. List the possible health benefits of dietary fiber.
8. Identify the food sources of each of the vitamins and minerals.
9. Describe the changes in nutrient needs as an individual ages.
10. Differentiate anorexia nervosa, bulimia, and binge eating disorder.
11. Discuss the different types of nutritional support.
12. Identify guidelines for the nutritional assessment.

PART I: MASTERING THE BASICS

A. Key Terms.

Match the definition in the numbered column with the most appropriate term in the lettered column.

1. _____ Lipid-wrapped proteins carried into the bloodstream; includes high-density and low-density lipoproteins, which carry cholesterol

2. _____ Small amounts of metals (calcium, sodium, and potassium) and nonmetals (chloride, phosphate) that are essential to the body; can build up

3. _____ Lipids composed of three fatty acid chains and a glycerol molecule

4. _____ Combination of incomplete proteins that provide all nine essential amino acids when consumed together

5. _____ Compounds that come chiefly from animal sources and are usually solid at room temperature; also coconut and palm oils

6. _____ Large organic compounds made of various combinations of amino acids; found in meat, milk, fish, and eggs

7. _____ Organic compounds supplied by food that the body requires for normal growth and development

8. _____ A group of 22 substances that can be bonded in different ways to make a variety of proteins; the body can manufacture sufficient amounts of these, provided the nine essential amino acids are derived from the diet

9. _____ Indigestible roughage found in plant cells; aids in stool formation and elimination

10. _____ Compounds that come from plants or fish and are generally liquid at room temperature; can be monounsaturated (olive, peanut, canola, and avocado oils) or polyunsaturated (corn, safflower, and sesame oils)

11. _____ Energy expended in the resting state; measured in the morning with the body at complete mental and physical rest, but not asleep

12. _____ Plant protein lacking one or more essential amino acids

13. _____ Fats in solid or liquid form; store energy, carry fat-soluble vitamins, and maintain healthy skin and hair; supply essential fatty acids and promote a feeling of fullness (satiety)

14. _____ Standard unit for measuring energy; the amount of heat needed to raise the temperature of 1 g of water at a standard temperature by 1° Celsius

15. _____ Measurement of energy expenditure taken at any time of the day and 3–4 hours after the last meal

16. _____ Protein containing all nine essential amino acids; usually of animal origin (e.g., meat, eggs)

A. Saturated fatty acids
B. Incomplete protein
C. Triglycerides
D. calorie
E. Vitamins
F. Lipids
G. Minerals
H. Basal metabolic rate (BMR)
I. Amino acids
J. Complementary protein
K. Complete protein
L. Insoluble fiber
M. Lipoproteins
N. Resting energy expenditure
O. Proteins
P. Unsaturated fatty acids

B. Macronutrients.
Which of the following are macronutrients? Select all that apply.
1. Minerals
2. Vitamins
3. Hormones
4. Carbohydrates
5. Lipids
6. Amino acids
7. Fluids
8. Vegetables
9. Proteins
10. Fluids

C. Basal Metabolic Rate.
Which are hormones that affect the BMR? Select all that apply.
1. Dopamine
2. Insulin
3. Estrogens
4. Growth hormone
5. Epinephrine
6. Aldosterone
7. Cortisol
8. Thyroxine

D. Basal Metabolic Rate.
Which are reasons why the BMR of a sleeping person is lower than that of an awake, alert person? Select all that apply.
1. Increased activity of the sympathetic nervous system
2. Muscle relaxation
3. Decreased thyroxine
4. Increased body temperature

E. Basal Metabolic Rate.
List the number of kcalories per gram provided by lipids, carbohydrates, and protein.

1. Lipids: _____

2. Carbohydrates: _____

3. Protein: _____

F. Basal Metabolic Rate.
How many kcalories are provided when a person consumes 2 grams of lipids, 4 grams of carbohydrates, and 4 grams of protein?

_____

G. Complete Protein.
Which are sources of complete proteins in foods? Select all that apply.
1. Fish
2. Milk
3. Dry beans
4. Eggs
5. Rice
6. Meat
7. Nuts
8. Cheese

H. MyPyramid Guides.

1. What are the six foods represented by the six colored bands on MyPyramid?

   _____

   _____

   _____

   _____

   _____

   _____

2. In addition to nutrition, what additional topic is included in MyPyramid?

   _____

3. Which of the following foods provide protein content? Select all that apply.
   1. Fish
   2. Potatoes
   3. Nuts
   4. Beans
   5. Meat
   6. Cheese
   7. Milk

4. Using Figure 9-4 (textbook p. 132), label the feeding tubes in the figure below using the following terms: nasogastric, nasoduodenal, nasojejunal, PEG

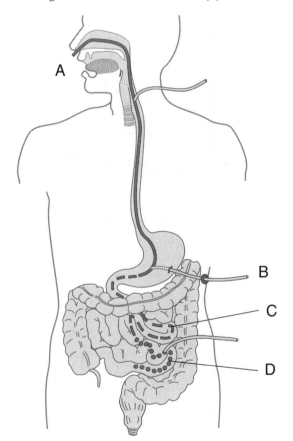

A. _____

B. _____

C. _____

D. _____

I.   Nutrition Labels.

Refer to Figure 9-2 (textbook p. 126) below. Read the nutrition label and fill in the blanks below.

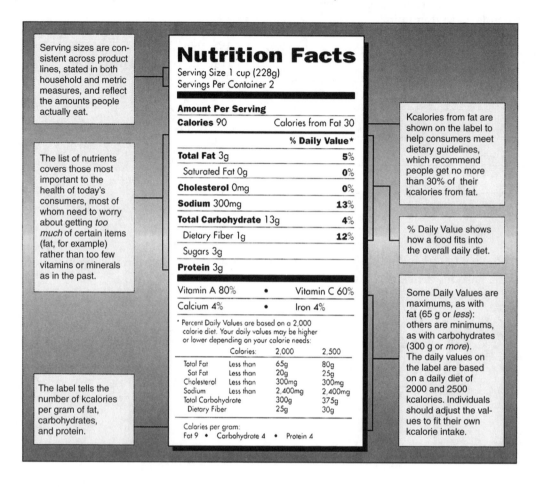

1.   How many Calories per serving are provided? _____

2.   How many servings are in this container? _____

3.   What is the size of one serving? _____

4.   What percentage of vitamin A is provided in one serving? _____

5.   How many Calories are provided in one container? _____

6.   Dietary guidelines recommend that people get no more than what percentage of their kilocalories from fat? _____

J.   Skin Measurement.

What is measured by skin calipers?

1.   Cholesterol
2.   Body surface area (BSA)
3.   Muscle tissue
4.   Subcutaneous fat tissue

K. Energy Requirement.

1. What are the energy requirements (number of kcal/day) for women (59 inches tall) with a BMI of 18.5 kg/in²?
   1. 1626 kcal
   2. 1762 kcal
   3. 1803 kcal
   4. 1956 kcal

2. What are the energy requirements for a very active man (65 inches tall) with a BMI of 24.99 kg/in²?
   1. 2490 kcal
   2. 2842 kcal
   3. 2880 kcal
   4. 3296 kcal

PART II: PUTTING IT ALL TOGETHER

L. Multiple Choice/Multiple Response.
Choose the most appropriate answer or select all that apply.

1. The stomach is normally emptied in:
   1. 30–60 minutes.
   2. 1–4 hours.
   3. 5–8 hours.
   4. 10–12 hours.

2. What is one type of carbohydrate that cannot be digested and is excreted unchanged in the feces?
   1. Fiber
   2. Glucose
   3. Glycogen
   4. Monosaccharide

3. What is the parasympathetic effect in the stomach carried by the vagus nerve in response to the sight or smell of food?
   1. Increases the appetite
   2. Increases gastric acid secretions
   3. Increases the feeling of fullness
   4. Speeds the movement of food through the intestines

4. Which lipoprotein increases the risk of atherosclerosis by contributing to plaque buildup on the artery walls?
   1. Triglycerides
   2. LDLs
   3. HDLs
   4. Phospholipids

5. Which food is the most easily digested?
   1. Raw carrots
   2. Cooked pasta
   3. Fried chicken
   4. Sandwich meats

6. For which body tissues are lipids NOT a source of energy?
   1. Bladder
   2. Stomach
   3. Heart
   4. Brain

7. A calorie is the amount of heat energy required to raise the temperature of 1 g of water at a standard initial temperature by:
   1. 1° C.
   2. 10° C.
   3. 25° C.
   4. 50° C.

8. Which are components of carbohydrates? Select all that apply.
   1. Nitrogen
   2. Oxygen
   3. Iron
   4. Calcium
   5. Hydrogen
   6. Oxygen

9. For immediate use by the body's cells, carbohydrates are converted primarily to:
   1. glycogen.
   2. glucose.
   3. sucrose.
   4. fructose.

10. What acts like a sponge to absorb many times its weight in water and helps provide a full feeling long after eating?
    1. Soluble fiber
    2. Monosaccharides
    3. Insoluble fiber
    4. Glycerols

11. Diets without at least 50–100 g of carbohydrates per day are likely to lead to:
    1. ketosis.
    2. alkalosis.
    3. hyperglycemia.
    4. hypernatremia.

12. Which of the following nutrients releases the most energy?
    1. Fiber
    2. Carbohydrates
    3. Protein
    4. Lipid

13. Where are most lipids carried to be converted to energy or used in the synthesis of new triglycerides?
    1. Gallbladder
    2. Liver
    3. Heart
    4. Kidney

14. Most nutritionists recommend that the daily fat intake should be what percentage of the daily caloric intake?
    1. 50% or less
    2. 30% or less
    3. 15% or less
    4. 10% or less

15. Which of the following foods has the highest protein content?
    1. Cereals
    2. Beans
    3. Poultry
    4. Lentils

16. How much water should adults drink daily?
    1. 500 ml
    2. 1000 ml
    3. 2500 ml
    4. 5000 ml

17. The diet for older adults should include:
    1. low-fat foods.
    2. low-sodium foods.
    3. all the food groups.
    4. high-protein foods.

18. For what deficiencies are older adults with chronic diseases at increased risk? Select all that apply.
    1. Protein deficiency
    2. Vitamin deficiency
    3. Mineral deficiency
    4. Carbohydrate deficiency
    5. Negative nitrogen balance

19. Overweight individuals are considered obese if their weight is what percent above the ideal body weight?
    1. 5% or more
    2. 10% or more
    3. 20% or more
    4. 30% or more

20. Which nutrient must be eaten daily, as it cannot be stored in the body?
    1. Carbohydrates
    2. Protein
    3. Lipids
    4. Minerals

21. What type of solution is administered through a Hickman- or Broviac-type catheter?
    1. Hypotonic
    2. Hypertonic
    3. Isotonic
    4. Glucose and sterile water

22. What is a complication of enteral tube feedings when viscous formulas and crushed medications are inadequately flushed?
    1. Dumping syndrome
    2. Diarrhea
    3. GI bleeding
    4. Tube blockage

23. When moving from enteral to oral feedings, the patient may experience:
    1. breathing difficulties.
    2. bleeding at the TPN site.
    3. heart palpitations.
    4. poor appetite.

24. Which grain product has the highest carbohydrate content?
    1. Tapioca
    2. Popcorn
    3. Crackers
    4. Macaroni

25. Which vegetable has the highest sodium content?
    1. Carrots
    2. Peas
    3. Tomatoes
    4. Cabbage

26. Which hormone increases the rate of glucose utilization?
    1. Insulin
    2. Glucagon
    3. Epinephrine
    4. Growth hormone

27. Which of the following foods has the highest dietary fiber content?
    1. Breads
    2. Vegetables
    3. Rice
    4. Pasta

28. Why is folate necessary for the human body?
    1. Aids in removal of CO_2
    2. Acts in metabolism of carbohydrates and amino acids
    3. Essential for normal metabolism of red blood cells
    4. Important in immune responses

29. How is vitamin C helpful for the human body?
    1. Enzyme development
    2. Wound healing
    3. Night vision
    4. Blood clotting

30. What nutrition-related metabolic change occurs in older adults?
    1. BMR decreases
    2. Lean body mass increases
    3. Plasma glucose levels decrease
    4. Tolerance to glucose increases

31. What nutrition-related change occurs in older adults?
    1. Appetite increases
    2. Salivary secretions increase
    3. Acid secretion increases
    4. Absorption of vitamin B_{12} decreases

32. What is the most common fluid and electrolyte disturbance in older adults?
    1. Hyponatremia
    2. Hypokalemia
    3. Dehydration
    4. Edema

33. Which of the following has over 25 g of fat?
    1. Bran muffin
    2. Hot dog
    3. Cheesecake
    4. Cheeseburger

34. Which has 0 g of fat?
    1. Angel food cake
    2. Chicken noodle soup
    3. Yogurt
    4. Sunflower seeds

35. Which contains the greatest amount of protein?
    1. Canned corn
    2. Bran cereal
    3. Navy beans, cooked
    4. French fries

PART III: CHALLENGE YOURSELF!

M. Getting Ready for NCLEX.

Choose the most appropriate answer or select all that apply.

1. Which of the following are grain products? Select all that apply.
    1. Oatmeal
    2. White bread
    3. Lima beans
    4. Saltine crackers
    5. Spaghetti

2. Which of the following foods contain high amounts of dietary fiber? Select all that apply.
    1. Macaroni
    2. Bagel
    3. Raisin bran cereal
    4. Lima beans
    5. Dried peas

3. The patient's family members ask the nurse about the intake of nutrients that should be kept as low as possible. Which are recommended in very small amounts? Select all that apply.
    1. Dietary cholesterol
    2. Dietary fiber
    3. Trans-fatty acids
    4. Saturated fatty acids

4. Which foods are high in calcium? Select all that apply.
    1. Poultry
    2. Milk
    3. Sardines
    4. Whole-grain cereals

5. Which foods are included in the meat and beans group of the food pyramid? Select all that apply.
    1. Milk
    2. Fish
    3. Egg
    4. Nuts
    5. Wheat bread
    6. Peanut butter

6. The patient with anemia asks the nurse about foods high in iron. Which of the following are high in iron? Select all that apply.
    1. Corn
    2. Spinach
    3. Egg yolk
    4. Milk
    5. Legumes
    6. Bananas

7. Rank in order (from 1 to 7) the following foods from those with the lowest amount of fat to those with the highest amount of fat. The lowest amount is marked 1 and the highest amount is 7.
    A. _____   Hot dog
    B. _____   Tuna
    C. _____   Cup of whole milk
    D. _____   Fruits and vegetables
    E. _____   Chicken pot pie
    F. _____   Macaroni with cheese
    G. _____   Popcorn

8. Rank in order (from 1 to 6) the following foods from those with the lowest protein content (1) to those with the highest protein content (6).
    A. _____   Egg, one
    B. _____   Hamburger
    C. _____   Bread
    D. _____   Peanuts
    E. _____   Butter
    F. _____   Potatoes

Developmental Processes

chapter
10

 Go to http://evolve.elsevier.com/Linton/medsurg/ for additional activities and exercises.

NCLEX CATEGORIES:

Health Promotion and Maintenance

Physiological Integrity: Physiological Adaptation

OBJECTIVES

1. List the developmental tasks for successful adulthood.
2. Identify the health problems specific to the adult age groups.
3. Discuss the health care needs of young, middle-aged, and older adults.

PART I: MASTERING THE BASICS

A. Developmental Stages.
Which of the following describe middle adulthood? Select all that apply.
1. Focus on marriage, childbearing, and work
2. "Sandwich" generation
3. Redirection of energy and talents to new roles and activities
4. Earn most of their money
5. Retirement
6. Establish career goals

B. Developmental Stages.
Which of the following describe young adulthood? Select all that apply.
1. Settling down to job and raising a family
2. Decreased short-term memory
3. Pay most taxes
4. Establish career goals

C. Developmental Stages.
Which of the following relate to older adulthood? Select all that apply.
1. Guidance of grown children
2. Home and time management
3. Learn to combine new dependency needs with the continuing need for independence
4. Help growing and grown children to become happy, responsible adults
5. Adjust to decreasing physical strength and health changes
6. Establish independence from parental home and financial aid
7. Accept role-reversal with aging parents
8. Adjust to loss of physical strength, illness, and one's own mortality

D. Developmental Tasks.
Match the health developmental task in the numbered column with the developmental stage in the lettered column.

1. _____ Generativity versus stagnation
2. _____ Intimacy versus isolation
3. _____ Ego integrity versus despair

A. Young adulthood
B. Middle adulthood
C. Older adulthood

E. Health Problems.

Which health problems are related to middle adulthood? Select all that apply.

1. Benign or malignant prostate enlargement
2. Bone mass begins to decrease
3. Smoking; alcohol and drug abuse
4. Injuries, frequently causing absence from work among men
5. Vehicular accidents and suicide
6. Stress related to managing a household
7. Perimenopausal period
8. Stress related to caregiving role for older parents

F. Age-Related Health Problems.

Which of the following health problems are related to older adults? Select all that apply.

1. Development of presbyopia
2. GI problems
3. Homicide and accidents
4. Arthritis
5. Obesity
6. Accidental falls
7. Emphysema
8. HIV infection
9. Alcoholism

G. Health Risks.

Match the harmful health practices in the numbered column with possible effects on health in the lettered column.

1. _____ Cigarette smoking
2. _____ Alcohol abuse
3. _____ Lack of physical activity
4. _____ Obesity

A. Osteoporosis
B. Degenerative joint disease
C. Cancer of the bladder
D. Malnutrition

PART II: PUTTING IT ALL TOGETHER

H. Multiple-Choice Questions.

Choose the most appropriate answer.

1. Establishing independence from parental home and financial aid is a developmental task of the:
    1. middle-aged adult.
    2. older adult.
    3. young adult.
    4. adolescent.

2. At what age is a baseline mammogram recommended for women?
    1. 20 years old
    2. 30 years old
    3. 40 years old
    4. 50 years old

3. Health promotion for people in their thirties includes:
    1. effective parenting, stress management.
    2. yearly blood pressure screening.
    3. influenza vaccinations.
    4. yearly mammograms.

4. What is the average life expectancy of a child born in 2005?
    1. 65.4 years
    2. 70.2 years
    3. 77.8 years
    4. 82.4 years

PART III: CHALLENGE YOURSELF!

I. Getting Ready for NCLEX.

Choose the most appropriate answer or select all that apply.

1. If older adults cannot adjust to the physical, psychological, and sociologic changes that occur as they age, they are at risk for:
    1. isolation.
    2. stagnation.
    3. generativity.
    4. despair.

2. To collect data about the developmental tasks of young adulthood, the nurse asks:
   1. whether the patient has meaningful, intimate relationships.
   2. what the patient does for leisure or recreation.
   3. what the patient does each day.
   4. what signs of depression the patient has.

3. Asking the patient about meaningful relationships is a way of monitoring the developmental task of:
   1. generativity versus stagnation.
   2. intimacy versus isolation.
   3. ego integrity versus despair.
   4. trust versus distrust.

4. Which health screening tests should begin in young adulthood? Select all that apply.
   1. Routine glucose testing
   2. Pelvic exams
   3. Pap smears
   4. Routine cholesterol
   5. Routine blood pressure screens
   6. Mammograms

5. Which health promotion and disease prevention programs are recommended for adults? Select all that apply.
   1. Reduce sedentary lifestyle
   2. Have annual Pap smears
   3. Maintain ideal weight
   4. Use stress-management programs
   5. Monitor blood pressure once a day

The Older Patient

chapter
11

 Go to http://evolve.elsevier.com/Linton/medsurg/ for additional activities and exercises.

NCLEX CATEGORIES:

Safe and Effective Care Environment:
Coordinated Care

Health Promotion and Maintenance

Psychosocial Integrity

Physiological Integrity: Pharmacological
Therapies, Reduction of Risk Potential,
Physiological Adaptation

OBJECTIVES

1. Describe the roles of the gerontological nurse.
2. Determine the extent to which selected myths and stereotypes about older adults are factual.
3. Describe biologic and physiologic factors associated with aging.
4. Explain psychosocial factors associated with aging.
5. Describe modifications needed for activities of daily living.
6. Explain why drug dosage adjustments may be needed for older persons.

PART I: MASTERING THE BASICS

A. Age-Related Changes.
Which of the following age-related changes decrease in older people? Select all that apply.
   1. Pain, touch, and tactile sensation
   2. Conduction speed in CNS
   3. Pulmonary blood flow
   4. Force of pulse
   5. Intellectual capability
   6. Sound judgment
   7. Cerebral blood flow

B. Age-Related Changes.
Which of the following age-related changes increase in older people? Select all that apply.
   1. Loss of neurons (brain cells)
   2. Functional ability of brain cells
   3. Conduction speed associated with synaptic transmission
   4. Heart size
   5. Vital capacity
   6. Long-term memory
   7. Chronic hypoxia of brain

PART II: PUTTING IT ALL TOGETHER

C. Multiple Choice/Multiple Response.
Choose the most appropriate answer or select all that apply.

1. Which system shows only a slight decline with age?
   1. Renal system
   2. Central nervous system
   3. Respiratory system
   4. Cardiovascular system

2. A frequent concern of older adults is:
   1. long-term memory loss.
   2. creativity loss.
   3. short-term memory loss.
   4. judgment loss.

3. Which of the following result in decreased vital capacity in older persons? Select all that apply.
   1. Vertebral loss of calcium
   2. Calcification of costal cartilage
   3. Decreased anteroposterior chest diameter
   4. Contractures
   5. Kyphosis

4. A frequent respiratory complaint of older adults is:
   1. orthostatic hypotension.
   2. inability to breathe.
   3. increased respirations.
   4. exertional dyspnea.

5. Standard components of respiratory care for the older adult include:
   1. coughing and deep-breathing exercises and range-of-motion exercises to facilitate lung expansion.
   2. frequent ambulation and auscultation of lungs.
   3. intake and output and postural drainage exercises.
   4. deep-breathing exercises and positioning to facilitate lung expansion and gas exchange.

6. With increasing age, a person's reduced tolerance for physical work may be due to the decreased:
   1. number of neurons in the brain.
   2. capacity of heart cells to utilize oxygen.
   3. size of the heart.
   4. resistance to blood flow in many organs.

7. Which change occurs in aging kidneys?
   1. Decreased filtration rate
   2. Increased extracellular fluid
   3. Increased cell mass
   4. Decreased residual urine

8. An age change that occurs due to loss of oils in the skin is:
   1. infection.
   2. itching.
   3. wrinkles.
   4. brown spots.

9. The leading cause of disability in old age is:
   1. urinary tract infection.
   2. macular degeneration
   3. pressure ulcers.
   4. arthritis.

10. The curvature of the thoracic spine that causes a bent-over appearance in some older adults is:
    1. kyphosis.
    2. arthritis.
    3. scoliosis.
    4. lordosis.

11. The term for hearing loss associated with age is:
    1. tinnitus.
    2. ototoxicity.
    3. presbyopia.
    4. presbycusis.

12. What percentage of older adults are hearing-impaired?
    1. 10%
    2. 25%
    3. 50%
    4. 75%

13. The leading cause of new cases of blindness in older people is age-related:
    1. glaucoma.
    2. cataracts.
    3. corneal abrasion.
    4. macular degeneration.

14. Which of the following is a normal aging change?
    1. Decreased secretion of saliva
    2. Increased acidity of saliva
    3. Increased peristalsis
    4. Decreased gastric emptying

15. The developmental challenge in old age is to:
    1. develop close relations with other people; to learn and experience love.
    2. find a vocation or hobby where the individual can help others or in some way contribute to society.
    3. establish trusting relationships with other people.
    4. review life and gain a feeling of accomplishment or fulfillment.

16. For effective gerontological care, the crucial basis for deciding care needs is:
    1. medical diagnosis.
    2. functional assessment.
    3. activities of daily living.
    4. community resources.

17. Which of the following age-related changes affect the inactivation of drugs in the body? Select all that apply.
    1. Decreased liver size
    2. Reduced blood flow through the liver
    3. Decreased body water
    4. Reduced liver enzyme activity
    5. Decreased renal function

18. Progressive slowing of responses and reflexes in older adults is due to:
    1. decreased impulse conduction speed.
    2. loss of neurons in the brain.
    3. inadequate tissue oxygenation.
    4. atherosclerosis and decreased cellular respiration.

PART III: CHALLENGE YOURSELF!

D. Getting Ready for NCLEX.

Choose the most appropriate answer.

1. A stressor, such as illness, may impair the older person's ability to compensate, resulting in:
   1. disorientation.
   2. hypotension.
   3. loss of brain neurons.
   4. sedation.

2. A 74-year-old man with cirrhosis is admitted to the hospital, and he has started taking a diuretic. Which age-related change may result in decreased drug clearance in this patient?
   1. Increased body fat
   2. Decreased body water
   3. Decreased hepatic blood flow
   4. Decreased serum albumin

3. Because older adults have a decreased number and sensitivity of sensory receptors and neurons, they should:
   1. avoid temperature extremes and accomplish tasks at a slower pace.
   2. do deep-breathing exercises and positioning to facilitate lung expansion.
   3. use mnemonics and rehearsal memory training to improve memory performance.
   4. use assistive devices for walking and preventing falls.

4. The nurse is taking care of a 70-year-old patient whose blood pressure is 150/90 mm Hg. What is an age-related cause of this blood pressure?
   1. Decreased neurons and conduction speed at synapses
   2. Decreased baroreceptor reflexes and inelasticity of vessel walls
   3. Chronic hypoxic state of the brain
   4. Decreased heart rate and stroke volume

5. The nurse is taking care of a 75-year-old patient whose resting cardiac output has fallen 40%. What is an explanation for this finding?
   1. Decreases in filtration and plasma flow rate
   2. Increased valvular rigidity
   3. Incomplete closure of the aortic and pulmonic valves
   4. Decreased heart rate and stroke volume

6. A chronic hypoxic state of the brain in older persons may result in:
   1. difficulty remembering planned events for the day.
   2. slow responses.
   3. decrease in creativity.
   4. inability to learn new material.

The Nursing Process and Critical Thinking

Go to http://evolve.elsevier.com/Linton/medsurg/ for additional activities and exercises.

NCLEX CATEGORIES:

Safe and Effective Care Environment:
Coordinated Care

Health Promotion and Maintenance

Physiological Integrity: Physiological Adaptation

OBJECTIVES

1. Describe the components of the nursing process.
2. Explain the role of the licensed practical nurse/licensed vocational nurse (LPN/LVN) in the nursing process.
3. Describe the proper documentation of the nursing process.
4. Describe the relationship of the nursing process with the process of documentation.
5. Explain the relationship between the nursing process and critical thinking.
6. Describe the characteristics of a critical thinker.
7. Describe how critical thinking skills are used in clinical practice.
8. Describe principles of setting priorities for nursing care.

PART I: MASTERING THE BASICS

A. Key Terms.
Match the definition in the numbered column with the most appropriate term in the lettered column.

1. _____ Method of recordkeeping that focuses on patient problems rather than on medical diagnoses

2. _____ Systematic, problem-solving approach to providing nursing care in an organized, scientific manner

3. _____ Tapping on the skin to assess the underlying tissues

4. _____ Method of physical examination that uses the sense of touch to assess various parts of the body

5. _____ Listening to sounds produced by the body, such as heart, lung, and intestinal sounds

6. _____ Purposeful observation or scrutiny of the person as a whole and then of each body system

7. _____ Actual or potential health problems derived from data gathered during the assessment of a patient or client

8. _____ Information reported by patients or family members

9. _____ Collection of data about the health status of a patient or client

10. _____ Information about the patient collected by the nurse or other members of the health care team

A. Auscultation
B. Objective data
C. Nursing diagnosis
D. Problem-oriented medical record
E. Subjective data
F. Nursing process
G. Percussion
H. Inspection
I. Assessment
J. Palpation

B. Nursing Process.

Match the definition in the numbered column with the most appropriate component of the nursing process in the lettered column. Answers may be used more than once.

1. _____ Putting the plan into action
2. _____ Systematic collection of data relating to patients and their problems
3. _____ Assessing the achievement of patient goals
4. _____ Setting goals
5. _____ Interpretation of the data for problem identification
6. _____ Identify health problems or potential health problems
7. _____ Determine priorities from the list of nursing diagnoses
8. _____ Collect data, including height, weight, and vital signs
9. _____ Obtain information through a health history by direct questioning
10. _____ Measure the patient's progress toward meeting goals
11. _____ Actual performance of nursing interventions identified in the care plan
12. _____ Set short-term and long-term goals to determine outcomes of care

A. Assessment
B. Nursing diagnosis
C. Planning
D. Intervention (implementation)
E. Evaluation

C. Objective Data.

Match the description in the numbered column (objective data) with the problem in the lettered column.

1. _____ A patient's disheveled appearance based on sight
2. _____ A patient's noisy and labored breathing based on hearing
3. _____ A fruity mouth odor based on smell
4. _____ Cold, clammy skin based on touch

A. Possible respiratory problems
B. Possible sign of diabetic ketoacidosis
C. May indicate that patient is in shock
D. May indicate inability to carry out self-care activities at home

D. Critical Thinking.

Match the description of critical thinking tools in the numbered column with the corresponding critical thinking tool in the lettered column.

1. _____ Deriving alternatives and drawing conclusions
2. _____ Clarifying the meaning of events and data
3. _____ Reconsidering conclusions and recognizing the need to make changes
4. _____ Presenting arguments for decisions and justifying
5. _____ Examining ideas and breaking them down into components
6. _____ Assessing possibilities, opinions, and usual practices

A. Interpretation
B. Analysis
C. Evaluation
D. Inference
E. Explanation
F. Self-regulation

E. Critical Thinking.

Which characteristics of critical thinking are related to analytical thinking? Select all that apply.

1. Willing to consider various alternatives
2. Examines parts and sees how they fit together
3. Recognizes that many variables are at work in patient situations
4. Uses an organized approach to problem-solving
5. The desire not just to know, but to understand, how to apply the knowledge
6. Applies knowledge from various disciplines

F. Nursing Diagnosis.

Choose the most appropriate answer.

1. A 75-year-old man is admitted to a long-term care facility with weight loss and diarrhea. Which nursing diagnosis is the highest priority for this patient?
   1. Complicated grieving
   2. Dysfunctional gastrointestinal motility
   3. Impaired individual resilience
   4. Ineffective self-care management
   5. Insomnia

2. A 72-year-old patient admitted to the hospital takes a diuretic, an antihypertensive drug, and an anticoagulant. Which nursing diagnosis is the highest priority for this patient?
   1. Risk for acute confusion
   2. Risk for bleeding
   3. Risk for complicated grieving
   4. Risk for compromised resilience

3. A postoperative patient has just been transferred from the recovery unit to his bed on the medical floor. Which diagnosis is the highest priority for this patient?
   1. Risk for shock
   2. Risk for infection
   3. Risk for loneliness
   4. Risk for powerlessness

G. Nursing Diagnosis.

Which of the following are nursing diagnoses? Select all that apply.
   1. Peptic ulcer
   2. Pneumonia
   3. Insomnia
   4. Myocardial infarction
   5. Readiness for enhanced hope
   6. Moral distress
   7. Risk for falls

H. Data Collection.

Which of the following are objective data? Select all that apply.
   1. A shooting pain in my arm
   2. Noisy, labored breathing
   3. Fruity mouth odor
   4. Cold, clammy skin
   5. Blood pressure of 120/80 mm Hg
   6. Headache
   7. Fear of surgery

I. Physical Assessment Techniques.

Match the condition to be assessed in the numbered column with the appropriate technique in the lettered column. Answers may be used more than once.

1. _____ Bowel sounds
2. _____ Pitting edema
3. _____ Mucous membranes
4. _____ Jaundice
5. _____ Blood pressure
6. _____ Radial pulse
7. _____ Lung sounds
8. _____ Cyanosis

A. Inspection
B. Percussion
C. Palpation
D. Auscultation

PART II: PUTTING IT ALL TOGETHER

J. Multiple-Response Questions.

Choose the most appropriate answer.

1. The goal of the nursing process is to:
   1. obtain information through observation, physical examination, or diagnostic testing.
   2. interview the patient or family in a goal-directed, orderly, and systematic way.
   3. record objective data, writing exactly what is observed.
   4. alleviate, minimize, or prevent real or potential health problems.

2. In the planning phase of the nursing process, which of the following actions occurs first?
   1. Set short-term goals to determine outcomes of care.
   2. Set long-term goals to determine outcomes of care.
   3. Develop objectives to meet goals.
   4. Determine priorities from the list of nursing diagnoses.

3. The role of the LPN in relation to the planning phase of the nursing process is to:
   1. perform a physical assessment.
   2. perform therapeutic nursing measures.
   3. assist with the development of nursing care plans.
   4. evaluate the nursing care given.

4. When admitting a patient with pneumonia, which step of the nursing process is done first?
   1. Implementation
   2. Determine outcome criteria
   3. Set short-term goals
   4. Collect data

5. Which step of the nursing process does the nurse use to determine whether outcome criteria have been met?
   1. Assessment
   2. Planning
   3. Implementation
   4. Evaluation

6. Why is auscultation done before percussion and palpation when doing a physical assessment of the abdomen?
   1. Auscultation aids in the palpation process.
   2. Palpation can alter auscultation findings.
   3. Auscultation can alter palpation findings.
   4. Auscultation findings determine where to perform percussion.

7. Which of the following describes critical thinking?
   1. Thinking based on learning many facts
   2. Reasonable thinking focused on deciding what to do
   3. Thinking based on the utilization of the nursing process
   4. Reflective thinking related to reading and gathering information

8. Auscultation is used to assess the:
   1. skin.
   2. joints.
   3. lungs.
   4. head.

9. Which of the following is the best method for obtaining objective data?
   1. Asking the patient about his pain
   2. Observing the patient to see if he is afraid
   3. Watching the patient for signs of fatigue
   4. Inspecting the color of the patient's skin

10. Which of the following short-term goals is incomplete?
    1. The patient will drink 1500 ml by 8:00 AM on 3/22.
    2. The patient will ambulate in the hall twice a day on 3/22.
    3. The patient will have less pain by 8:00 AM on 3/22.
    4. The patient will cough and deep-breathe every 4 hours on 3/22.

11. Which critical thinking tool is utilized when considering possible outcomes of each nursing action and choosing one intervention?
    1. Interpretation: identifying data
    2. Evaluation: assessing possibilities
    3. Inference: drawing conclusions
    4. Self-regulation: reconsidering conclusions

PART III: CHALLENGE YOURSELF!

K. Getting Ready for NCLEX.

Choose the most appropriate answer.

1. The statement, "Does not turn self in bed; 2 cm, stage 2 pressure ulcer on sacrum," refers to which component of documentation?
   1. Subjective information
   2. Assessment
   3. Plan
   4. Objective information

2. The statement, "Turn from side to side every 2 hours. Get out of bed at least twice a day. Begin ambulating as tolerated," refers to which component of documentation?
   1. Plan
   2. Assessment
   3. Evaluation
   4. Objective information

3. Which would the nurse chart under objective data?
   1. Lumbar back pain
   2. Nausea
   3. No shortness of breath
   4. Pupils equal and reactive

4. Which is a correct recording of observational data?
   1. The skin is cool and clammy.
   2. The skin looks good.
   3. The patient states, "My skin is cool and clammy."
   4. The patient's skin has improved.

5. Which of the following observations about the patient is documented as subjective data?
   1. Patient is 6' 3" tall and weighs 180 pounds.
   2. Patient's skin is jaundiced.
   3. Patient has pain associated with taking deep breaths.
   4. Patient's blood pressure is 130/80 mm Hg.

6. A new patient is admitted to the hospital with the following nursing diagnoses: Fatigue, Nausea, Ineffective individual coping, and Ineffective breathing pattern. Which diagnosis requires immediate attention?
   1. Fatigue
   2. Nausea
   3. Ineffective individual coping
   4. Ineffective breathing pattern

7. The care plan states that the nurse is supposed to give the patient a bath. The patient states that he feels "wobbly" when he stands up. The nurse checks his blood pressure, which is 90/60 mm Hg and his pulse is 120 and weak. What is the best nursing action?
   1. Try again to get him up
   2. Give him a bed bath
   3. Let him rest and see how he feels later
   4. Exercise his legs before letting him stand

8. Into what level of Maslow's hierarchy does the nursing diagnosis of Disturbed body image fall?
   1. Physiological
   2. Safety
   3. Love and belonging
   4. Self-esteem

9. A patient, Mrs. C., had a radical mastectomy of her left breast. Mrs. C.'s husband was not supportive of her surgery, and Mrs. C. needed his support to cope with her surgery. What is the priority initial nursing intervention for Mrs. C.?
   1. Assist Mrs. C. to discuss changes caused by illness and surgery.
   2. Monitor frequency of Mrs. C.'s statements of self-criticism.
   3. Determine patient's and family's perception of Mrs. C.'s alteration in body image vs. reality.
   4. Identify support groups available to Mrs. C.

Inflammation, Infection, and Immunity

 Go to http://evolve.elsevier.com/Linton/medsurg/ for additional activities and exercises.

NCLEX CATEGORIES:

Safe and Effective Care Environment:
Coordinated Care, Safety and Infection Control

Health Promotion and Maintenance

Physiological Integrity: Reduction of Risk Potential, Physiological Adaptation

OBJECTIVES

1. Describe physical and chemical barriers.
2. Describe how inflammatory changes act as bodily defense mechanisms.
3. Identify the signs and symptoms of inflammation.
4. Discuss the process of repair and healing.
5. Differentiate infection from inflammation.
6. Discuss the actions of commonly found infectious agents.
7. Describe the ways that infections are transmitted.
8. Identify the signs and symptoms of infection.
9. Compare community-acquired and health care–associated infections.
10. Discuss the nursing care of patients with infections.
11. Describe the Centers for Disease Control (CDC) Standard Precautions guidelines for infection prevention and control.
12. Describe the Centers for Disease Control isolation guidelines for Airborne, Droplet, and Contact (Transmission-Based) Precautions.
13. Describe the CDC isolation guidelines for a Protective Environment.
14. Describe the immune response.
15. Identify organs involved in immunity.
16. Compare natural and acquired immunity.
17. Differentiate between humoral (antibody-mediated) and cell-mediated immunity.
18. Describe the nursing care of patients with immunodeficiency and of those with allergies.
19. Describe the process of autoimmunity.

PART I: MASTERING THE BASICS

A. Key Terms.

Match the definition in the numbered column with the most appropriate term in the lettered column.

1. _____ An antigen that causes a hypersensitive reaction
2. _____ A protein that is created in response to a specific antigen
3. _____ Vegetable-like organisms that feed on organic matter and are capable of producing disease
4. _____ A substance, usually a protein, that is capable of stimulating a response from the immune system
5. _____ One-celled organisms capable of multiplying rapidly and causing illness
6. _____ Infectious microorganisms that can live and reproduce only within living cells; capable of causing illness, inflammation, and cell destruction
7. _____ Microorganisms that are resistant to one or more classes of antimicrobial agents

A. Allergen
B. Antibody
C. Antigen
D. Bacteria
E. Fungi
F. Multi-drug resistant organisms
G. Viruses

B. Key Terms.

Match the definition in the numbered column with the most appropriate term in the lettered column.

1. _____ Limiting the spread of microorganisms; often called *clean technique*

2. _____ Elimination of microorganisms from any object that comes in contact with the patient; often called *sterile technique*

3. _____ Nonspecific immune response that occurs in response to bodily injury; condition in which the body is invaded by infectious organisms that multiply, causing injury and inflammatory response

4. _____ Hospital-acquired infections (infections that were not present at the time of admission)

5. _____ Presence of an infectious organism on a body surface or an object

6. _____ A condition in which the body is invaded by infectious organisms that multiply, causing injury

7. _____ A condition in which the body is unable to distinguish self from nonself, causing the immune system to react and destroy its own tissues

8. _____ Illness caused by infectious organisms or their toxins that can be transmitted, either directly or indirectly, from one person to another

9. _____ Condition in which the immune system is unable to defend the body against organisms

10. _____ Resistance to or protection from a disease

A. Autoimmunity
B. Communicable disease
C. Contamination
D Immunity
E. Immunodeficiency
F. Infection
G. Inflammation
H. Medical asepsis
I. Health care–associated infection
J. Surgical asepsis

C. Infectious Agents.

Which of the following are infectious agents? Select all that apply.

1. Helminths
2. Protozoa
3. Macrophages
4. Fungi
5. Allergens
6. Viruses

D. Signs of Infection.

Which of the following are observable signs (objective data) of infection? Select all that apply.

1. Redness
2. Pus
3. Pain
4. Swelling
5. Discoloration
6. Heat
7. Decreased skin turgor

E. Age-Related Changes.

What reasons explain why the healing process can be delayed in older adults? Select all that apply.

1. Decreased tissue elasticity
2. Decreased lean muscle mass
3. Decreased blood supply to tissues
4. Decreased renal function

F. Chain of Infection.

Place the six factors of the chain of infection in sequence. (Note: Begin by numbering causation agent as 1).

A. _____ Portal of entry
B. _____ Reservoir
C. _____ Susceptible host
D. _____ Mode of transmission
E. _____ Portal of exit
F. _____ Causation agent

G. Allergies.
Match each common allergic reaction in the numbered column with the most appropriate causative agent in the lettered column.

1. _____ Asthma
2. _____ Anaphylaxis
3. _____ Urticaria (hives)
4. _____ Atopic dermatitis (eczema)
5. _____ Allergic contact dermatitis

A. Food
B. Latex gloves, plants (poison ivy)
C. Pollens, dust
D. Soaps
E. Insect venom, antibiotics

H. Resistance.
Which of the following are reasons for the development of resistant bacterial strains? Select all that apply.
1. Bacterial cells develop mutations.
2. Overuse of antibiotics.
3. Introduction of allergens.
4. Exposure to cigarette smoke.

I. Prevention of Antimicrobial Resistance.
Which nursing considerations are recommended by CDC to prevent antimicrobial resistance in long-term care patients? Select all that apply.
1. Encourage patients to have annual influenza vaccine.
2. Monitor blood glucose.
3. Monitor body temperature.
4. Prevent aspiration and pressure ulcers.
5. Use proper technique for catheter insertion and care.

J. Standard Precautions.
Contact with which substances require the use of Standard Precautions when the nurse is performing procedures? Select all that apply.
1. Patient's blood
2. Sweat and perspiration
3. Mucous membranes
4. Intact skin
5. Body fluids

K. Standard Precautions.
For each disease or condition in the numbered column, indicate all of the appropriate types of precautions in the lettered column.

1. _____ Mumps
2. _____ Scabies
3. _____ Influenza
4. _____ Impetigo
5. _____ Rubeola (measles)
6. _____ Respiratory syncytial virus (RSV)
7. _____ Varicella (chickenpox)
8. _____ Rubella
9. _____ Tuberculosis
10. _____ Diphtheria (pharyngeal)

A. Airborne precautions
B. Droplet precautions
C. Contact precautions

L. Lab Tests.
Which of the following are laboratory tests used to screen patients for infection? Select all that apply.
1. White blood cell differentiated count
2. Liver function
3. Electrolytes
4. Blood cultures
5. Platelet count

M. Hyperbaric Oxygen Therapy.
Which of the following are complications for which the nurse monitors the patient during hyperbaric oxygen therapy? Select all that apply.
1. Ear pain
2. Eye pain
3. Seizures
4. Bradycardia
5. Chest pain
6. Allergic reaction

N. Immune System.

Which of the following are factors that can compromise the immune system? Select all that apply.

1. Aging
2. Disease
3. Stress
4. Use of antihypertensives
5. Use of steroids

O. Antigens.

Which of the following are antigens? Select all that apply.

1. Microorganisms
2. White blood cells
3. Environmental substances
4. Platelets
5. Dust

P. Immune System Organs.

Which body organs are involved in immunity? Select all that apply.

1. Bone marrow
2. Heart
3. Lungs
4. Lymph nodes
5. Spleen
6. Thyroid gland

Q. Drug Therapy.

Which classifications of medications often place patients at risk for infection? Select all that apply.

1. Antibiotics
2. Antihypertensives
3. Steroids
4. Antineoplastics
5. Diuretics
6. Cholesterol-lowering drugs

R. Allergens.

Which of the following are common allergens? Select all that apply.

1. Animal dander
2. Molds
3. Foods
4. Viruses
5. Bacteria
6. Pollens
7. Cigarette smoke
8. Fungi
9. Latex gloves
10. Pus

S. Anaphylaxis.

Which of the following are effects of histamine on the body when it is released during anaphylaxis? Select all that apply.

1. Shock from hypervolemia
2. Decreased vascular permeability
3. Edema
4. Bronchospasm
5. Vasoconstriction

T. Inflammatory Response.

Indicate the stages of the antiinflammatory response following tissue injury outlined in Figure 13-1 (textbook p. 175) using the letters A–D.

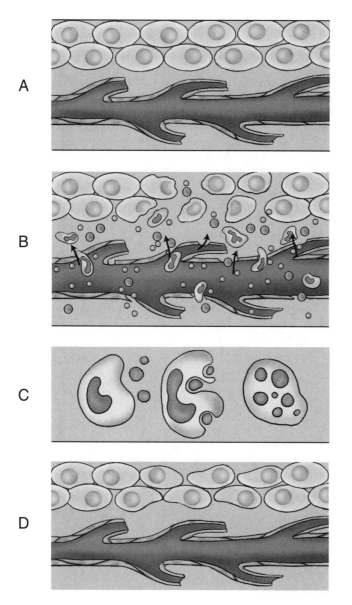

1. _____ Release of chemical mediators
2. _____ Ingestion and destruction of foreign agents
3. _____ Repair and regeneration
4. _____ Intact cells
5. _____ Movement of proteins, water, and white blood cells out of capillaries into injured tissues
6. _____ Exudate formation
7. _____ Normal blood vessel
8. _____ Phagocytic lymphocytes enter area of injury
9. _____ Dilated blood vessels and increased capillary permeability

A. Normal tissue
B. Stage I
C. Stage 2
D. Stage 3

U. Immune System Organs.
Using Figure 13-5 (p. 190) below, label organs involved in immunity (A–G).

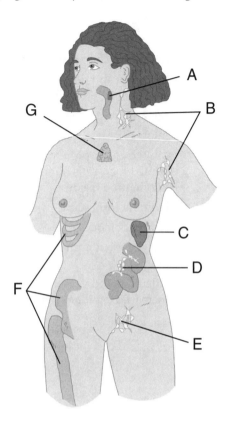

A. _____

B. _____

C. _____

D. _____

E. _____

F. _____

G. _____

V. Autoimmune Disorders.
Match the autoimmune disorders in the numbered column with the most appropriate targets in the lettered column.

1. _____ Diabetes mellitus type 1

2. _____ Addison's disease

3. _____ Multiple sclerosis

4. _____ Myasthenia gravis

5. _____ Rheumatic fever

6. _____ Ulcerative colitis

7. _____ Crohn's disease

8. _____ Rheumatoid arthritis

9. _____ Autoimmune thrombocytopenic purpura

A. Colon
B. Adrenal gland
C. Ileum
D. Joints
E. Brain and spinal cord
F. Pancreas
G. Neuromuscular junction
H. Heart
I. Platelets

PART II: PUTTING IT ALL TOGETHER

W. Multiple Choice/Multiple Response.

Choose the most appropriate answer or select all that apply.

1. Prostaglandins, histamine, and leukotrienes are examples of:
   1. hormonal factors.
   2. chemical mediators.
   3. erythrocytes.
   4. thrombocytes.

2. A hormone produced by the adrenal cortex that is antiinflammatory is:
   1. epinephrine.
   2. cortisol.
   3. aldosterone.
   4. thyroxine.

3. Cells that are produced to clean up inflammatory debris are called:
   1. fibroblasts.
   2. platelets.
   3. neutrophils.
   4. macrophages.

4. Which of the following is a sign of local infection?
   1. Fever
   2. Chills
   3. Warm skin
   4. Pale skin

5. Many childhood illnesses such as measles and chickenpox and some forms of hepatitis are caused by:
   1. viruses.
   2. bacteria.
   3. protozoa.
   4. fungi.

6. It is seldom possible to kill viruses because:
   1. replication of the virus occurs within the host cell.
   2. the cell wall can be destroyed with drugs.
   3. the cell wall requires oxygen for functions.
   4. the host cell is separate from the virus.

7. Ringworm (tinea corporis) and athlete's foot (tinea pedis) are examples of disease caused by:
   1. bacteria.
   2. viruses.
   3. fungi.
   4. protozoa.

8. Which type of patients are most susceptible to hospital-acquired infections? Select all that apply.
   1. Patients with pneumonia
   2. Patients requiring insulin
   3. Patients with myocardial infarction
   4. Patients with AIDS
   5. Cancer patients receiving chemotherapy
   6. Patients with emphysema

9. The overgrowth of a second microorganism that can cause illness following antibiotic therapy for one microorganism is called:
   1. thrombophlebitis.
   2. superinfection.
   3. sexually transmitted infection.
   4. septicemia.

10. The most basic and effective method of preventing cross-contamination is:
    1. hand hygiene.
    2. antibiotics.
    3. isolation.
    4. use of gown and gloves.

11. The primary cause of health care–associated infections is:
    1. soiled hands.
    2. faulty equipment.
    3. airborne droplets.
    4. open wounds.

12. The elimination of microorganisms from any object that comes in contact with the patient is called:
    1. medical asepsis.
    2. clean technique.
    3. isolation technique.
    4. surgical asepsis.

13. How much fluid is required by patients with infection?
    1. 1 liter/day
    2. 2 liters/day
    3. 5 liters/day
    4. 10 liters/day

14. Patient teaching for people undergoing hyperbaric oxygen therapy includes:
    1. do not take aspirin 1 week before.
    2. do not wear watches.
    3. swallow first to prevent pressure buildup.
    4. wear everyday clothes.

15. An advantage of home health care for infected patients is that the patient is:
    1. exposed to fewer health care–associated infections.
    2. not capable of spreading infections to others.
    3. not susceptible to poorly prepared food.
    4. vulnerable to poor hygiene.

16. Which type of precaution is used to treat methicillin-resistant *Staphylococcus aureus* (MRSA) infections?
    1. Airborne
    2. Droplet
    3. Respiratory
    4. Contact

17. People with generalized infections become dehydrated because of:
    1. poor skin turgor and dry mouth.
    2. dry mucous membranes and decreased metabolism.
    3. inflammation and pain.
    4. fever and anorexia.

18. A diet recommended for patients with infection is:
    1. low sodium.
    2. high fiber.
    3. high protein.
    4. low potassium.

19. A common side effect of broad-spectrum antibiotics is:
    1. superinfection.
    2. hemorrhage.
    3. hypotension.
    4. hypokalemia.

20. Food-borne illness is a common community-acquired infectious disease often caused by:
    1. pseudomonas.
    2. diphtheria.
    3. streptococcus.
    4. salmonella.

21. What percentage of the U.S. population suffers from allergies of some sort?
    1. Under 5%
    2. 20–25%
    3. 40–45%
    4. 50–75%

22. Antigens that cause hypersensitivity reactions are called:
    1. antibodies.
    2. complement.
    3. allergens.
    4. interferon.

23. Allergy testing is performed by injecting small amounts of allergen:
    1. intradermally.
    2. intramuscularly.
    3. intravenously.
    4. interstitially.

24. In anaphylaxis, what are the effects of histamine? Select all that apply.
    1. Bronchospasm
    2. Vasoconstriction
    3. Phagocytosis
    4. Increased vascular permeability

25. Which drugs are used in the treatment of anaphylaxis? Select all that apply.
    1. Atropine
    2. Diphenhydramine
    3. Corticosteroids
    4. Propranolol
    5. Aminophylline
    6. Epinephrine

26. A 36-year-old female has multiple sclerosis. Which tissues and organs are affected?
    1. Heart and kidney tissue
    2. White matter of brain and spinal cord
    3. Lung tissue and liver cells
    4. Spleen tissue and thymus gland

27. What are common portals of entry for flu and cold viruses? Select all that apply.
    1. Mouth
    2. Skin
    3. Nose
    4. Conjunctiva
    5. Lungs
    6. Outer ear canal

28. It is now necessary to give two or more drugs to tuberculosis patients because:
    1. they prolong the effects of each drug.
    2. they potentiate the effect of each drug.
    3. strains of bacteria resistant to drugs have developed.
    4. more people are susceptible to tuberculosis.

29. A common protozoal infection that occurs as an opportunistic infection in persons who are HIV-positive is:
    1. pneumocystic pneumonia.
    2. Rocky Mountain spotted fever.
    3. thrush.
    4. conjunctivitis.

30. Any items that have been touched or cross-contaminated by the host, such as bed linens or side rails, are:
    1. vectors.
    2. common vehicles.
    3. pathogens.
    4. fomites.

PART III: CHALLENGE YOURSELF!

X. Getting Ready for NCLEX.

Choose the most appropriate answer.

1. Which of the following are considered to be autoimmune disorders? Select all that apply.
   1. Pneumonia
   2. Graves' disease (hyperthyroid disease)
   3. Crohn's disease
   4. Tuberculosis
   5. Hypertension
   6. Multiple sclerosis

2. Which of the following are common reportable diseases? Select all that apply.
   1. Syphilis
   2. Crohn's disease
   3. Hypertension
   4. Encephalitis
   5. Diabetes mellitus
   6. Gonorrhea
   7. Hepatitis
   8. AIDS
   9. Pneumonia

3. Which of the following illnesses require the use of airborne precautions? Select all that apply.
   1. Pneumonia
   2. Measles
   3. Tuberculosis
   4. Pertussis
   5. Meningitis
   6. Varicella

4. Which of the following require contact precautions? Select all that apply.
   1. Tuberculosis
   2. Influenza
   3. Impetigo
   4. Wound infection
   5. Viral conjunctivitis

5. What general health practices can help to slow the development of a patient with multi-drug resistant organisms (MDROs)? Select all that apply.
   1. Encourage vaccinations for communicable diseases.
   2. Reserve antibiotics for serious infections.
   3. Wear gown and gloves at all times when working with patients who have MDROs.
   4. Remove gown and gloves immediately after leaving the patient's room.
   5. Place the patient in a private room.

6. Which are common nursing diagnoses in patients with infections? Select all that apply.
   1. Chronic pain
   2. Decreased cardiac output
   3. Risk for injury
   4. Impaired tissue integrity
   5. Social isolation
   6. Excess fluid volume

Fluids and Electrolytes

chapter

14

 Go to http://evolve.elsevier.com/Linton/medsurg/ for additional activities and exercises.

NCLEX CATEGORIES:

Health Promotion and Maintenance

Physiological Integrity: Basic Care and Comfort, Pharmacological Therapies, Reduction of Risk Potential, Physiological Adaptation

OBJECTIVES

1. Describe the extracellular and intracellular fluid compartments.
2. Describe the composition of the extracellular and intracellular body fluid compartments.
3. Discuss the mechanisms of fluid transport and fluid balance.
4. Identify the causes, signs and symptoms, and treatment of fluid imbalances.
5. Describe the major functions of the major electrolytes—sodium, potassium, calcium, magnesium, and chloride.
6. Identify the causes, signs and symptoms, and treatment of electrolyte imbalances.
7. List data to be collected in assessing fluid and electrolyte status.
8. Discuss the medical treatment and nursing management of people with fluid and electrolyte imbalances.
9. Explain why older adults are at increased risk for fluid and electrolyte imbalances.
10. List the four types of acid-base imbalances.
11. Identify the major causes of each acid-base imbalance.
12. Explain the management of acid-base imbalances.

PART I: MASTERING THE BASICS

A. Body Water.

Select the correct word to complete each sentence.

1. With increasing age, body water (increases/decreases).

2. Fat cells contain (more/less) water than other cells.

3. Females have (higher/lower) body water percentages than males.

4. An obese person has a (higher/lower) percentage of body water than a thin person.

B. Electrolytes.

Which of the following are electrolytes? Select all that apply.

1. Bilirubin
2. Urea
3. Magnesium
4. Phosphate
5. Creatinine
6. Sodium
7. Potassium
8. Protein
9. Chloride
10. Calcium

C. Fluid Balance.

Which of the following conditions have great potential for altering fluid balance? Select all that apply.

1. Burns
2. Multiple sclerosis
3. Ulcerative colitis
4. Dyspnea
5. Vomiting
6. Kidney disease
7. Tachycardia
8. Hypothermia
9. Diarrhea
10. Congestive heart failure

D. Skin Turgor.

What are locations where skin turgor is best measured? Select all that apply.

1. Wrist
2. Sternum
3. Inner aspects of thighs
4. Cheeks
5. Forehead
6. Fingertips

E. Edema Measurement.

What are common parts of the body against which skin is pressed to test for edema? Select all that apply.

1. Radius
2. Ankle
3. Tibia
4. Fibula
5. Femur
6. Sternum
7. Sacrum

F. Fluid Balance.

Which of the following are related to fluid volume excess (hypervolemia)? Select all that apply.

1. Stimulates thirst
2. Dilute urine
3. Decreased urination
4. Stimulates aldosterone
5. Inhibits ADH

G. Regulation of Body Fluid Volume.

Match the condition in the numbered column with the most appropriate effect in the lettered column. Answers may be used more than once or not at all.

1. Hyperkalemia
2. Increased plasma osmolality
3. Hyponatremia
4. Decreased plasma osmolality

A. Stimulates ADH release
B. Inhibits ADH release
C. Stimulates aldosterone release
D. Inhibits aldosterone release

H. Fluid and Electrolyte Changes.

Which of the following vital sign changes (assessment) are related to fluid volume deficit? Select all that apply.

1. Bounding pulse
2. Increased blood pressure
3. Deep, fast respirations
4. Fall in systolic blood pressure >20 mm Hg from lying to standing
5. Fever
6. Increased respiratory rate
7. Subnormal body temperature
8. Increased pulse rate

I. Blood Gas Values.

Refer to Table 14-7 in the textbook. Add arrows (↑, ↓) or Normal in the table below.

Arterial Blood Gas Values with Uncompensated Respiratory and Metabolic Acidosis and Alkalosis				
CONDITION	CAUSE	pH	HCO_3	$PaCO_2$
Respiratory acidosis	Hypoventilation			
Respiratory alkalosis	Hyperventilation			
Metabolic acidosis	Diabetic ketoacidosis Lactic acidosis Diarrhea Renal insufficiency			
Metabolic alkalosis	Vomiting HCO_3 retention Volume depletion K^+ depletion			

J. Fluid and Electrolyte Imbalances.

What respiratory changes occur with metabolic alkalosis? Select all that apply.

1. Deep, rapid respirations
2. Slow, shallow respirations
3. Dyspnea
4. Intermittent apnea
5. Tachypnea

PART II: PUTTING IT ALL TOGETHER

K. Multiple Choice/Multiple Response.

Choose the most appropriate answer or select all that apply.

1. The major electrolytes in extracellular fluid are:
   1. sodium and chloride.
   2. potassium and phosphate.
   3. calcium and bicarbonate.
   4. magnesium and phosphate.

2. Which of the following are anions? Select all that apply.
   1. Sodium
   2. Potassium
   3. Chloride
   4. Bicarbonate
   5. Phosphate

3. The concentration of electrolytes in a solution or body fluid compartment is measured in:
   1. milligrams (mg).
   2. grams (g).
   3. milliliters (ml).
   4. milliequivalents (mEq).

4. In what type of environment does water loss via the skin and lungs increase?
   1. Hot, moist environment
   2. Hot, dry environment
   3. Cool, dry environment
   4. Cool, moist environment

5. Because the retention of sodium causes water retention, aldosterone acts as a regulator of:
   1. acid balance.
   2. base balance.
   3. blood pH.
   4. blood volume.

6. One way the body tries to compensate for fluid volume deficits is to:
   1. increase heart rate.
   2. decrease heart rate.
   3. increase blood pressure.
   4. decrease ADH.

7. ADH is decreased in response to:
   1. fluid volume deficit.
   2. fluid volume excess.
   3. decreased urination.
   4. concentrated urine.

8. The body tries to compensate for fluid volume excess by:
   1. inhibiting aldosterone.
   2. stimulating ADH.
   3. inhibiting epinephrine.
   4. stimulating thirst.

9. Which electrolytes cause a majority of health problems when there is an electrolyte imbalance? Select all that apply.
   1. Potassium
   2. Chloride
   3. Magnesium
   4. Bicarbonate
   5. Sodium

10. When the body goes without fluid intake, which hormone increases water reabsorption?
    1. Thyroxine
    2. Epinephrine
    3. ADH
    4. Aldosterone

11. Which of the following disturbances are a result of low levels of serum potassium? Select all that apply.
    1. Metabolic function
    2. Neuromuscular function
    3. Cardiac function
    4. Bone structure
    5. Acid-base balance

12. Which of the following drugs cause hypokalemia? Select all that apply.
    1. Narcotics
    2. Anticholinergics
    3. Diuretics
    4. Calcium channel blockers
    5. Corticosteroids

13. If more calcium is needed in the bones, it is taken from the blood as well as being reabsorbed through the:
    1. lungs.
    2. kidneys.
    3. heart.
    4. liver.

14. One liter of fluid retention equals a weight gain of:
    1. 1 pound.
    2. 2.2 pounds.
    3. 5.4 pounds.
    4. 10 pounds.

15. Puffy eyelids and fuller cheeks suggest:
    1. fluid volume excess.
    2. fluid volume deficit.
    3. potassium excess.
    4. potassium deficit.

16. If a depression remains in the tissue after pressure is applied with a fingertip, the edema is described as:
    1. excessive.
    2. pitting.
    3. depressed.
    4. minimal.

17. A deep and persistent pit that is approximately 1 inch deep is described as:
    1. 1+.
    2. 2+.
    3. 3+.
    4. 4+.

18. If the veins take longer than 3 to 5 seconds to fill when placed in a dependent position, the patient may have:
    1. hypokalemia.
    2. hyperkalemia.
    3. hypovolemia.
    4. hypervolemia.

19. Weakness and muscle cramps are symptoms of:
    1. hyponatremia.
    2. hypokalemia.
    3. fluid volume deficit.
    4. respiratory acidosis.

20. The normal range for urine pH is:
    1. 2.0–7.0.
    2. 4.0–12.0.
    3. 4.6–8.0.
    4. 7.8–12.0.

21. A urine specimen that is not tested within 4 hours of collection may become:
    1. alkaline.
    2. acidic.
    3. more concentrated.
    4. less concentrated.

22. A measure of the kidneys' ability to dilute or concentrate urine is called:
    1. pH.
    2. urine potassium.
    3. creatinine clearance.
    4. specific gravity.

23. In most instances, normal urine specific gravity is between:
    1. 1.010 and 1.025.
    2. 2.001 and 4.035.
    3. 4.001 and 6.035.
    4. 5.0 and 7.0.

24. A 24-hour urine specimen is required for:
    1. creatinine clearance.
    2. pH.
    3. specific gravity.
    4. osmolality.

25. BUN provides a measure of:
    1. blood volume.
    2. renal function.
    3. cardiac function.
    4. liver function.

26. Which one of the following is a symptom of hyponatremia?
    1. Palpitations
    2. Hypertension
    3. Confusion
    4. Insomnia

27. What amount of fluid per day is needed by the average person for adequate hydration?
    1. 500–700 ml/day
    2. 800–1000 ml/day
    3. 1500–2000 ml/day
    4. 3500–5000 ml/day

28. To prevent hyponatremia in patients with feeding tubes, what should be used for irrigation?
    1. Sterile water
    2. Normal glucose
    3. Normal saline
    4. Sterile dextrose

29. The heart rate of patients on digitalis should be closely watched because hypokalemia can contribute to:
    1. congestive heart failure.
    2. pericarditis.
    3. digitalis toxicity.
    4. diuresis.

30. In order to prevent gastrointestinal irritation, oral potassium supplements should be given with:
    1. meals.
    2. a full glass of water or fruit juice.
    3. a full glass of milk.
    4. a teaspoon of applesauce.

31. When the respiratory system fails to eliminate the appropriate amount of carbon dioxide to maintain the normal acid-base balance, what occurs?
    1. Respiratory alkalosis
    2. Respiratory acidosis
    3. Metabolic acidosis
    4. Metabolic alkalosis

32. The most common cause of respiratory alkalosis is:
    1. hypoventilation.
    2. hyperventilation.
    3. drowning.
    4. obesity.

33. Patients may develop high levels of magnesium in their blood if they are taking:
    1. diuretics.
    2. antihypertensives.
    3. antacids.
    4. salicylates.

34. Which patient should be encouraged to breathe slowly into a paper bag?
    1. Patient who is hyperventilating
    2. Patient with emphysema
    3. Patient with respiratory acidosis
    4. Patient with hypokalemia

35. When the body retains too many hydrogen ions or loses too many bicarbonate ions, what occurs?
    1. Respiratory acidosis
    2. Respiratory alkalosis
    3. Metabolic acidosis
    4. Metabolic alkalosis

36. Potassium is a critical factor for the transmission of nerve impulses because it is necessary for:
    1. muscular activity.
    2. acid-base balance.
    3. fluid balance.
    4. membrane excitability.

37. In addition to its role in regulating fluid balance, sodium is also necessary for:
    1. nerve impulse conduction.
    2. bone structure.
    3. protein structure.
    4. breakdown of glycogen.

38. The most common cause of hypocalcemia is related to problems with which hormone?
    1. ADH
    2. Aldosterone
    3. Thyroxine
    4. PTH

39. What is the normal total daily intake of fluids?
    1. 1000 ml
    2. 1200 ml
    3. 1500 ml
    4. 2500 ml

40. What is the best position for the patient who is experiencing dyspnea?
    1. Keep the bed flat.
    2. Elevate the head of the bed 30 degrees.
    3. Elevate the head of the bed 60 degrees.
    4. Elevate the head of the bed 90 degrees.

41. A bounding pulse occurs in patients with:
    1. dehydration.
    2. hypovolemia.
    3. circulatory overload.
    4. hyperthermia.

42. What is the patient at risk for when the total intake is substantially less than the total output?
    1. Fluid volume excess
    2. Fluid volume deficit
    3. Hypoventilation
    4. Hyperventilation

43. What is the normal hourly adult urine output?
    1. 30–40 ml/hour
    2. 40–80 ml/hour
    3. 50–60 ml/hour
    4. 100 ml/hour

44. A rapid weight gain of 8% is considered to be:
    1. minimal.
    2. mild.
    3. moderate.
    4. severe.

45. If the patient has a rapid weight loss of 2 kilograms, what is the equivalent loss of fluid?
    1. 1 liter
    2. 2 liters
    3. 4 liters
    4. 6 liters

PART III: CHALLENGE YOURSELF!

L. Getting Ready for NCLEX.

Choose the most appropriate answer or select all that apply.

1. Which electrolytes are present in greater amounts in the extracellular fluid (ECF) than in the intracellular fluid (ICF)? Select all that apply.
   1. Sodium (Na)
   2. Potassium (K)
   3. Chloride (Cl)
   4. Bicarbonate (HCO_3)
   5. Calcium (Ca^{++})
   6. Magnesium (Mg)
   7. Phosphate (HPO_4)

2. Which factors are related to causes of hypovolemia? Select all that apply.
   1. Decreased oral fluid intake
   2. Vomiting
   3. Decreased ADH production
   4. High fever
   5. Diarrhea
   6. Excessive sweating

3. Which of the following are indicators of dehydration? Select all that apply.
   1. Hypotension
   2. Decreased pulse
   3. Decreased respirations
   4. Increased temperature
   5. Weight loss
   6. Decreased hematocrit (Hct) and hemoglobin (Hgb)

4. What are signs of fluid volume excess in a patient being treated for dehydration who receives excessive fluid replacement? Select all that apply.
   1. Increased pulse
   2. Decreased blood pressure
   3. Dyspnea
   4. Decreased respirations

5. What are indicators of fluid volume excess? Select all that apply.
   1. Increased blood pressure
   2. Bounding pulse
   3. Decreased respirations
   4. Weight loss
   5. Irritability

6. What is the treatment for fluid volume excess? Select all that apply.
   1. Restrict sodium intake
   2. Increase water intake
   3. Give diuretics
   4. Give antiemetics

7. Which of the following are nursing interventions for the patient with fluid volume excess? Select all that apply.
   1. Offer ice chips
   2. Offer clear liquids
   3. Use small fluid containers
   4. Turn every 2 hours
   5. Inspect skin for breakdown
   6. Check temperature

8. A patient has been admitted to a long-term care facility with fluid volume deficit. Which nursing diagnoses would the nurse expect with this patient? Select all that apply.
   1. Acute confusion
   2. Risk for impaired tissue integrity
   3. Constipation
   4. Diarrhea
   5. Impaired swallowing

9. Which aspects of the health and physical exam are important in determining the fluid and electrolyte status of a patient? Select all that apply.
   1. Numbness
   2. Seizures
   3. Vomiting
   4. Use of diuretics
   5. Use of salicylates
   6. Dyspnea
   7. Skin turgor

10. Which foods are high in sodium? Select all that apply.
    1. Natural cheese
    2. Sausage
    3. Cooked oatmeal
    4. Fresh chicken
    5. Pizza
    6. Frozen peas

11. Which foods are high in potassium? Select all that apply.
    1. Lima beans
    2. Fresh apricots
    3. Broccoli
    4. Banana
    5. Ginger ale
    6. Fresh apple
    7. Corn
    8. Watermelon

12. Which of the following are manifestations of acid-base imbalance? Select all that apply.
    1. Dyspnea
    2. Confusion
    3. Vomiting
    4. Muscle weakness
    5. Numbness
    6. Decreased skin turgor

13. Which of the following are reasons older people are at high risk for fluid and electrolyte imbalance? Select all that apply.
    1. Decreased renal response
    2. Decreased lean muscle mass
    3. Decreased sense of thirst
    4. Increased total body water

14. Which assessment finding is the *least* reliable indicator of fluid status in an 80-year-old person?
    1. Pitting peripheral edema
    2. Poor tissue turgor
    3. Intake and output
    4. Mucous membrane moisture

15. When the blood is more concentrated in a patient with fluid volume deficit, which blood study result is expected? Select all that apply.
    1. Increased blood urea nitrogen (BUN)
    2. Increased creatinine
    3. Increased hematocrit
    4. Decreased hemoglobin

16. When breathing problems occur in a patient with fluid volume excess, the patient should:
    1. lie flat in bed.
    2. have head of bed elevated 30 degrees.
    3. ambulate frequently.
    4. be in side-lying position.

17. The patient with heart failure has fluid volume excess with pitting edema. What is the priority nursing intervention for this patient?
    1. Turn the patient every 2 hours.
    2. Have the patient cough and deep-breathe every 2 hours.
    3. Ambulate the patient every 2 hours.
    4. Check the blood pressure every 2 hours.

18. The nurse is taking care of a patient with hypokalemia. Which of the following are nursing interventions for this patient? Select all that apply.
    1. Monitor serum potassium levels.
    2. Monitor arterial blood gas results.
    3. Record intake and output.
    4. Monitor heart rate and rhythms.
    5. Encourage green, leafy vegetables in the diet.
    6. Encourage oranges and bananas in the diet.

19. What is the best way to decrease the incidence of serious fluid and electrolyte imbalances?
    1. Monitor blood pressure carefully.
    2. Monitor temperature carefully.
    3. Monitor rate and rhythm of the pulse carefully.
    4. Monitor records of fluid intake and output carefully.

20. A patient has fluid volume excess. Which nursing diagnoses would the nurse expect with this patient? Select all that apply.
    1. Acute confusion related to cerebral edema
    2. Acute confusion related to decreased cerebral tissue perfusion
    3. Ineffective tissue perfusion related to reduced cardiac output with heart failure
    4. Ineffective tissue perfusion related to decreased cardiac output secondary to blood volume
    5. Risk for impaired skin integrity related to poor tissue turgor
    6. Risk for impaired skin integrity related to edema

Pain Management

 Go to http://evolve.elsevier.com/Linton/medsurg/ for additional activities and exercises.

NCLEX CATEGORIES:

Safe and Effective Care Environment:
Coordinated Care, Safety and Infection Control

Psychosocial Integrity

Physiological Integrity: Pharmacological Therapies, Reduction of Risk Potential, Physiological Adaptation

OBJECTIVES

1. Define pain.
2. Explain the physiologic basis for pain.
3. Identify situations in which patients are likely to experience pain.
4. Explain the relationships among past pain experiences, anticipation, culture, anxiety, and a patient's response to pain.
5. Identify differences in the duration of pain and patient responses to acute and chronic pain.
6. Explain the special needs of older adult patients with pain.
7. List the data to be collected in assessing pain.
8. Describe interventions used in the management of pain.
9. Describe the nursing care of patients receiving opioid and nonopioid analgesics for pain.
10. List the factors that should be considered when pain is not relieved with analgesic medications.

PART I: MASTERING THE BASICS

A. Key Terms.

Match the definition in the numbered column with the most appropriate term in the lettered column.

1. _____ Process of pain transmission

2. _____ Unpleasant sensory and emotional experience associated with actual or potential tissue damage, existing whenever the person says it does

3. _____ Drug that acts on the nervous system to relieve or reduce the suffering or intensity of pain

4. _____ A physiologic result of repeated doses of an opioid where the same dose is no longer effective in achieving the same analgesic effect

5. _____ Behavioral pattern of compulsive drug use characterized by craving for an opioid and obtaining and using the drug for effects other than pain relief

6. _____ Physiologic adaptation of the body to an opioid so that a person exhibits withdrawal symptoms when the opioid is stopped abruptly after repeated administration

7. _____ Amount of pain a person is willing to endure before taking action to relieve pain

8. _____ Pain that lasts longer than 6 months

9. _____ Point at which a stimulus causes the sensation of pain

10. _____ Pain that occurs after injury to tissues from surgery, trauma, or disease

A. Pain
B. Addiction
C. Acute pain
D. Pain tolerance
E. Nociception
F. Physical dependence
G. Tolerance
H. Chronic pain
I. Pain threshold
J. Analgesic

B. Gate Control Theory.

Which of the following are factors that close the gate, according to the gate control theory? Select all that apply.
  1. Distraction
  2. Massage
  3. Position change
  4. Fear of pain
  5. Guided imagery
  6. Heat application

C. Patient Situation.

A 42-year-old male with multiple fractures in the right arm used the numeric scale from 1 to 10 for rating pain. The patient complained of throbbing in his right arm and a backache. He rated the intensity of both pains at 7 on the scale at 8:00 PM. The nurse applied heat to the lower back as ordered, massaged his back, and administered 10 mg of morphine intramuscularly. At 9:00 PM, the patient rated intensity of both pains at 2 and stated that the pain was slowly going away.

What evidence indicates that the pain was relieved? Select all that apply.
  1. Morphine 10 mg was given IM.
  2. Patient stated that the pain was slowly going away.
  3. Heat was applied to his lower back as ordered.
  4. Pain intensity rated by the patient decreased from 7 to 2.
  5. No further complaints of throbbing in his arm.

D. Pain Nursing Diagnoses.

List seven possible nursing diagnoses for patients who have pain.

1. _____

2. _____

3. _____

4. _____

5. _____

6. _____

7. _____

E. Pain Key Terms.

Which of the following describe addiction? Select all that apply.
  1. Physiologic changes that occur from repeated doses of opioids
  2. Compulsive obtaining and use of drug for psychic effects
  3. Withdrawal symptoms may occur if the opioid is stopped abruptly (e.g., irritability, chills, sweating, nausea)
  4. Psychological dependence characterized by continued craving for opioid for other than pain relief
  5. The need for higher doses to achieve pain relief

F. Pain Response.

Which of the following are physical factors that influence response to pain? Select all that apply.
  1. Age
  2. Type of surgery
  3. Pain tolerance
  4. Endocrine system activity
  5. Body temperature
  6. Physical activity
  7. Blood pressure

PART II: PUTTING IT ALL TOGETHER

G. Multiple-Response Questions.

Choose the most appropriate answer.

1. One difference between acute and chronic pain is that a patient with acute pain:
   1. often becomes depressed.
   2. shows little facial expression.
   3. feels isolated.
   4. has a fast heart rate.

2. Which of the following are physical factors that influence the response to pain? Select all that apply.
   1. Age
   2. Type of surgery
   3. Culture
   4. Religion
   5. Pain tolerance
   6. Pain threshold
   7. Anxiety

3. When the pain threshold is lowered, the person experiences pain:
   1. less easily.
   2. more easily.
   3. as excruciating.
   4. as mild.

4. Which age group tends to report their pain as much less severe than it really is?
   1. Older adults
   2. Middle-aged adults
   3. Young adults
   4. Adolescents

5. Surgery in which area is reported to be the most painful for patients?
   1. Skull region
   2. Thoracic region
   3. Upper abdominal region
   4. Lower abdominal region

6. Dilated pupils, perspiration, and pallor are results of which nervous system response to pain?
   1. Voluntary
   2. Somatic
   3. Parasympathetic
   4. Sympathetic

7. Postoperative pain and pain in childbirth are examples of:
   1. chronic pain.
   2. permanent pain.
   3. acute pain.
   4. nonmalignant pain.

8. An example of acute pain with recurrent episodes is pain associated with:
   1. low back pain.
   2. migraine headaches.
   3. rheumatoid arthritis.
   4. cancer pain.

9. A pain that cannot be explained or that persists after healing has taken place is:
   1. acute benign pain.
   2. acute metastatic pain.
   3. chronic benign pain.
   4. chronic metastatic pain.

10. When possible, the information about pain should obtained from the:
    1. nurse.
    2. patient.
    3. doctor.
    4. patient's family.

11. Which are examples of cutaneous stimulation methods for pain control? Select all that apply.
    1. Guided imagery
    2. Application of heat
    3. Application of cold
    4. Listening to music
    5. TENS
    6. Massage
    7. Anxiety reduction

12. The longest time a cold application can be used without tissue injury would be:
    1. 3 minutes.
    2. 15 minutes.
    3. 30 minutes.
    4. 60 minutes.

13. Fentanyl (Duragesic) transdermal patches are used to treat chronic pain by delivering:
    1. NSAIDs.
    2. salicylates.
    3. opioids.
    4. steroids.

14. Relaxation is most effective for:
    1. delusional pain.
    2. mild to moderate pain.
    3. moderate to severe pain.
    4. severe pain.

15. When pain is unpredictable, analgesics are more effective when given:
    1. once a day.
    2. twice a day.
    3. around the clock.
    4. PRN.

16. The initial treatment choice for mild pain is:
    1. opioid analgesics.
    2. nonopioid analgesics.
    3. narcotics.
    4. anesthetics.

17. Aspirin, acetaminophen, and NSAIDs are examples of:
    1. opioid analgesics.
    2. nonopioid analgesics.
    3. narcotics.
    4. anesthetics.

18. Ketorolac tromethamine (Toradol) is generally used for the short-term management of:
    1. cancer pain.
    2. heart failure.
    3. urinary tract infection.
    4. postoperative pain.

19. Drugs, such as nonopioids, that do not improve analgesia beyond a certain dosage are said to have a:
    1. peak effect.
    2. duration effect.
    3. ceiling effect.
    4. onset effect.

20. Nonopioids tend to block pain transmission:
    1. at the central nervous system.
    2. during cell wall synthesis.
    3. at the myocardium.
    4. on the peripheral nervous system.

21. Nalbuphine (Nubain), butorphanol (Stadol), and pentazocine (Talwin) are examples of:
    1. nonopioid analgesics.
    2. anticholinergics.
    3. opioid agonist-antagonists.
    4. opioid agonists.

22. A patient receiving 10 mg morphine IM for pain will be given what dose PO to receive an equianalgesic dose?
    1. 10 mg
    2. 30 mg
    3. 60 mg
    4. 80 mg

23. If the patient is nauseated or has difficulty swallowing, which route is useful for administering opioids?
    1. Oral
    2. Rectal
    3. Topical
    4. Intradermal

24. To evaluate the patient for constipation, the nurse monitors the patient for:
    1. black, tarry stools and anorexia.
    2. decreased blood pressure, itching, and respiratory distress.
    3. abdominal distention, cramping, and abdominal pain.
    4. intake and output, nausea and vomiting.

25. Which nonpharmacologic pain intervention increases the pain threshold and reduces muscle spasm?
    1. Jaw relaxation
    2. Simple imagery
    3. Music
    4. TENS

26. When a pain medication order states 10–20 mg IM prn for pain, what will the nurse do when 10 mg have been given and it is not effective?
    1. Adjust the next dose up as ordered until pain is relieved with minimal or no side effects.
    2. Give an additional 10 mg as soon as possible.
    3. Wait 4 hours, and give 20 mg the next time.
    4. Determine if the patient has developed pain tolerance.

PART III: CHALLENGE YOURSELF!

H. Getting Ready for NCLEX.

Choose the most appropriate answer or select all that apply.

1. Which of the following are characteristics of chronic pain? Select all that apply.
   1. Lasts 3–6 months
   2. Responds to analgesics
   3. Pain is a sign of tissue injury
   4. Normal heart rate and blood pressure
   5. Oral route is preferred route
   6. Minimal facial expression
   7. Restlessness
   8. Grimacing

2. Which of the following are examples of conditions that cause acute pain? Select all that apply.
   1. Low back pain
   2. Rheumatoid arthritis
   3. Neuralgia (herpes zoster)
   4. Sickle cell crisis
   5. Phantom limb pain
   6. Migraine headaches

3. Which of the following are adjuvant analgesics and medications for the treatment of pain? Select all that apply.
   1. Antidepressants
   2. Muscle relaxants
   3. Anticonvulsants
   4. Antipsychotics
   5. Diuretics

4. Which of the following are parasympathetic responses to pain? Select all that apply.
   1. Constipation
   2. Increased blood pressure
   3. Dilated pupils
   4. Urinary retention
   5. Perspiration

5. What are common pain behaviors in cognitively impaired older adults? Select all that apply.
   1. Grimacing
   2. Crying
   3. Decreased wandering
   4. Increased appetite
   5. Noisy breathing

6. A 46-year-old patient has received nitrous oxide during surgery and says he does not have pain postoperatively. Which factor best explains his response to pain?
   1. Pain threshold
   2. Religious beliefs
   3. Age
   4. Anesthetic

7. A stoic 75-year-old Asian woman who has been experiencing back pain states that she does not want to bother the nurse. Which factors best explain her response to pain? Select all that apply.
   1. Age
   2. Fear
   3. Anxiety
   4. Culture
   5. Pain tolerance

8. Which factors affect the pain threshold? Select all that apply.
   1. Age
   2. Anger
   3. Fatigue
   4. Depression
   5. Insomnia
   6. Religion

9. List in the proper sequence the steps in pain management. Use 1 as the first step and 6 as the last step.
   A. _____ Determine the status of the pain.
   B. _____ Describe the pain (location, quality, intensity, aggravating factors).
   C. _____ Identify coping methods.
   D. _____ Accept the patient's report of pain.
   E. _____ Examine the site.
   F. _____ Record assessment, interventions, and evaluation.

10. The application of cold is contraindicated in patients with:
    1. hip fracture.
    2. muscle sprain.
    3. allergic reaction.
    4. peripheral vascular disease.

11. Which effect of opioids is not potentiated by the use of promethazine (Phenergan)?
    1. Sedation
    2. Respiratory depression
    3. Hypotension
    4. Analgesia

12. A drug classification that is effective in treating neuropathic pain is:
    1. muscle relaxants.
    2. benzodiazepines.
    3. antidepressants.
    4. corticosteroids.

13. A patient who has had back surgery complains of muscle spasms. Which drug may be most effective in relieving his pain?
    1. Muscle relaxant
    2. Opioid
    3. NSAID
    4. Aspirin

14. When observing sedation in a patient, which stage would the nurse consider to be an emergency?
    1. Sleeping, but arouses when called
    2. Drowsy, but easily aroused
    3. Frequently drowsy to drifting off to sleep during conversations
    4. Minimal response to physical stimulation

First Aid, Emergency Care, and Disaster Management

Ⓔ Go to http://evolve.elsevier.com/Linton/medsurg/ for additional activities and exercises.

NCLEX CATEGORIES:

Safe and Effective Care Environment:
Coordinated Care, Safety and Infection Control

Physiological Integrity: Reduction of Risk
Potential, Physiological Adaptation

OBJECTIVES

1. List the principles of emergency and first-aid care.
2. List the steps of the initial assessment and interventions for the person requiring emergency care.
3. Describe the components of the nursing assessment of the person requiring emergency care.
4. Outline the steps of the nursing process for emergency or first-aid treatment of victims of cardiopulmonary arrest, choking, shock, hemorrhage, traumatic injury, burns, heat or cold exposure, poisoning, bites, and stings.
5. Discuss the roles of nurses and nursing students in relation to bioterrorism and natural disasters.
6. Explain the legal implications of administering first-aid in emergency situations.
7. Explain the implications of the Good Samaritan Law doctrine.

PART I: MASTERING THE BASICS

A. Key Terms.

Match the definition in the numbered column with the most appropriate term in the lettered column.

1. _____ Tearing away of tissue
2. _____ Presence of air in the pleural cavity that causes the lung on the affected side to collapse
3. _____ Loss of a large amount of blood
4. _____ An injury to muscle tissue or the tendons that attach them to bones, or both
5. _____ A severe, potentially fatal, allergic reaction characterized by hypotension and bronchial constriction
6. _____ Presence of blood in the pleural cavity causing the lung on the affected side to collapse
7. _____ Elevation of body core temperature above 99° F
8. _____ Blood in the pericardial sac that causes decreased cardiac output
9. _____ Nosebleed
10. _____ Decrease in body core temperature below 95° F
11. _____ An injury to a ligament
12. _____ Any substance that, in small quantities, is capable of causing illness or harm following ingestion, inhalation, injection, or contact with the skin
13. _____ Absence of breathing
14. _____ Protrusion of internal organs through a wound
15. _____ Absence of heartbeat and breathing
16. _____ Loss of support of chest wall where several adjacent ribs are broken in more than one place
17. _____ Acute circulatory failure that can lead to death

A. Shock
B. Hypothermia
C. Cardiopulmonary arrest
D. Hemothorax
E. Flail chest
F. Sprain
G. Evisceration
H. Avulsion
I. Hemorrhage
J. Hyperthermia
K. Strain
L. Poison
M. Respiratory arrest
N. Pneumothorax
O. Anaphylactic shock
P. Cardiac tamponade
Q. Epistaxis

B. Emergency Care.

List, in sequence, the five steps in the initial assessment and immediate intervention in emergency care.

A. _____   Look for uncontrolled bleeding.

B. _____   Initiate CPR or rescue breathing as needed.

C. _____   Look for medical alert tag.

D. _____   Assess the ABCs: airway, breathing, and circulation.

E. _____   Examine for injuries.

C. First-aid.

What are general guidelines for first-aid treatment of emergency patients? Select all that apply.

1. Splint injured parts in the position they are found.
2. Prevent chilling, and do not add excessive heat.
3. Remove any penetrating objects.
4. Give the unconscious person sips of water.
5. Stay with the injured person until help arrives.

D. Cardiopulmonary Arrest.

Which of the following are nursing diagnoses for patients in cardiopulmonary arrest? Select all that apply.

1. Ineffective airway clearance
2. Ineffective peripheral tissue perfusion
3. Increased cardiac output
4. Ineffective breathing pattern
5. Risk for suffocation

E. Burns.

Match the type of burn in the numbered column with the emergency intervention in the lettered column.

1. _____   Superficial, minor burn

2. _____   Sunburn

3. _____   Extensive burns

4. _____   Chemical burns

A. Cover burns with a clean, dry dressing or cloth.
B. Immerse the injured body part in cool water for 2–5 minutes.
C. Remove contaminated clothing and then flush skin with water for 30 minutes.
D. Apply topical preparations with benzocaine.

F. Bites.

Match the intervention in the numbered column with the type of bite in the lettered column. Answers may be used more than once.

1. _____   Immobilize the body part with the bite and keep it at or below the heart, to minimize absorption of venom.

2. _____   Clean thoroughly and apply a dressing. Seek medical attention for antibiotic therapy.

3. _____   Clean the wound thoroughly and apply a bulky dressing.

4. _____   Calamine lotion or a paste of baking soda or meat tenderizer is soothing.

5. _____   The patient with severe allergies may be given epinephrine, Benadryl, aminophylline, or hydrocortisone.

6. _____   Try to keep the patient still.

7. _____   Advise the patient to have a tetanus booster if immunizations are not current.

8. _____   Remove the stinger with a scraping motion.

A. Snake bite
B. Insect bite or sting
C. Animal bite
D. Human bite

G. Fractures.

Match the definition in the numbered column with the appropriate term in the lettered column.

1. _____ A fracture that does not break the skin

2. _____ A fracture in which the ends of the broken bone protrude through the skin

3. _____ A fracture in which the broken ends are separated

4. _____ A fracture in which the bone ends are not separated

A. Complete
B. Incomplete
C. Simple
D. Compound

PART II: PUTTING IT ALL TOGETHER

H. Multiple-Response Questions.

Choose the most appropriate answer.

1. General guidelines for first-aid treatment of emergency patients include:
   1. cover with wool blanket to prevent chills.
   2. remove penetrating objects.
   3. splint injured parts in the position they are found.
   4. give orange juice with sugar if unconscious.

2. The first assessment priorities must be:
   1. observation of uncontrolled bleeding or shock.
   2. systematic head-to-toe assessment.
   3. airway, breathing, and circulation.
   4. palpation of carotid and peripheral pulses.

3. In most cases, the brain begins to die after 4 minutes without oxygen due to hypoxia of:
   1. heart tissue.
   2. nerve tissue.
   3. lung tissue.
   4. blood vessels.

4. Prompt recognition and treatment of cardiopulmonary arrest are important due to the need to maintain the oxygen supply to the:
   1. heart.
   2. brain.
   3. lungs.
   4. blood vessels.

5. Grabbing the throat with one or both hands is the universal sign for:
   1. heart attack.
   2. choking.
   3. danger.
   4. loss of consciousness.

6. If the choking victim is conscious, the rescuer performs:
   1. the Heimlich maneuver.
   2. CPR.
   3. 15 chest compressions.
   4. assessment of breathing.

7. If a choking victim loses consciousness, list the steps for assistance in order from 1 to 4. Use 1 for the first action and 4 for the fourth action.
   A. _____ Open the airway and inspect for an object that could be causing the obstruction.
   B. _____ Begin CPR.
   C. _____ Remove any visible object.
   D. _____ Activate the emergency response system.

8. Choking deaths can be prevented by:
   1. not talking while chewing.
   2. lowering blood pressure.
   3. decreasing weight.
   4. increasing exercise.

9. In an adult, what amount of blood loss may result in hypovolemic shock?
   1. 30 ml or more
   2. 1 pint or more
   3. 1 liter or more
   4. 10 liters or more

10. Immediate treatment for external bleeding is:
    1. application of ice.
    2. elevate the site of bleeding.
    3. direct, continuous pressure.
    4. check vital signs.

11. The primary symptom of fracture is:
    1. numbness.
    2. tingling.
    3. pain.
    4 hemorrhage.

12. The key to emergency management of fractures is:
    1. application of cold.
    2. elevation of injury.
    3. immobilization.
    4. application of heat.

13. Emergency treatment for sprains and strains include:
    1. direct wound pressure.
    2. immobilization.
    3. application of heat.
    4. application of splint.

14. Change in behavior, increased blood pressure, and unequal pupils are signs of:
    1. anaphylactic shock.
    2. altered breathing.
    3. increased intracranial pressure.
    4. spinal cord injury.

15. When there is a neck or spinal injury, the nurse first assesses:
    1. blood loss and level of consciousness.
    2. breathing and circulation.
    3. movement of extremities.
    4. sensation in extremities.

16. After a diving injury, while removing the victim from the water, efforts are made to:
    1. immobilize the extremities.
    2. immobilize the neck and back.
    3. turn the victim in a prone position.
    4. turn the victim in a supine position.

17. The priority goal for the patient with a neck or spinal injury is to:
    1. provide adequate ventilation.
    2. increase cardiac output.
    3. reduce fear.
    4. decrease risk of additional injury.

18. When chemicals come in contact with the eye, the nurse should:
    1. cover the eye with a loose dressing.
    2. flush with water to irrigate the eye for 30 minutes.
    3. apply pressure with a sterile cloth.
    4. place patient in shower under cold water.

19. The abnormal chest wall movement in flail chest would be described as what sort of motion?
    1. Sawing
    2. Paradoxical
    3. Pulsating
    4. Sucking

20. The abnormal chest wall action in flail chest causes:
    1. altered tissue perfusion.
    2. increased cardiac output.
    3. increased pulse strength.
    4. impaired gas exchange.

21. Outcome criteria for evaluating emergency nursing care of the patient with an abdominal wound includes:
    1. protection of injured (eviscerated) tissue.
    2. control of bleeding.
    3. restoration of a strong pulse.
    4. reduction of fear.

22. First-aid for minor superficial burns is to:
    1. apply butter to the burn.
    2. apply petroleum jelly to the burn.
    3. cover the burn with a cloth.
    4. immerse the injured body part in cool water.

23. When a large body surface area is burned or any area is severely burned, the nurse should:
    1. apply medications to the burn.
    2. cover the burn with a clean dry dressing or cloth.
    3. cover the burn with a cool wet dressing or cloth.
    4. apply ice to the burn.

24. Heat exhaustion is treated by:
    1. pushing fluids with caffeine.
    2. ambulating the victim.
    3. cooling and hydrating the victim.
    4. placing victim in ice.

25. Patients with heat exhaustion would be considered stable when they exhibit:
    1. urine output of at least 10 ml/hr and pulse rate of 100 bpm or more.
    2. ability to take a regular diet without nausea.
    3. below-normal body temperature and normal pulse rate.
    4. lowered body temperature and intake and retention of fluids.

26. The skin is red, hot, and dry and perspiration is absent in:
    1. heatstroke.
    2. heat exhaustion.
    3. hyperthermia.
    4. hypothermia.

27. The immediate treatment of mild cold injury is:
    1. rapid rewarming.
    2. massaging to increase circulation.
    3. covering with dressing.
    4. immersing in tepid water.

28. Carbon monoxide poisoning occurs because carbon monoxide:
    1. is blown off too rapidly during exhalation.
    2. binds to hemoglobin and occupies sites needed to transport oxygen to the cells.
    3. binds to white blood cells and causes infection.
    4. is retained and prevents oxygen from being inhaled in adequate amounts.

29. The primary nursing diagnosis for the victim of carbon monoxide poisoning is:
    1. Impaired gas exchange.
    2. Ineffective breathing pattern.
    3. Risk for aspiration.
    4. Anxiety related to ineffective breathing pattern.

30. The primary nursing diagnosis for the victim of drug or chemical poisoning is:
    1. Altered thought processes.
    2. Risk for infection.
    3. Risk for injury.
    4. Risk for suffocation.

31. Flu-like symptoms following a tick bite may be symptoms of:
    1. poisoning.
    2. Lyme disease.
    3. staph infection.
    4. hypersensitivity.

32. Which of the following are local effects of venom on blood and blood vessels? Select all that apply.
    1. Skin breakdown
    2. Petechiae
    3. Discoloration
    4. Pain
    5. Coolness of extremities
    6. Edema
    7. Brittle nails, hair loss, and cellulitis

33. What is the danger of too-rapid rewarming as the treatment for a patient with severe hypothermia?
    1. Cardiac dysrhythmias
    2. Heatstroke
    3. Tingling and numbness of extremities
    4. Muscle cramps

34. What is the first nursing action for any chemical eye injury?
    1. Gently touch the eye with the corner of a clean cloth.
    2. Flush the eye for 30 minutes.
    3. Tape an inverted paper cup over the eye.
    4. Apply a loose dressing to the eye.

PART III: CHALLENGE YOURSELF!

I. Getting Ready for NCLEX.

Choose the most appropriate answer or select all that apply.

1. Which of the following are common signs and symptoms of heat exhaustion? Select all that apply.
    1. Dizziness
    2. Muscle cramps
    3. Pale, damp skin
    4. Hot, dry skin
    5. Absent perspiration
    6. Seizures

2. Following a severe allergic reaction to an insect bite, which drugs are indicated to prevent anaphylaxis? Select all that apply.
    1. Demerol
    2. Epinephrine
    3. Hydrocortisone
    4. Ibuprofen
    5. Benadryl

3. Which of the following are local effects of snake bites? Select all that apply.
   1. Local itching
   2. Pain
   3. Mild to moderate edema
   4. Urticaria
   5. Discoloration

4. Which of the following are nursing diagnoses for a patient who is choking? Select all that apply.
   1. Ineffective airway clearance
   2. Decreased cardiac output
   3. Ineffective tissue perfusion
   4. Risk for suffocation

5. Which of the following are goals and outcome criteria for a patient with cardiopulmonary arrest? Select all that apply.
   1. Decreased coughing
   2. Improving skin color
   3. Spontaneous respirations
   4. Patent airway
   5. Palpable pulse

6. Which of the following are nursing diagnoses for a patient with hemorrhage? Select all that apply.
   1. Ineffective tissue perfusion
   2. Decreased cardiac output
   3. Fear
   4. Ineffective breathing patterns

7. Which of the following are goals and outcome criteria for a patient with hemorrhage? Select all that apply.
   1. Skin warm and dry
   2. Patent airway with normal respirations
   3. Adequate oxygenation
   4. Blood pressure within normal range

8. Which of the following are nursing diagnoses for a patient with a head injury? Select all that apply.
   1. Risk for injury
   2. Risk for suffocation
   3. Ineffective breathing pattern
   4. Decreased cardiac output

9. Which of the following are manifestations that will aid in the prompt recognition of a patient with a head injury? Select all that apply.
   1. Numbness and tingling
   2. Unequal pupils
   3. Changes in behavior, agitation, and confusion
   4. Pain
   5. Abnormal response of pupils to light

10. Nursing diagnoses that might apply to the patient with a head injury during the emergency phase of treatment include:
    1. Decreased cardiac output related to hypovolemia and fear related to possible impending death.
    2. Ineffective tissue perfusion related to cessation of heartbeat and decreased cardiac output.
    3. Ineffective breathing pattern related to neurologic trauma and risk for injury related to increasing intracranial pressure.
    4. Risk for trauma related to improper movements of the spine.

11. Outcome criteria for the patient with a neck or spinal injury is based on:
    1. continuous monitoring for signs of increased intracranial pressure and oxygenation.
    2. continuous immobilization of the back and spine and transport for medical care.
    3. prevention of aspiration and maintenance of circulation.
    4. prevention of skin breakdown and shock.

12. If bleeding is under control, the priority nursing diagnosis for a traumatic injury to the auricle is:
    1. Impaired body image related to injury.
    2. Anemia related to blood loss.
    3. Impaired tissue integrity related to trauma.
    4. Decreased cardiac output related to blood loss.

13. Which of the following are outcome criteria for emergency care of the burn victim? Select all that apply.
    1. Improved gas exchange
    2. Absence of symptoms of shock
    3. Burned areas covered
    4. Skin surfaces free from burning materials
    5. Pain reduced
    6. No symptoms of ileus

14. The priority nursing diagnosis for the victim of frostbite is:
    1. Sensory/perceptual alterations related to decreased circulation.
    2. Risk for impaired skin integrity related to vascular changes.
    3. Risk for infection related to tissue damage.
    4. Risk for disuse syndrome related to vascular changes.

15. Which drugs increase the risk of heatstroke by affecting the body's heat-reducing mechanisms?
    1. Adrenergics and bronchodilators
    2. Diuretics and anticholinergics
    3. Steroids and salicylates
    4. Anticoagulants and antihistamines

16. Which outcomes indicate that a victim of a snakebite is improved? Select all that apply.
    1. Wound is free from debris.
    2. Patient is sleepy but able to be aroused.
    3. Specific toxic effects are absent.
    4. Patient is alert without dyspnea.

17. For a minor superficial burn, what is the immediate nursing care?
    1. Apply butter to the injured body part.
    2. Apply topical preparations with benzocaine.
    3. Immerse the injured body part in cool water for 2–5 minutes.
    4. Cover the burn with a clean, dry dressing or cloth.

18. List in sequential order the steps the nurse follows when approaching an emergency situation.
    A. _____ Try to determine the nature of the emergency. (How was the injury caused?)
    B. _____ Look for hazards to the victim and to the rescuer.
    C. _____ Ask the victim his name to see whether he can speak.
    D. _____ Approach the victim so he does not have to move his head to see you.

19. During the initial survey of an emergency situation, what is the process to be followed? Place the steps in sequential order.
    A. _____ Look for uncontrolled bleeding, identify the source, and apply pressure.
    B. _____ Systematically examine for injuries from head to feet; immobilize the spine, if needed.
    C. _____ Assess airway, breathing, and circulation.
    D. _____ Look for medical alert tag.
    E. _____ Initiate CPR or rescue breathing, if needed.

Surgical Care

chapter
17

 Go to http://evolve.elsevier.com/Linton/medsurg/ for additional activities and exercises.

NCLEX CATEGORIES:

Safe and Effective Care Environment:
Coordinated Care, Safety and Infection Control

Physiological Integrity: Pharmacological Therapies, Reduction of Risk Potential, Physiological Adaptation

OBJECTIVES

1. State the purpose of each type of surgery: diagnostic, exploratory, curative, palliative, and cosmetic.
2. List data to be included in the nursing assessment of the preoperative patient.
3. Identify the nursing diagnoses, goals and outcome criteria, and interventions during the preoperative phase of the surgical experience.
4. Outline a preoperative teaching plan.
5. List the responsibilities of each member of the surgical team.
6. Explain the nursing implications of each type of anesthesia.
7. Explain how the nurse can help prevent postoperative complications.
8. List data to be included in the nursing assessment of the postoperative patient.
9. Identify nursing diagnoses, goals and outcome criteria, and interventions for the postoperative patient.
10. Explain patient needs to be considered in discharge planning.

PART I: MASTERING THE BASICS

A. Age-Related Surgical Outcomes.

Which of the following are reasons that older adults are often at greater risk for surgical complications? Select all that apply.

1. Secretions are more copious.
2. Impaired healing and recovery, if chronic illness is present.
3. Takes longer to regain strength following periods of inactivity.
4. Ciliary activity is less effective.
5. Age-related changes in the heart and brain.

B. Pulmonary Complications.

Which of the following are reasons that smoking increases the risk of pulmonary complications? Select all that apply.

1. Ineffective breathing patterns
2. Risk for suffocation
3. More tenacious secretions
4. Less effective ciliary activity

C. Lab Studies.

Which are diagnostic tests that are done preoperatively? Select all that apply.

1. ECG
2. Urine tests
3. Culture and sensitivity tests
4. Chest radiograph
5. Thyroid function tests

D. Informed Consent.

Which of the following are components of a consent form for surgery? Select all that apply.
1. Patient must be informed about the procedure to be done.
2. Results of preoperative work-up are explained.
3. Alternative treatments are discussed.
4. Discharge instructions are included.
5. Risks involved are mentioned.
6. Patient agrees to procedure.

E. Drug Therapy.

Which drugs increase effects of general anesthetics? Select all that apply.
1. Anticonvulsants
2. Antihistamines
3. Barbiturates
4. Antihypertensives
5. Potassium-wasting diuretics
6. Atropine
7. Aminoglycosides
8. Muscle relaxants

F. Preoperative Medications.

Which are safety nursing interventions following administration of the preoperative medication? Select all that apply.
1. Instruct patient to remain in bed.
2. Have the consent form signed.
3. Raise the side rails of the bed.
4. Have the patient void.

G. Complications/Local Anesthesia.

Which are complications of local anesthesia? Select all that apply.
1. Allergic responses
2. Seizures
3. Hypotension
4. Local tissue damage
5. Respiratory depression
6. Muscle relaxation

H. General Anesthesia.

Which of the following are methods by which general anesthetic agents can be given? Select all that apply.
1. Inhalation
2. Intravenous infusion
3. Oral administration
4. Rectal administration
5. Intramuscular injection

I. Drug Therapy.

Which are classifications of preoperative and operative drugs that depress respiratory function and cause pulmonary secretions to be drier and thicker during the postoperative phase? Select all that apply.
1. Preoperative anticholinergics
2. Opioid analgesics
3. Corticosteroids
4. General anesthetics
5. Antihypertensives

J. Wound Complications.

Which of the following are complications of wound healing? Select all that apply.
1. Dehiscence
2. Evisceration
3. Infection
4. Hypotension
5. Bradycardia

K. Impaired Peristalsis.

Which are factors that may cause peristalsis to be impaired after surgery? Select all that apply.
1. Hypertension
2. Opioid analgesics
3. Immobility
4. Inability to cough
5. Nausea

L. Surgical Complications.

What are causes of urinary retention following surgery? Select all that apply.
1. Altered tissue perfusion
2. Decreased cardiac output
3. Anxiety about voiding
4. Trauma to the urinary tract

M. Safety Precautions.
What safety precautions should be taken when patients are transferred to their own beds on the nursing unit? Select all that apply.
1. Lower the bed.
2. Place call button within reach.
3. Take vital signs every 4 hours.
4. Place head of bed in high Fowler's position.

N. Postoperative Care/Coughing.
Which of the following are types of surgeries in which coughing is contraindicated? Select all that apply.
1. Appendectomy
2. Cataracts
3. Brain surgery
4. Mastectomy
5. Hip replacement
6. Hernias
7. Hemoptysis

O. Paralytic Ileus.
Which are characteristics of paralytic ileus? Select all that apply.
1. Abdominal pain
2. Presence of bowel sounds
3. Increased temperature
4. Increased blood pressure
5. Abdominal distention
6. Likely to happen when there is excessive strain on the suture line

P. Drug Therapy/Preoperative Medications.
Match the preoperative drug in the numbered column with the most appropriate classification for use with preoperative surgical patients in the lettered column. Some answers may be used more than once.

1. _____ Glycopyrrolate (Robinul)
2. _____ Chloral hydrate (Noctec)
3. _____ Promethazine hydrochloride (Phenergan)
4. _____ Pentobarbital sodium (Nembutal Sodium)
5. _____ Diazepam (Valium)
6. _____ Atropine sulfate
7. _____ Meperidine hydrochloride (Demerol HCl)

8. _____ Secobarbital sodium (Seconal sodium)
9. _____ Morphine sulfate (MS Contin, Duramorph)

A. Tranquilizer
B. Analgesic
C. Anticholinergic
D. Sedative or hypnotic
E. Antiemetic
F. Skeletal muscle relaxant

Q. Surgical Complications.
Match the treatment in the numbered column with the complication it is used for in the lettered column. Some complications may be used more than once, and some treatments may match more than one complication.

1. _____ Administer oxygen.
2. _____ Pour warm water over perineum.
3. _____ Give intravenous (IV) fluids as ordered; encourage oral intake when allowed.
4. _____ Ambulate frequently when permitted; laxatives or enemas, or both, as ordered.
5. _____ Vasopressors (drugs to raise blood pressure) as ordered.
6. _____ Position to promote effective ventilation.
7. _____ Cover the open wound with a sterile dressing; if organs protrude, saturate the dressing with normal saline, notify physician, and keep patient still and quiet.
8. _____ Antiemetic drugs as ordered.
9. _____ Encourage deep-breathing and coughing.
10. _____ Bedrest; anticoagulant therapy as ordered.
11. _____ Rectal tube, heat to abdomen, bisacodyl suppositories as ordered; position on right side; nasogastric intubation with suction as ordered.
12. _____ Fluid or blood replacement.
13. _____ Rest; oxygen and antibiotics as ordered.

14. _____   Additional surgery to control bleeding.

15. _____   Suction as necessary.

A. Fluid and electrolyte imbalances
B. Altered elimination
C. Impaired wound healing
D. Shock
E. Nausea and vomiting
F. Hypoxia
G. Thrombophlebitis
H. Inadequate oxygenation
I. Abdominal distention
J. "Gas" pains/constipation

PART II: PUTTING IT ALL TOGETHER

R. Multiple Choice/Multiple Response.

Choose the most appropriate answer or select all that apply.

1. Which of the following are reasons why there is a risk of shock in the immediate postoperative period? Select all that apply.
   1. Loss of blood
   2. Ineffective breathing patterns
   3. Altered tissue perfusion
   4. Effect of anesthesia

2. Which of the following are reasons why hypoxia may occur in the immediate postoperative period? Select all that apply.
   1. Tongue falls back and blocks the airway.
   2. Secretions are more copious.
   3. Cough and swallowing reflexes are depressed by anesthesia.
   4. Ciliary activity is less effective.
   5. Risk of laryngospasm or bronchospasm.

3. Which measures are taken to prevent the postoperative complication of shock? Select all that apply.
   1. Observe wound dressing.
   2. Report excessive drainage or bleeding.
   3. Adequate fluids and nutrition.
   4. Assist to cough and deep-breathe.
   5. Monitor intake and output.
   6. Note early changes in vital signs.
   7. Withhold oral fluids until nausea subsides.
   8. Splint incision during activity.

4. Which of the following are criteria that determine when the patient can be moved from the recovery room to the nursing unit? Select all that apply.
   1. Patient is able to void.
   2. Gag reflex is present.
   3. Patient is able to ambulate.
   4. Vital signs are stable.
   5. Patient has minimal pain.
   6. Patient can be awakened easily.

5. What measures are used to prevent thrombophlebitis and related pulmonary emboli? Select all that apply.
   1. Early ambulation
   2. Leg exercises
   3. Coughing and deep-breathing
   4. Monitor vital signs
   5. Antiembolic stockings

6. Which are signs and symptoms that would alert the nurse to possible pulmonary emboli? Select all that apply.
   1. Hypotension
   2. Decreased respiratory rate
   3. Chest pain
   4. Dyspnea

7. Which criteria are used for evaluating the outcomes of nursing goals related to risk of infection? Select all that apply.
   1. Absence of fever
   2. Intact wound margins
   3. Minimal swelling
   4. Patient statement of pain relief

8. Label each method of wound closure (A–C).

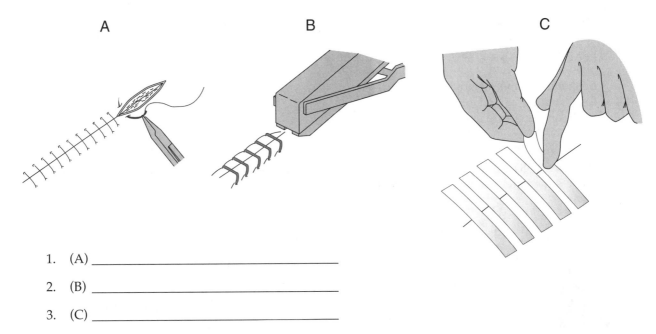

A   B   C

1. (A) _____

2. (B) _____

3. (C) _____

9. Label each complication of wound healing (A and B).

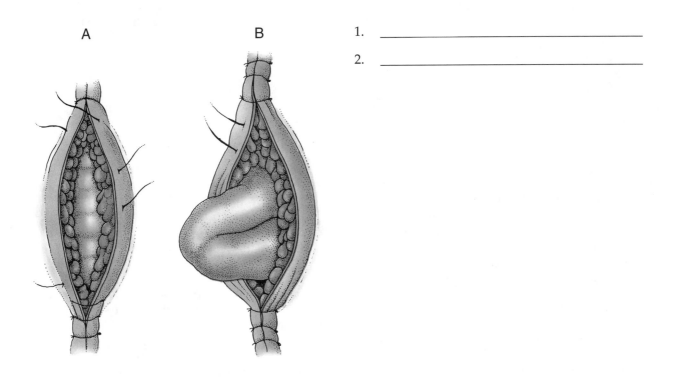

A   B   1. _____

2. _____

10. Which of the following descriptions refer to dehiscence? Select all that apply.
    1. Most likely to occur between the 5th and 12th postoperative days
    2. Protrusion of body organs through the open wound
    3. Reopening of the surgical wound
    4. Likely to happen when there is excessive strain on the suture line

11. Using Figure 17-8 below (p. 276 in the textbook), answer the questions that follow and specify by listing the letter. Some letters may be used more than once.

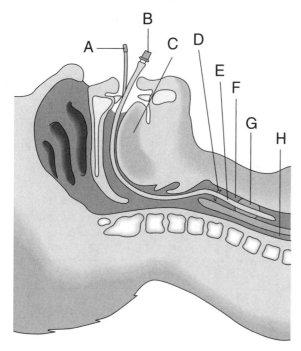

1. Which letter shows the endotracheal tube?
   _____

2. Which part of the figure shows the inflated cuff? _____

3. Through which tube is inhalation administered? _____

4. What prevents aspiration of gastric contents while the patient is unconscious? _____

5. Which part of the drawing shows the part that prevents leakage during mechanical ventilation? _____

12. Which postoperative problems are obese surgical patients more likely to have?
    1. Infection and increased temperature
    2. Excessive bleeding and hemorrhage
    3. Headache and bradycardia
    4. Respiratory and wound healing complications

13. Electrolyte imbalances may predispose the surgical patient to:
    1. cardiac arrhythmias.
    2. lung complications.
    3. liver malfunction.
    4. bone tissue loss.

14. If the patient is a minor, who signs the surgical consent form?
    1. Physician
    2. Registered nurse
    3. Parent or guardian
    4. Close relative

15. Shaving the skin in preparation for surgery is often delayed until shortly before surgery in order to:
    1. improve wound healing.
    2. control bleeding.
    3. allow less time for organisms to multiply.
    4. prevent postoperative edema.

16. The use of local anesthetics that block the conduction of nerve impulses in a specific area is called:
    1. general anesthesia.
    2. sedative anesthesia.
    3. anticonvulsant anesthesia.
    4. regional anesthesia.

17. The injection of an anesthetic agent into and under the skin around the area of treatment is called:
    1. local infiltration.
    2. topical administration.
    3. nerve block technique.
    4. intravenous infusion.

18. One complication of spinal anesthesia is:
    1. tachycardia.
    2. hemorrhage.
    3. headache.
    4. shock.

19. Postspinal headache can be relieved by:
    1. elevating the head of the bed.
    2. lying flat.
    3. early ambulation.
    4. coughing and deep-breathing.

20. A "blood patch" may help treat:
    1. hemorrhage.
    2. postspinal headache.
    3. shock.
    4. tachycardia.

21. Which of the following adverse effects of anesthetic agents may be reduced by giving pre-anesthetic medications?
    1. Tachycardia
    2. Dry mouth
    3. Urinary retention
    4. Vomiting

22. Which are characteristics of the life-threatening complication of inhalation anesthesia, malignant hyperthermia? Select all that apply.
    1. Increased metabolic rate
    2. Hypertension
    3. Cyanosis
    4. Muscle rigidity
    5. Bradycardia

23. When peristalsis is slow and there is increased gas buildup, what is the result?
    1. Abdominal cramping and distention
    2. Diarrhea and tachycardia
    3. Fever and infection
    4. Nausea and vomiting

24. "Gas pains" typically occur:
    1. during surgery.
    2. immediately after surgery.
    3. 6 hours after surgery.
    4. on second or third day after surgery.

25. An outcome criterion related to absence of thrombophlebitis is:
    1. adequate oxygenation.
    2. normal arterial blood gases.
    3. negative Homans sign.
    4. normal wound healing.

26. What is used to monitor the oxygenation of the blood?
    1. Sphygmomanometer
    2. Incentive spirometer
    3. Oximeter
    4. Stethoscope

27. When regional block anesthesia is used during surgery, the nurse must remember that after surgery:
    1. sensation in the area is impaired.
    2. circulation in the area is impaired.
    3. infection is likely to occur.
    4. fever may make the patient drowsy.

28. Once the immediate postoperative phase has passed, which risks lessen?
    1. Fever and infection
    2. Pneumonia and atelectasis
    3. Shock and hemorrhage
    4. Thrombophlebitis and decubitus ulcer

29. Clean sutured incisions heal by:
    1. first intention.
    2. second intention.
    3. third intention.
    4. fourth intention.

30. A soft tube that permits passive movement of fluids from the wound is called a(n):
    1. active drain.
    2. Hemovac.
    3. Penrose drain.
    4. Jackson-Pratt drain.

31. In the postoperative phase, place the colors of the wound drainage in order. Place 1 by the immediate postoperative phase, and 4 when the amount of blood in the drainage decreases.
    A. _____ Straw-colored
    B. _____ Clear
    C. _____ Bright red
    D. _____ Pink

32. Which sudden change in condition may precede wound dehiscence?
    1. Decrease in wound drainage
    2. Increase in wound drainage
    3. Increase in temperature
    4. Increase of purulent drainage

33. If evisceration occurs, the usual practice is to cover the wound with:
    1. dry sterile dressings.
    2. saline-soaked gauze with a dry dressing over it.
    3. antibiotic ointment and dry dressings.
    4. steroid ointment and dry dressings.

34. Signs and symptoms of wound infection usually do not develop until:
    1. the first hour after surgery.
    2. 12 hours after surgery.
    3. the first and second days after surgery.
    4. the third to fifth day after surgery.

35. A postoperative patient complains of pain, fever, swelling, and purulent drainage. These signs and symptoms are indications of:
    1. thrombophlebitis.
    2. evisceration.
    3. dehiscence.
    4. wound infection.

36. Pulmonary emboli usually originate from thrombi that develop in veins of the:
    1. chest.
    2. arms and shoulders.
    3. legs and pelvis.
    4. abdomen.

37. Emboli may be treated with:
    1. phenytoin (Dilantin) and anticonvulsants.
    2. morphine and analgesics.
    3. heparin and thrombolytic agents.
    4. furosemide (Lasix) and diuretics.

38. Catheterization is usually done postoperatively if the patient does not void in:
    1. 2 hours.
    2. 4 hours.
    3. 8 hours.
    4. 10 hours.

39. When a patient passes small amounts of urine frequently without feeling relief of fullness, this indicates:
    1. retention with overflow.
    2. stress incontinence.
    3. urge incontinence.
    4. kidney failure.

40. Some agencies have policies that limit the amount of urine that can be drained from a full bladder at one time; these limits are usually:
    1. 5–10 ml.
    2. 50–100 ml.
    3. 400–500 ml.
    4. 750–1000 ml.

41. When do most patients pass flatus?
    1. 15 minutes after surgery
    2. 1 hour after surgery
    3. 48 hours after surgery
    4. 1 week after surgery

42. Which surgical drain works by creating negative pressure when the receptacle is compressed?
    1. Penrose
    2. Urinary
    3. Hemovac
    4. Passive

43. Which drug supplements the effects of local anesthetics?
    1. Propranolol (Inderal)
    2. Atropine
    3. Morphine
    4. Epinephrine

44. A patient states that his wound feels as if it is "pulling apart." This is an indication of:
    1. healing by first intention.
    2. dehiscence.
    3. evisceration.
    4. singultus.

45. Which of the following postoperative drugs causes urinary retention?
    1. Antibiotics
    2. Thrombolytics
    3. Opioid analgesics
    4. Anticoagulants

46. The use of IV drugs to reduce pain intensity or awareness without loss of reflexes is called:
    1. regional anesthesia.
    2. conscious sedation.
    3. general anesthesia.
    4. balanced anesthesia.

47. Which is a commonly used IV drug for conscious sedation?
    1. Succinylcholine
    2. Isoflurane
    3. Nitrous oxide
    4. Midazolam (Versed)

48. Enflurane (Ethrane) and nitrous oxide are administered by:
    1. inhalation.
    2. IV infusion.
    3. intramuscular (IM) injection.
    4. rectal insertion.

PART III: CHALLENGE YOURSELF!

S. Getting Ready for NCLEX.

Choose the most appropriate answer or select all that apply.

1. The surgical patient who is malnourished is at risk for:
    1. excessive bleeding and hemorrhage.
    2. drug toxicity and ineffective metabolism.
    3. cardiac complications and dyspnea.
    4. poor wound healing and infection.

2. The patient develops rupture of the suture line and states: "My incision is breaking open." Which of the following actions should the nurse take to prevent complications in this patient?
    1. Keep the patient in bed.
    2. Administer opioid analgesics as ordered.
    3. Have the patient cough and deep-breathe every 2 hours.
    4. Auscultate breath sounds.

3. After the first 24 hours following surgery, which finding should be reported to the physician if it is observed?
    1. Respirations of 20/minute
    2. Temperature of 98.8° F
    3. Blood pressure of 110/70 mm Hg
    4. Continued or excessive bleeding

4. Which finding in a postoperative patient should be reported to the physician?
    1. Redness that spreads to the surrounding area
    2. Redness at the wound suture site
    3. Low-grade fever
    4. Serosanguineous drainage

5. A week after surgery, the patient develops pain, fever, swelling, and purulent drainage around the wound site. Which of the following actions should the nurse take to prevent complications?
    1. Keep the patient in bed
    2. Early, frequent ambulation
    3. Monitor intake and output
    4. Good hand hygiene

6. What is the priority nursing diagnosis during the immediate postoperative period?
    1. Acute pain
    2. Impaired tissue integrity
    3. Shock
    4. Urinary retention

7. What are four essential components for transferring primary responsibility of care from one health care provider to another? Select all that apply.
    1. Assessment
    2. Recommendation
    3. Care Plan
    4. Background
    5. Teaching Plan
    6. Situation

8. Which are minimal information reports that must be communicated about a surgical procedure during a "hand off"? Select all that apply.
    1. Any medication given
    2. Latest vital signs
    3. Lab tests ordered
    4. Blood administered
    5. Any drains in place
    6. Discharge instructions

9. What are causes of shock during the postoperative period? Select all that apply.
   1. Effect of anesthesia
   2. Loss of blood
   3. Dehydration without adequate replacement
   4. High blood volume
   5. Opioid administration before anesthesia is worn off

Intravenous Therapy

chapter

18

 Go to http://evolve.elsevier.com/Linton/medsurg/ for additional activities and exercises.

NCLEX CATEGORIES:

Safe and Effective Care Environment: Safety and Infection Control

Physiological Integrity: Pharmacological Therapies, Reduction of Risk Potential, Physiological Adaptation

OBJECTIVES

1. List the indications for intravenous fluid therapy.
2. Describe the types of fluids used for intravenous fluid therapy.
3. Describe the types of venous access devices and other equipment used for intravenous therapy.
4. Given the prescribed hourly flow rate, calculate the correct drop rate for an intravenous fluid.
5. Explain the causes, signs and symptoms, and nursing implications of the complications of intravenous fluid or drug therapy.
6. Explain the nursing responsibilities when a patient is receiving intravenous therapy.
7. Identify intravenous medications that require dilution because they are vesicants or irritants.

PART I: MASTERING THE BASICS

A. Key Terms.
Match the definition in the numbered column with the most appropriate term in the lettered column. Not all answers may be used.

1. _____ A liquid containing one or more dissolved substances

2. _____ A term used to describe a solution that has a higher concentration of electrolytes than normal body fluids

3. _____ A term used to describe a solution that has the same concentration of electrolytes as normal body fluids

4. _____ A term used to describe a solution that has a lower concentration of electrolytes than normal body fluids

5. _____ A measure of the concentration of electrolytes in a fluid

6. _____ Escape of fluid or blood from a blood vessel into body tissue

A. Hypotonic
B. Cannula
C. Solution
D. Hypertonic
E. Extravasation
F. Isotonic
G. Tonicity

B. Key Terms. Complications.
Match the definition or description in the numbered column with the most appropriate term in the lettered column.

1. _____ Leakage of fluid from a blood vessel

2. _____ Piece of catheter breaks off in vein

3. _____ Skin torn or irritated by tape or insertion of cannula

4. _____ Attached blood clot

5. _____ Obstruction caused by trapped embolus

6. _____ Collection of infused fluid in tissue surrounding the cannula

7. _____ Unattached blood clot

8. _____ Inflammation of the vein

A. Deep vein thrombus
B. Embolism
C. Infiltration
D. Catheter embolus
E. Embolus
F. Trauma
G. Phlebitis
H. Extravasation

C. Nursing Diagnoses.

Which of the following are nursing diagnoses for patients receiving intravenous therapy? Select all that apply.

1. Decreased cardiac output
2. Risk for injury
3. Fluid volume excess
4. Altered tissue perfusion
5. Impaired gas exchange
6. Risk for infection
7. Risk for imbalanced fluid volume

PART II: PUTTING IT ALL TOGETHER

D. Multiple Choice/Multiple Response.

Choose the most appropriate answer or select all that apply.

1. Irrigation of an occluded IV cannula is not recommended because:
   1. the IV cannula may become infiltrated.
   2. clots may be forced into the bloodstream.
   3. the IV cannula may become dislodged.
   4. thrombophlebitis may occur.

2. An IV solution of 0.45% sodium chloride is given if the patient has experienced:
   1. excessive water loss.
   2. cerebral edema.
   3. excessive sodium loss.
   4. burns.

3. In which position should the nurse place a patient if air accidentally enters a central line?
   1. On the left side
   2. On the right side
   3. Semi-Fowler's
   4. Fowler's

4. Which of the following are advantages of peripherally inserted central catheters (PICCs) over other central catheters? Select all that apply.
   1. Smaller needle
   2. Easier insertion
   3 Cost savings
   4. Reduced risk of infection
   5. Fewer dressing changes
   6. Less traumatic to vein
   7. No restriction of arm movement

5. The nurse notices that the IV on the patient is running too fast. To slow the rate down, the nurse:
   1. vents the IV container.
   2. splints the arm with an armboard.
   3. turns the arm so that the IV site is free.
   4. lowers the fluid container.

6. Which are symptoms of an air embolus? Select all that apply.
   1. Pulmonary edema
   2. Frothy, pink sputum
   3. Shortness of breath
   4. Chest pain
   5. Hypertension
   6. Possible shock
   7. Nausea

7. Edema, coolness, and pain at the IV insertion site are indications of:
   1. thrombophlebitis.
   2. infection.
   3. air embolus.
   4. infiltration.

8. Which IV complication is characterized by redness, swelling, and warmth?
   1. Phlebitis
   2. Infiltration
   3. Hemorrhage
   4. Catheter embolus

9. A patient's IV has been running too fast over the past hour. Which are signs of fluid volume excess? Select all that apply.
   1. Confusion
   2. Bounding pulse
   3. Inflammation
   4. Redness
   5. Increased blood pressure
   6. Dyspnea

10. If signs of fluid volume excess occur, the nurse should:
    1. turn the patient to the right side.
    2. elevate the head of the bed.
    3. check the vital signs.
    4. lower the head of the bed.

11. The patient with an air embolus is placed on the left side to trap air in the:
    1. left atrium so that it can be gradually absorbed.
    2. right ventricle so that it is not transferred to the lungs.
    3. left ventricle so that it is not transferred to the lungs.
    4. right atrium so that it can be gradually absorbed.

12. Which nursing intervention may prevent fluid volume excess during IV therapy?
    1. Encourage the patient to ambulate.
    2. Encourage the patient to cough.
    3. Time-tape the IV bag and monitor closely.
    4. Keep an accurate intake and output record.

13. What does a "drop factor of 15" mean?
    1. The infusion set will deliver 15 ml of fluid for every drop.
    2. The infusion set will deliver 1 ml of fluid for every 15 drops.
    3. The infusion set will deliver 1 ml of fluid in 15 minutes.
    4. The infusion set will deliver 15 ml of fluid in 1 minute.

14. How much air does it take to cause an air embolism in an adult?
    1. 5 cc
    2. 10 cc
    3. 15 cc
    4. 25 cc

15. An IV fluid container should not be used for more than:
    1. 12 hours.
    2. 24 hours.
    3. 48 hours.
    4. 72 hours.

16. A cannula with a clot in it should not be irrigated because it could cause:
    1. extravasation.
    2. infiltration.
    3. air embolism.
    4. pulmonary embolism.

PART III: CHALLENGE YOURSELF!

E. Getting Ready for NCLEX.

Choose the most appropriate answer or select all that apply.

1. Which is the outcome criteria for a patient with decreased cardiac output related to blood loss through a disrupted intravenous line?
   1. Pulse and blood pressure within normal limits
   2. Patient activities completed without disruption of intravenous therapy
   3. Normal body temperature; no purulent drainage or redness at venipuncture site
   4. Fluid output equal to intake; no dyspnea or edema

2. The absence of which outcome criteria are used for evaluating the nursing care of a patient with an IV? Select all that apply.
   1. Palpitations
   2. Cyanosis
   3. Blood return
   4. Edema
   5. Redness
   6. Swelling at the infusion site

3. As the nurse is making rounds at 7:00 AM, he notes that the patient's IV has 900 ml and is running at 75 ml/hour as ordered. When he checks the IV on his 10:00 AM rounds, the nurse notes that there is only 100 ml remaining. Which signs and symptoms does the nurse need to be alert for with this patient?
   1. Flushing of the face
   2. Nausea and vomiting
   3. Bounding pulse
   4. Diarrhea

4. A patient complains of crushing chest pain and difficulty breathing and has a rapid, thready pulse. The nurse suspects that he is experiencing an air embolism. Which interventions are appropriate?
   1. Turn the patient onto his left side, raise the head of the bed, and notify the charge nurse or physician.
   2. Turn the patient onto his left side, lower the head of the bed, and notify the charge nurse or physician.
   3. Place the patient on his back, lower the head of the bed, and notify the charge nurse.
   4. Ambulate the patient for 15 minutes and notify the charge nurse.

5. The nurse checks a patient's IV site and finds that her vein is cord-like. The IV is running well, but the site is red; the patient tells the nurse that the site is "sore when touched." These are signs of:
   1. infiltration.
   2. catheter embolus.
   3. air embolus.
   4. phlebitis.

6. The nurse checked the patient's IV 1 hour ago, and it was running at the correct rate of 50 ml/ hour. Now the IV is running at 100 ml/hour. What may be the cause of this increased rate?
   1. The tubing has a kink in it.
   2. The clamp has slipped.
   3. The fluid container is too low.
   4. The filter is blocked.

7. Because older people often have less efficient cardiac function, the nurse should monitor an older person with an IV for:
   1. fluid volume excess.
   2. bleeding.
   3. infection.
   4. infiltration.

8. An older patient is receiving IV fluids to treat dehydration. When he complains of pain and a burning sensation at the IV site, assessment reveals that the IV site is pale, puffy, and cool. Which complication does the nurse suspect?
   1. Phlebitis
   2. Infiltration
   3. Fluid volume excess
   4. Embolism

9. The patient is an 80-year-old male with a history of high blood pressure. When the nurse comes in to give him a bath, she notices that his IV of D_5W, which was hung 1 hour before she came into his room, contains 500 ml. 1000 ml was ordered to run in over 8 hours. The nurse should observe him for signs of:
   1. infection.
   2. shock.
   3. hemorrhage.
   4. heart failure.

10. While Mr. E. is receiving his IV, his BP is 145/90 mm Hg, his pulse is 110 bpm and bounding, and he reports difficulty breathing. After the nurse slows the infusion, what nursing intervention is appropriate?
    1. Monitor his vital signs hourly.
    2. Inspect the infusion site for swelling and bleeding.
    3. Elevate the head of his bed.
    4. Check connections to be sure they are secure.

11. Mr. E. was admitted for nausea and vomiting of 3 days' duration. Intravenous fluids were begun at 150 ml/hour via a 21-gauge cannula. His IV was started at 1:00 PM. How much fluid should have been administered by 3:30 PM that same day? _____

12. The nurse has an order to discontinue Mr. E.'s IV after 24 hours. There were no complications of IV therapy. What must be recorded after discontinuing his IV? Select all that apply.
    1. Size of cannula
    2. Appearance of IV site
    3. Blood pressure
    4. Weight
    5. How Mr. E. tolerated the procedure
    6. Respirations

13. Which statements are true about factors affecting the IV infusion rate? Select all that apply.
    1. When the fluid container is raised, the fluid flows slower.
    2. As the fluid container empties, the rate slows down.
    3. Thin fluids flow faster than thick fluids.
    4. By straightening out the extremity, the fluid flows slower.

14. Which are descriptions of the best sites for IV insertion? Select all that apply.
    1. Use the least restrictive site.
    2. Use a small vein that is in good condition.
    3. Use a soft, straight vein.
    4. Use the nondominant arm.
    5. Begin with the most proximal vein, and move distally as needed.

15. Which of the following assignments can the LPN make to the CNA?
    1. Ask the CNA to slow the infusion rate when it is flowing too fast.
    2. Ask the CNA to determine the best site.
    3. Ask the CNA to start the IV.
    4. Ask the CNA to protect the IV infusion, while providing basic care.

Shock

 Go to http://evolve.elsevier.com/Linton/medsurg/ for additional activities and exercises.

NCLEX CATEGORIES:

Safe and Effective Care Environment:
Coordinated Care, Safety and Infection Control

Psychosocial Integrity

Physiological Integrity: Pharmacological Therapies, Reduction of Risk Potential, Physiological Adaptation

OBJECTIVES

1. List the types of shock.
2. Describe the pathophysiologic features of each type of shock.
3. List the signs and symptoms of each stage of shock.
4. Explain the first-aid emergency treatment of shock outside the medical facility.
5. Identify general medical and nursing interventions for shock.
6. Explain the rationale for medical-surgical treatment of shock.
7. Assist in developing care plans for patients in each type of shock.

PART I: MASTERING THE BASICS

A. Key Terms.
Match the definition in the numbered column with the correct term in the lettered column.

1. _____ Presence of systemic inflammatory response syndrome (SIRS) with a confirmed infection

2. _____ Generalized inflammatory condition that follows serious physiologic threat; characterized by damage to vascular endothelium and hypermetabolic state

3. _____ Deficiency of blood flow

4. _____ Failure of more than one organ as a result of SIRS

5. _____ A state of acute circulatory failure and impaired tissue perfusion

6. _____ A pathologic condition associated with an increase in acid relative to bicarbonate content; increased hydrogen ion concentration

A. Ischemia
B. Metabolic acidosis
C. Multiple organ dysfunction syndrome (MODS)
D. Sepsis
E. Shock
F. Systemic inflammatory response syndrome (SIRS)

B. Types of Shock.
Select all that apply.

1. Which of the following descriptions are related to hypovolemic shock? Select all that apply.
   1. Caused by hemorrhage, severe diarrhea or vomiting, and excessive perspiration
   2. Complicated by increased capillary permeability
   3. Occurs with physical impairment of blood flow
   4. Associated with pulmonary embolism and tension pneumothorax
   5. Occurs when the circulating blood volume is inadequate to maintain the supply of oxygen and nutrients to tissue

2. Which of the following descriptions relate to vasogenic shock? Select all that apply.
   1. Fluid pools in dependent areas of the body
   2. Related to excessive blood or fluid loss, inadequate fluid intake, or a shift of plasma from blood into body tissues
   3. Occurs when heart fails as a pump
   4. Problem is with excessive dilation of blood vessels
   5. Related to burns, peritonitis, and intestinal obstruction
   6. Associated with congestive heart failure (CHF), acute myocardial infarction (MI), and heart rhythm disturbances

3. Which are three types of vasogenic shock? Select all that apply.
   1. Hypovolemic
   2. Cardiogenic
   3. Anaphylactic
   4. Septic
   5. Obstructive
   6. Neurogenic

C. Drug Therapy.
Which medications are commonly used in the treatment of cardiogenic shock? Select all that apply.
   1. Inotropics
   2. Vasopressors
   3. Corticosteroids
   4. Histamine 1 blockers
   5. Venodilators
   6. Antimicrobials
   7. Vasodilators
   8. Vasoconstrictors

PART II: PUTTING IT ALL TOGETHER

D. Multiple Choice/Multiple Response.
Choose the most appropriate answer or select all that apply.

1. Which are compensatory mechanisms in shock related to the sympathetic nervous system response? Select all that apply.
   1. Decreased heart rate
   2. Peripheral vasodilation
   3. Constriction of renal arteries
   4. Renin-angiotensin-aldosterone system activated
   5. Increased ADH secretion
   6. Increased water excretion

2. Following an automobile accident, a 35-year-old man experienced severe hemorrhage. This type of shock is classified as:
   1. hypovolemic.
   2. cardiogenic.
   3. obstructive.
   4. distributive.

3. A woman experiences burns over 80% of her body. The nurse suspects she has:
   1. hypovolemic shock.
   2. cardiogenic shock.
   3. obstructive shock.
   4. distributive shock.

4. A person has a severe allergic reaction that results in bronchoconstriction and increased capillary permeability. This type of shock is:
   1. anaphylactic.
   2. cardiogenic.
   3. hypovolemic.
   4. septic.

5. Which type of shock occurs suddenly, following exposure to a substance for which the patient had already developed antibodies?
   1. Neurogenic
   2. Septic
   3. Anaphylactic
   4. Cardiogenic

6. The body of a patient with neurogenic shock is unable to compensate with vasoconstriction because:
   1. the vasomotor center is incapacitated.
   2. chemicals released as a result of tissue ischemia depress the myocardium.
   3. bronchoconstriction and airway obstruction occur.
   4. systemic inflammatory response syndrome occurs.

7. One of the effects of shock on the neuroendocrine system is:
   1. release of catecholamines.
   2. decreased ADH.
   3. increased cerebral blood flow.
   4. decreased aldosterone.

8. One of the effects of shock on the respiratory system is:
   1. metabolic alkalosis.
   2. tissue hypoxia.
   3. depressed immune system.
   4. bronchodilation.

9. Assessment findings in the compensatory stage are likely to include:
   1. drowsiness.
   2. slightly increased blood pressure.
   3. increased blood glucose.
   4. increased bowel sounds.

10. Which assessment data would the nurse expect to find in a patient in the progressive stage of shock?
    1. Increased pulse pressure
    2. Weak, thready pulse
    3. Warm, flushed skin
    4. Increased blood pressure

11. The stage of shock in which death is imminent is known as:
    1. compensatory.
    2. refractory.
    3. progressive.
    4. hypovolemic.

12. The purpose of giving blood and fluids to improve cardiac output in a patient with cardiogenic shock is to:
    1. promote delivery of oxygen to cells.
    2. correct acid-base imbalances.
    3. improve fluid and electrolyte imbalances.
    4. decrease the incidence of infection.

13. Which type of shock does *not* have replacement of fluid as a priority?
    1. Distributive
    2. Neurogenic
    3. Hypovolemic
    4. Cardiogenic

14. Vasopressin is given to patients with septic shock because it is a:
    1. vasoconstrictor.
    2. vasodilator.
    3. bronchodilator.
    4. positive inotropic.

15. For which type of shock are antimicrobials prescribed?
    1. Hypovolemic
    2. Cardiogenic
    3. Distributive
    4. Septic

16. Why is atropine prescribed for neurogenic shock?
    1. Raise heart rate
    2. Raise blood pressure
    3. Treat pain
    4. Dilate blood vessels

17. For which type of shock are inotropic and anti-dysrhythmic agents ordered?
    1. Neurogenic
    2. Distributive
    3. Cardiogenic
    4. Anaphylactic

18. Hypermetabolism in shock causes which type of malnutrition?
    1. Decreased carbohydrate
    2. Decreased protein
    3. Decreased glucose
    4. Increased nitrogen

19. Which assessment finding would the nurse expect to see in a patient with septic shock that would not be present in a patient with hypovolemic shock?
    1. Cool skin
    2. Fever
    3. Low blood pressure
    4. Dizziness

PART III: CHALLENGE YOURSELF!

E. Getting Ready for NCLEX.

Choose the most appropriate answer.

First Aid for Shock.

1. List in order of priority the steps to be taken in the first-aid treatment for a patient in shock.
    A. _____ Control external bleeding with direct pressure or pressure dressing.
    B. _____ Keep the patient in a flat position, with legs elevated (unless further injury could be caused by raising legs).
    C. _____ Summon medical assistance.
    D. _____ Protect the patient from cold but do not overheat.
    E. _____ Establish/maintain patent airway.

2. Following a spinal cord injury, a 24-year-old man develops hypotension and bradycardia. This type of shock is:
    1. hypovolemic.
    2. septic.
    3. anaphylactic.
    4. neurogenic.

3. A priority in shock treatment is to:
    1. correct acid-base imbalances.
    2. manage cardiac dysrhythmias.
    3. administer antishock drugs.
    4. improve blood flow and oxygen supply to vital organs.

4. Which position is best to maintain blood flow to vital organs for a patient with shock?
    1. Supine with head lowered
    2. Fowler's
    3. Supine with legs elevated 45 degrees
    4. Left side-lying

5. Why is improving blood flow and oxygen supply to the vital organs a priority in shock treatment?
    1. Brain cells begin to die after 4 minutes without oxygen.
    2. Cells resort to anaerobic metabolism, producing lactic acid immediately.
    3. Acidosis has a depressant effect on myocardial cells.
    4. If compensatory mechanisms are effective, the blood pressure will remain normal.

6. A patient in shock has a pulse of 120 bpm, BP of 80/40 mm Hg, and respirations of 28. These signs represent:
    1. deficient fluid volume.
    2. ineffective tissue perfusion.
    3. decreased cardiac output.
    4. electrolyte imbalance.

Falls

chapter
20

 Go to http://evolve.elsevier.com/Linton/medsurg/ for additional activities and exercises.

NCLEX CATEGORIES:

Safe and Effective Care Environment: Safety and Infection Control

Physiological Integrity: Basic Care and Comfort, Pharmacological Therapies, Physiological Adaptation

OBJECTIVES

1. Define *falls*.
2. State the incidence of falls
3. Describe factors that increase the risk of falls.
4. Discuss the relationship between restraint use and falls, types of restraints, and regulations for restraint use.
5. Describe fall prevention techniques.
6. Describe nursing interventions to use when a fall occurs.
7. Explain what is meant by "least restrictive" interventions for fall prevention.

PART I: MASTERING THE BASICS

A. Key Terms.

Match the definition in the numbered column with the most appropriate term in the lettered column.

1. _____ Anything that restricts movement

2. _____ Circumstance in which one unintentionally falls to the ground or hits an object such as a chair or stair

3. _____ Factors related to the internal functioning of an individual, such as the aging process or physical illness that can cause falls

4. _____ Psychotropic medication given to subdue agitated or confused patients

5. _____ Law enacted in 1987 to protect patients from unnecessary restraints in nursing homes

6. _____ Factors in the environment that can cause falls

A. Chemical restraints
B. Extrinsic factors
C. Fall
D. Omnibus Reconciliation Act (OBRA)
E. Physical restraint
F. Intrinsic factors

B. Risk Factors.

Which of the following are factors associated with people at greatest risk for injury from falls? Select all that apply.

1. Peripheral neuropathy
2. Pneumonia
3. Kidney disease
4. Confusion
5. Hypertension
6. Osteoporosis
7. Benzodiazepine use
8. Antibiotic therapy
9. Sensory impairment
10. Gait disorders
11. Short-term memory loss
12. Balance disorders

C. Restraints.

Which of the following are damaging psychological effects of restraints on older patients? Select all that apply.

1. Decreased dependency
2. Anger
3. Increased confusion
4. Decreased disorientation
5. Withdrawal
6. Aggressive behavior
7. Loss of self-image
8. Fear
9. Security

D. Nursing Interventions.

Match each risk factor in the numbered column with the most appropriate intervention in the lettered column.

1. _____ Musculoskeletal disorders
2. _____ Impaired adaptation to the dark
3. _____ Balance disorders
4. _____ Stroke
5. _____ Reduced visual acuity
6. _____ Postural hypotension
7. _____ Impacted cerumen (earwax)
8. _____ Peripheral neuropathy
9. _____ Impaired color perception
10. _____ Foot disorders
11. _____ Presbycusis

A. Maintain adequate lighting; reduce glare from shiny floors and allow time for eyes to adjust to light levels (e.g., from a dark room to outside); use night-light in bedroom and bathroom.
B. Trim toenails; use appropriate footwear.
C. Speak slowly; use low voice; decrease background noise; encourage use of hearing aid.
D. Remove earwax.
E. Use bright colors as markers, especially orange, yellow, and red.
F. Be sure that individual wears glasses, if appropriate; keep glasses clean; encourage regular eye examinations.
G. Use correctly sized footwear with firm soles.
H. Encourage balance, gait training, and muscle-strengthening exercises.
I. Encourage dorsiflexion exercises; use pressure-graded stockings; elevate head of bed; teach individual to get up from chair or bed slowly to avoid tipping head backward.
J. Encourage balance exercises.
K. Place call bell in visual field and within reach of arm that has use; anticipate needs for toileting, dressing, eating, and bathing; assist with transfer; provide passive range of motion exercises to improve functional ability.

E. Prevention.

Which of the following are basic strategies for reducing all types of falls? Select all that apply.

1. Decrease physical activities.
2. Increase exercise.
3. Modify the environment.
4. Reduce visual impairment.

F. Documentation.

What factors are important to document at the time when a fall occurs? Select all that apply.

1. What the patient was doing
2. Vital signs of the patient at the time of the fall
3. Mental status of the patient
4. Nutritional status of the patient
5. Environmental factors

G. Nursing Interventions.

What are interventions to prevent falls for a patient with impaired dark adaptation? Select all that apply.

1. Be sure the patient wears glasses, if appropriate.
2. Maintain adequate lighting.
3. Reduce glare from shiny floors.
4. Allow time to adjust to light levels (as patient moves from a dark room to outside).
5. Keep glasses clean.
6. Encourage regular eye examinations.
7. Use a night-light in the bathroom.

H. Intrinsic Risk Factors.

Which are intrinsic risk factors for falling? Select all that apply.

1. Impaired hearing
2. Balance and gait problems
3. Environmental factors
4. Loose rugs
5. Foot disorders
6. Postural hypotension
7. Glare from shiny floors

I. Prevention.

Which are environment-oriented fall prevention techniques used in long-term care facilities? Select all that apply.

1. Assist patient to void every 4 hours.
2. Check for proper fit of slippers and footwear.
3. Keep rooms and hallways free from clutter.
4. Place TV controls within reach.
5. Clean up spills, including urine.
6. Encourage exercise to strengthen muscles and prevent weakness.

J. Prevention in Home Setting.

Which are fall prevention guidelines for the home? Select all that apply.

1. Watch for pets underfoot and scattered pet food.
2. Check for even, nonglare lighting in every room.
3. Use 60 watt lightbulbs to provide proper lighting in rooms.
4. Make sure there is a telephone in the room next to the bedroom.

PART II: PUTTING IT ALL TOGETHER

K. Multiple-Response Questions.

Choose the most appropriate answer.

1. What is the estimated ratio of people aged 65 or older who fall in a given year?
   1. 1 in 3
   2. 1 in 10
   3. 1 in 20
   4. 1 in 100

2. After what age does there appear to be a steady increase in the number of falls?
   1. 40
   2. 65
   3. 75
   4. 85

3. Of the total number of deaths due to falls, which percentage of the victims are elderly?
   1. 10%
   2. 20%
   3. 50%
   4. 72%

4. Which percentage of deaths due to falls does the U.S. Public Health Service state are preventable?
   1. one-fifth
   2. one-third
   3. one-half
   4. two-thirds

5. Of all reported falls, what percentage does not result in injury?
   1. 10%
   2. 25%
   3. 50%
   4. 75%

6. What is the most frequent type of injury from falls, occurring in 25–30% of all falls?
   1. Deep tissue damage
   2. Contusions, cuts, or lacerations
   3. Concussion
   4. Fractures

7. Older patients are more likely than younger patients to be physically restrained because of their greater likelihood of:
   1. mental decline and weight loss.
   2. chronic illness and physical decline.
   3. heart disease and insomnia.
   4. falling and confusion.

8. Physical restraints should be removed and released for 10 minutes every:
   1. hour.
   2. 2 hours.
   3. 4 hours.
   4. 8 hours.

9. Psychoactive drugs should never be used for the purpose of:
   1. relief of headaches.
   2. insomnia.
   3. discipline.
   4. hallucinations.

10. Why are older adults at particular risk for injury from their accidents?
    1. They are more confused.
    2. They are more disoriented.
    3. They are likely to have poorer clinical outcomes.
    4. They are not as coordinated.

11. What percentage of falls result in fractures in older adults?
    1. 1%
    2. 5%
    3. 20%
    4. 30%

PART III: CHALLENGE YOURSELF!

L. Getting Ready for NCLEX.

Choose the most appropriate answer or select all that apply.

Case Study: The Patient with a History of Falls.

A 75-year-old woman resides in a long-term care facility because of chronic health problems, including hypertension, emphysema, and mild dementia. She has a history of several falls at home, including one that resulted in a wrist fracture that led to the admission to the LTC facility. *Refer to this case study to answer questions 1-3.*

1. Which factor in her health history put this patient most at risk for a fracture from a fall?
   1. Emphysema
   2. Dementia
   3. High blood pressure
   4. History of several falls at home

2. What is the priority intervention for this patient to prevent her from falling?
   1. Discuss possible environmental hazards and measures to reduce risks with the patient.
   2. Keep bed at lowest level.
   3. Orient patient frequently to person, place, and time.
   4. Remove restraints at least every 2 hours for 10 minutes for range of motion exercises.

3. Which are interventions related to this patient's risk for falls related to postural hypotension? Select all that apply.
   1. Provide nurse call button and respond quickly.
   2. Keep bed at lowest level.
   3. Suggest elastic stockings to improve venous return.
   4. Teach patient to change positions slowly.
   5. Encourage adequate fluids to prevent dehydration.

4. What are major complications from using physical restraints? Select all that apply.
   1. sedation from medications administered and accidental aspiration.
   2. falls from wheelchairs and beds (when patients are able to untie restraints or wriggle out of them) and accidental strangulation.
   3. fatigue from fighting the restraints and confusion resulting from fatigue.
   4. skin breakdown from friction and wound development.

5. Keeping the bed at the lowest level and using the least restrictive restraints are interventions related to:
   1. Impaired skin integrity.
   2. Risk for injury.
   3. Altered urinary function.
   4. Risk for infection.

6. The first step in preventing falls and injury is to determine:
   1. which medications the patient is taking.
   2. the hazards in the environmental setting.
   3. who is at greatest risk.
   4. whether the patient has alcohol or drug problems.

7. Which interventions are recommended to reduce the risk of falls? Select all that apply.
    1. Calcium and vitamin D for susceptible patients
    2. Exercises to improve balance
    3. Frequent ambulation
    4. Muscle strengthening exercises
    5. High-protein diet

8. Which nursing interventions are recommended for a patient with impaired hearing who is at risk for falls? Select all that apply.
    1. Maintain adequate lighting.
    2. Encourage balance and gait training.
    3. Speak slowly.
    4. Use a loud voice.
    5. Decrease background noises.
    6. Provide passive range of motion exercise.

Immobility

 Go to http://evolve.elsevier.com/Linton/medsurg/ for additional activities and exercises.

NCLEX CATEGORIES:

Safe and Effective Care Environment: Safety and Infection Control

Health Promotion and Maintenance

Physiological Integrity: Basic Care and Comfort, Reduction of Risk Potential, Physiological Adaptation

OBJECTIVES

1. Describe common problems associated with immobility.
2. Discuss the impact of exercise and positioning on preventing complications related to immobility.
3. Identify the risk factors for pressure ulcers.
4. Describe the stages of pressure ulcers.
5. Describe methods of preventing and treating pressure ulcers.
6. Discuss the effects of immobility on respiratory status, nutrition, and elimination.

PART I: MASTERING THE BASICS

A. Key Terms.
Match the definition in the numbered column with the most appropriate term in the lettered column.

1. _____ The inability to move; imposed restriction on entire body

2. _____ Exercise in which each joint is moved in various directions to the farthest possible extreme

3. _____ Exercise of the patient that is carried out by the therapist or nurse without the assistance of the patient

4. _____ Muscle contraction without movement used to maintain muscle tone

5. _____ Exercise carried out by the patient

6. _____ Redness of the skin; usually a sign that capillaries have become congested because of impaired blood flow

7. _____ Shortening of the muscles and tendons

8. _____ Two contacting parts sliding on each other

9. _____ An open wound caused by pressure on a bony prominence; also called a "bed sore" or "decubitus ulcer"

A. Erythema
B. Pressure ulcer
C. Isometric exercise
D. Immobility
E. Range of motion exercise
F. Active exercise
G. Contracture
H. Shearing forces
I. Passive exercise

B. Preventing Pressure Ulcers.

Which of the following are elements of a pressure sore prevention protocol? Select all that apply.

1. Reposition patient on bedrest at least every 4 hours.
2. Apply sheepskin boots to prevent shearing forces.
3. Utilize trapeze bars to enhance patient mobility.
4. Teach wheelchair patients to shift their weight every 15 minutes if able.
5. Position patients so that they are resting on pressure points of the skin.
6. When the patient is in bed, keep the head raised as much as possible to reduce shearing force.
7. Do not massage or use rubber rings to elevate heels or sacral areas.

C. Pressure Ulcers.

Select all that apply.

1. Which of the following characteristics are related to stage I pressure ulcers? Select all that apply.
   1. Irregular, ill-defined area of pressure reflecting the shape of the object creating the pressure
   2. Some skin loss in the epidermis and/or dermis
   3. Nonblanchable erythema
   4. Ulcer is surrounded by a broad, indistinct, painful, reddened area that is hot or warmer than normal
   5. Little destruction of tissue; condition is reversible
   6. Pain and tenderness may be present, with swelling and hardening of the skin and associated heat

2. Which of the following characteristics are related to stage III pressure ulcers? Select all that apply.
   1. A shallow ulcer develops and appears blistered, cracked, or abraded
   2. Crater-like sore with a distinct outer margin
   3. Wound may be infected and is usually open and draining
   4. Ulcer is usually infected and may appear black with exudation, foul odor, and purulent drainage

5. Full-thickness skin loss involving damage or necrosis of the dermis and subcutaneous tissues
6. Full-thickness skin loss with extensive destruction of the deeper underlying muscle and possible bone tissue

D. Consequences of Immobility.

Match the consequences of immobility in the numbered column with the body system in the lettered column. Answers may be used more than once.

1. _____ Increased risk of atelectasis and infection
2. _____ Decreased glomerular filtration rate
3. _____ Decreased tactile stimulation
4. _____ Thickening of joint capsule
5. _____ Pressure ulcers
6. _____ Constipation
7. _____ Increased storage of fat
8. _____ Increased peripheral resistance
9. _____ Decreased glucose tolerance
10. _____ Loss of smoothness of cartilage surface

A. Integumentary
B. Gastrointestinal
C. Musculoskeletal
D. Pulmonary
E. Urinary
F. Metabolic
G. Sensory
H. Cardiovascular

E. Pressure Ulcer Locations.

Refer to the figure below, Possible Locations of Pressure Ulcers (Figure 21-1, p. 337). Label the bony prominences (A–Z).

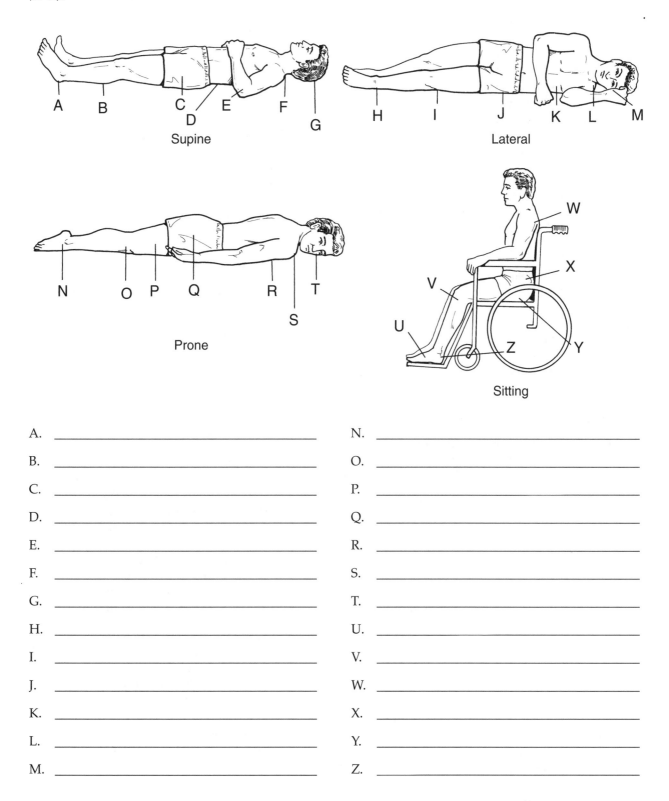

Supine

Lateral

Prone

Sitting

A. _____	N. _____
B. _____	O. _____
C. _____	P. _____
D. _____	Q. _____
E. _____	R. _____
F. _____	S. _____
G. _____	T. _____
H. _____	U. _____
I. _____	V. _____
J. _____	W. _____
K. _____	X. _____
L. _____	Y. _____
M. _____	Z. _____

F. Aging and Immobility.
Select all that apply.

1. Which common aging changes place the older adult at risk for immobility and its consequences? Select all that apply.
    1. Decreased flexibility
    2. Decreased strength
    3. Changes in posture
    4. Changes in gait
    5. Decreased kidney function
    6. Decreased neurons in brain
    7. Likelihood of having one or more chronic illnesses

2. Which of the following common medical illnesses place the older person at risk for immobility and its consequences? Select all that apply.
    1. Arthritis
    2. Cardiovascular disease
    3. Diabetes mellitus
    4. Stroke
    5. Anemia
    6. Thyroid disorders
    7. Parkinson disease
    8. Foot disorders

PART II: PUTTING IT ALL TOGETHER

G. Multiple Choice/Multiple Response.
Choose the most appropriate answer or select all that apply.

1. What is the result of little or no motion of the joints?
    1. Contractures
    2. Tendonitis
    3. Bursitis
    4. Skin breakdown

2. What is the most frequent site of skin breakdown?
    1. Ischial tuberosities
    2. Sacrum
    3. Heels
    4. Trochanter

3. The best preventive measure for pressure ulcers is:
    1. a high-protein diet.
    2. deep-breathing.
    3. frequent position changes.
    4. moderate exercise.

4. Which characteristics of patients with circulatory disease result in erythema progressing rapidly to an ulcerated stage? Select all that apply.
    1. Skin infection
    2. Poor skin turgor
    3. Malnourishment
    4. Obesity
    5. Lacerations
    6. Old age

5. Which of the following conditions result from pressure ulcers? Select all that apply.
    1. Falls
    2. Longer hospital stays
    3. Confusion
    4. Likelihood of long-term care facility placement
    5. Increased need for oxygen therapy
    6. Increased mortality

6. Which of the following are contraindicated in the care of patients with pressure ulcers? Select all that apply.
    1. Sheepskin
    2. Massage
    3. Egg-crate mattress
    4. Trapeze bars
    5. Rubber ring
    6. Heat lamp
    7. Use of moisturizers

7. A 65-year-old patient with heart failure is on bedrest and refuses to take deep breaths. Which of the following is most likely to occur to the respiratory status of this patient?
    1. An accumulation of carbon dioxide that collects in the alveoli
    2. An accumulation of thick secretions that pool in the lower respiratory structures
    3. Decreased circulation to the lungs
    4. Decreased oxygen entering the lungs

8. A 60-year-old patient with pneumonia has thick secretions pooled in the lower respiratory structures. These secretions interfere with the:
    1. exchange of white blood cells and red blood cells in the capillaries.
    2. circulation of blood to the extremities.
    3. detoxification process in the liver.
    4. exchange of oxygen and carbon dioxide in the lungs.

9. What is the most common problem associated with immobility in relation to food and fluid intake?
    1. Hypoproteinemia
    2. Hypokalemia
    3. Anorexia
    4. Nausea

10. For patients with pressure ulcers, the diet should be high in:
    1. potassium.
    2. fiber.
    3. protein.
    4. vitamins.

11. Which are causes of constipation in patients with pressure ulcers? Select all that apply.
    1. Anorexia
    2. Nausea
    3. Inactivity
    4. Decreased fluid intake
    5. Lack of fiber in diet

12. Which of the following is recommended for the treatment of stage I ulcers?
    1. Disinfectants
    2. Mild soap
    3. Alcohol
    4. Powder

13. What is the most effective way to prevent urinary incontinence associated with immobility?
    1. High-protein diet
    2. Coughing and deep-breathing program
    3. Restriction of fluid intake
    4. Schedule for toiletings

14. Which of the following are therapeutic reasons for immobility? Select all that apply.
    1. Reduce the workload of the heart in a cardiac condition
    2. Prevent atelectasis and hypostatic pneumonia
    3. Treat urinary incontinence
    4. Promote healing and repair
    5. Prevent further injury of a body part
    6. Obtain relief from joint contractures

15. Which side effects of drugs may contribute to factors causing immobility? Select all that apply.
    1. Vertigo
    2. Hypertension
    3. Loss of sensory function
    4. Hyperglycemia
    5. Tachycardia

PART III: CHALLENGE YOURSELF!

H. Getting Ready for NCLEX.

Choose the most appropriate answer or select all that apply.

1. A patient is slumped down while sitting in bed. Which action does the nurse take to prevent shearing? Select all that apply.
    1. Use moisturizers to prevent friction.
    2. Avoid friction when moving the patient to prevent damage to the uppermost layers of the skin.
    3. Reposition the patient in bed at least every 2 hours.
    4. Position the patient so that he is not resting on pressure points of the skin.
    5. Gently cleanse the skin when soiled.
    6. Keep the head of the bed lowered as much as possible to prevent the patient from sliding down in the bed.

2. What is the first step in the prevention of pressure ulcers?
    1. Reposition the patient in bed at least every 2 hours.
    2. Keep bed linens dry, smooth, and free of wrinkles.
    3. Use a special mattress or bed designed to reduce pressure.
    4. Identify patients at risk for developing pressure ulcers.

3. Which are ways to assist the immobile patient to gain independence? Select all that apply.
    1. Use of slip-on shoes
    2. Pressure-reducing pad for wheelchair
    3. Loose pullover shirts
    4. Velcro closures
    5. Increase fluid intake

Case Study: Immobility (Box 21-1 in textbook)

An 84-year-old woman, has resided in an intermediate care facility for 2 years. She was admitted to the facility because she had been living at home alone and was unable to shop and cook for herself after falling and breaking her wrist. She had previously been active in the community, but in the residential home she remained confined to her room and was not interested in interacting with other people. She preferred to stay in bed or in a chair most of the time. She had fallen many times, usually on her way to the dining room to eat. *Refer to this case study to answer questions 4 and 5.*

4. The team identified the following problems for this patient: risk for falls, risk for impaired skin integrity, and ineffective coping. Which additional problems is this patient likely to have? Select all that apply.
    1. Disturbed sleep pattern
    2. Risk for compromised human dignity
    3. Impaired gas exchange
    4. Sedentary lifestyle
    5. Risk for loneliness
    6. Complicated grieving
    7. Risk for bleeding

5. Which factors in the assessment of this patient put her at risk for injury? Select all that apply.
    1. Age
    2. Previous falls
    3. Keeps to herself
    4. Stays in bed or chair most of the time

Confusion

 Go to http://evolve.elsevier.com/Linton/medsurg/ for additional activities and exercises.

NCLEX CATEGORIES:

Safe and Effective Care Environment:
Coordinated Care, Safety and Infection Control

Health Promotion and Maintenance

Psychosocial Integrity

Physiological Integrity: Pharmacological Therapies, Reduction of Risk Potential, Physiological Adaptation

OBJECTIVES

1. Define delirium, dementia, and mild cognitive impairment.
2. Identify the causes of acute confusion.
3. Explain the differences between delirium and dementia.
4. Explain drug therapy for delirium and dementia.
5. Discuss nursing assessment and interventions related to delirium and dementia.

PART I: MASTERING THE BASICS

A. Key Terms.
Select all that apply.

1. Which of the following descriptions are related to delirium? Select all that apply.
   1. Short-term confusional state
   2. Often irreversible confusion
   3. Acute confusional state
   4. Chronic confusion
   5. Often reversible confusion
   6. Characterized by disturbances in attention, thinking, and perception

2. Which of the following descriptions are related to dementia? Select all that apply.
   1. Characterized by impaired intellectual function
   2. Caused by some underlying illness
   3. Develops over a short period of time
   4. Clearly defined hallucinations may be present
   5. Flat or indifferent affect
   6. Intermittent fear, perplexity, or bewilderment

B. Dementia.
Which of the following are general medical illnesses or conditions that may have dementia as a result? Select all that apply.
   1. Alzheimer disease
   2. Postoperative status
   3. Trauma
   4. Huntington disease
   5. HIV infection
   6. Parkinson disease

C. Dementia.
Which concepts should be used as a basis for providing care for patients with dementia? Select all that apply.
   1. Patients usually forget things relatively quickly.
   2. Orient the patients to time and person with clocks and calendars.
   3. Patients are usually unable to learn new things.
   4. Break down tasks into individual steps to be done one at a time.

D. Delirium.

Which are underlying medical illnesses or conditions that may cause delirium? Select all that apply.

1. Dehydration
2. Overmedication
3. Alzheimer disease
4. Parkinson disease
5. Infection

E. Disturbed Sleep Patterns.

Which of the following are related to dementia? Select all that apply.

1. Disturbed sleep pattern related to agitation
2. Disturbed sleep pattern related to drugs
3. Disturbed sleep pattern related to neurologic changes
4. Disturbed sleep pattern related to altered perceptions
5. Disturbed sleep pattern related to mood alterations

F. Risk for Injury.

Which of the following are related to delirium? Select all that apply.

1. Risk for injury related to disorientation
2. Risk for injury related to unfamiliar setting
3. Risk for injury related to poor judgment
4. Risk for injury related to physical decline
5. Risk for injury related to agitation
6. Risk for injury related to sensorimotor changes

G. Chronic Confusion.

Which of the following are related to dementia? Select all that apply.

1. Chronic confusion related to drugs
2. Chronic confusion related to infection
3. Chronic confusion related to memory loss
4. Chronic confusion related to altered perception

PART II: PUTTING IT ALL TOGETHER

H. Multiple-Choice Questions.

Choose the most appropriate answer.

1. A patient with delirium is having trouble falling asleep. Which is the most appropriate nursing intervention to help this patient fall asleep?
   1. A walk followed by a shower
   2. Pain medication and watching a movie
   3. A backrub, a glass of warm milk, and soothing conversation
   4. A sedative and reality orientation

2. The use of physical restraints should be avoided with patients with delirium because restraints tend to:
   1. increase anxiety.
   2. disturb thought processes.
   3. increase impaired thinking.
   4. disturb sleep patterns.

3. When a patient with dementia resists activities such as bathing or dressing, the nurse should:
   1. orient the patient to reality.
   2. avoid confrontations.
   3. state clearly what needs to be done.
   4. offer a variety of choices to encourage decision-making.

4. Patients with dementia should be offered:
   1. three full meals a day.
   2. low-fiber foods.
   3. a diet low in salt.
   4. finger foods high in protein and carbohydrates.

5. When the nurse is taking care of patients with dementia, it is helpful to remember that they usually:
   1. benefit from reality orientation.
   2. forget things quickly.
   3. do not forget things quickly.
   4. are able to learn new things.

6. Which approach may agitate patients with dementia?
   1. A nonconfrontational manner
   2. Use of calm, gentle mannerisms
   3. Reality orientation
   4. Use of simple, direct communication

7. When caring for a patient with delirium, the nurse should:
   1. provide frequent, routine toileting.
   2. provide frequent orientation to surroundings.
   3. cut the food into small portions.
   4. break tasks down into individual steps to be done one at a time.

8. Which of the following drugs may cause delirium? Select all that apply.
   1. Analgesics
   2. Antihistamines
   3. Benzodiazepines
   4. Antithyroids
   5. Antidepressants
   6. Steroids

PART III: CHALLENGE YOURSELF!

I. Getting Ready for NCLEX.

Choose the most appropriate answer.

1. What is the first step in collecting data about a confused person?
   1. Observe the behavior of the patient.
   2. List any known acute or chronic illnesses.
   3. List all medications the patient is taking.
   4. Collect data about the nutritional status of the patient.

2. When the nurse is caring for a delirious patient who is experiencing hallucinations, the best response of the nurse would be:
   1. "What is it that you are seeing on the wall?"
   2. "You are sick in the hospital, and what you are seeing is part of the illness."
   3. "The time is 2:00 PM and the day of the week is Monday."
   4. "Tell me what you are seeing."

3. If patients with dementia start to become very restless or agitated, an effective nursing intervention is to:
   1. discuss the cause of their discomfort with them.
   2. speak calmly and reassure them constantly.
   3. orient them to time and place.
   4. divert their attention and gently guide them to a new activity.

4. If a patient with dementia tells the nurse that he is afraid of bathtubs, the nurse should:
   1. reassure the patient that there is nothing to be afraid of.
   2. explain the reason for taking a bath in the bathtub.
   3. offer a variety of choices to the patient about taking a bath.
   4. arrange another way to give personal care.

Nursing Care Plan.

Read the following situation and answer questions 5-6. For more information, refer to Nursing Care Plan, The Patient with Delirium, p. 348 in your textbook.

An 81-year-old man was admitted for hip replacement surgery 2 days ago. Before his surgery he lived alone and cared for himself. He was active, alert, and independent. However, since his surgery, he has been combative with the nurses. His physician believes that he is suffering from delirium related to the anesthesia from surgery, and that it should resolve within a few days.

5. What is the first priority of nursing interventions for this patient?
   1. State clearly what needs to be done.
   2. Speak calmly and reassure the patient constantly.
   3. Provide reality orientation frequently.
   4. Provide safety and reduce anxiety.

6. What is the most appropriate nursing diagnosis for this type of delirium?
   1. Acute confusion
   2. Chronic confusion
   3. Risk for acute confusion
   4. Altered thought process

Nursing Care Plan.

Read the following situation and answer questions 7-8. For more information, refer to Nursing Care Plan, The Patient with Dementia, p. 350 in your textbook.

A 75-year-old woman is admitted to a long-term care facility by her daughter because she has been unsafe living alone at home. Her daughter reports she has been in good health, but during the past 5 years she has resisted taking a bath or changing her clothes. Sometimes she does not recognize her daughter and sometimes she forgets to eat. Recently, she has begun wandering. Her physician has diagnosed probable Alzheimer disease.

7. Which concept is used as a basis for breaking down self-care tasks for this patient?
   1. Patients can learn new things with repetition.
   2. Patients usually forget things quickly.
   3. Patients should be reoriented frequently and consistently.
   4. Patients should have family members stay with them.

8. Why is this patient at risk for injury?
   1. Poor judgment
   2. Impaired verbal communication
   3. Anxiety
   4. Agitation and mood alterations

Incontinence

 Go to http://evolve.elsevier.com/Linton/medsurg/ for additional activities and exercises.

NCLEX CATEGORIES:

Safe and Effective Care Environment: Safety and Infection Control

Physiological Integrity: Basic Care and Comfort, Pharmacological Therapies, Reduction of Risk Potential, Physiological Adaptation

OBJECTIVES

1. Identify the types of urinary and fecal incontinence.
2. Explain the pathophysiologic characteristics and treatment of specific types of incontinence.
3. Identify common therapeutic measures used for the patient with incontinence.
4. List nursing assessment data needed to assist in the evaluation and treatment of incontinence.
5. Assist in developing a nursing care plan for the patient with incontinence.

PART I: MASTERING THE BASICS

A. Key Terms.
Match the definition in the numbered column with the most appropriate type of urinary incontinence in the lettered column.

1. _____ Involuntary loss of urine during physical exertion

2. _____ Loss of urine due to reflexive contraction

3. _____ Inappropriate voiding in the presence of normal bladder and urethral function

4. _____ Involuntary loss of urine associated with a full bladder

5. _____ The inability to control the passage of urine

6. _____ Involuntary loss of urine, usually shortly after a strong urge to void

A. Functional urinary incontinence
B. Overflow urinary incontinence
C. Reflex urinary incontinence
D. Total urinary incontinence
E. Urge urinary incontinence
F. Stress urinary incontinence

B. Voiding.
Which factors are required for normal controlled voiding? Select all that apply.
1. Patent urethra
2. Underactive detrusor muscle
3. Mental alertness
4. Constricted bladder sphincter
5. Nerve impulse transmission

C. Urinary Urge Incontinence.
Which methods of treatment are used for urinary urge incontinence? Select all that apply.
1. Anticholinergics
2. Adrenergic drugs
3. Tricyclic antidepressants
4. Catheterization
5. Behavior modification

D. Overflow Incontinence.

Which factors contribute to overflow incontinence? Select all that apply.
1. Urethral obstruction
2. Spinal cord injury
3. Overactive detrusor muscle
4. Impaired nerve impulse transmission
5. Postanesthesia
6. Dementia

E. Drug Therapy.

Which drugs may cause urinary retention? Select all that apply.
1. Sedatives or hypnotics
2. Antipsychotics
3. Anticholinergics
4. Antihistamines
5. Theophylline (xanthines)
6. Epinephrine

F. Intermittent Catheterization.

Which type of patient usually requires intermittent catheterization only once or twice before normal bladder function returns? Select all that apply.
1. Postoperative patient
2. Spinal cord injury patient
3. Alzheimer patient
4. Postpartum patient

G. Stress Incontinence.

1. Which activities may lead to stress incontinence? Select all that apply.
   1. Coughing
   2. Laughing
   3. Lifting
   4. Nervous system disorder
   5. Urethral obstruction
   6. Sneezing

2. Which are contributing factors to stress incontinence? Select all that apply.
   1. Postpartum pelvic floor muscle relaxation
   2. Spinal cord injury
   3. Postanesthesia
   4. Obesity
   5. Aging

3. Which of the following are methods of treatment for a person with stress incontinence? Select all that apply.
   1. Scheduled voiding
   2. Pelvic muscle exercises
   3. Decreased fluid intake
   4. Avoid fluids with caffeine
   5. Use of Contigen (collagens)

H. Therapeutic Measures.

Match the definition or description in the numbered column with the most appropriate therapeutic measure in the lettered column.

1. _____ Intended to help the patient recognize incontinence and to ask caregivers for help with toileting
2. _____ Voiding schedule based on the patient's usual pattern
3. _____ Includes anticholinergics and smooth muscle relaxants
4. _____ Uses patient education, scheduled voiding, and positive reinforcement
5. _____ Sometimes employed by people with spinal cord injury
6. _____ Uses electronic or mechanical sensors to give feedback about physiologic activity
7. _____ Commonly called *Kegel exercises*
8. _____ Retained in the vagina to strengthen muscles of pelvic floor

A. Pelvic muscle exercises
B. Vaginal cones
C. Bladder training
D. Habit training
E. Drug therapy
F. Biofeedback
G. Prompted voiding
H. Reflex training

I. Nursing Diagnoses.

Match the nursing diagnosis in the numbered column with the most appropriate cause in the lettered column.

1. _____ Functional incontinence
2. _____ Reflex incontinence
3. _____ Risk for infection

A. Neurologic impairment
B. Chronic bladder distention or catheterization
C. Physical, cognitive, or environmental barriers

J. Drug Therapy.

1. Which types of drugs are commonly used to treat urge and reflex incontinence? Select all that apply.
   1. Antispasmodics
   2. Cholinergics
   3. Beta-adrenergic blockers
   4. Anticholinergics
   5. Alpha-adrenergic agonists
   6. Propranolol (Inderal)

2. Which types of drugs are used to treat overflow incontinence? Select all that apply.
   1. Bethanechol chloride (Urecholine)
   2. Doxazosin (Cardura)
   3. Ephedrine
   4. Oxybutynin (Ditropan)
   5. Propantheline bromide (Pro-Banthine)
   6. Finasteride (Proscar)
   7. Collagen (Contigen)

K. Types of Urinary Incontinence.

Match the cause of incontinence in the numbered column with the type of incontinence in the lettered column. Answers may be used more than once.

1. _____ Urinary tract infection
2. _____ Spinal cord injury above T10
3. _____ Relaxation of pelvic floor muscles
4. _____ Dementia
5. _____ Cerebrovascular accident
6. _____ Urethral trauma
7. _____ Postanesthesia

A. Urge
B. Overflow
C. Reflex
D. Stress
E. Functional

PART II: PUTTING IT ALL TOGETHER

L. Multiple-Choice Questions.

Choose the most appropriate answer.

1. Drugs that may cause urinary retention include:
   1. chlorothiazides and loop diuretics.
   2. antihypertensives and insulin.
   3. anticholinergics and epinephrine.
   4. antibiotics and antiviral drugs.

2. The amount of urine remaining in the bladder after voiding is called the:
   1. urodynamic series.
   2. clean catch.
   3. voiding duration.
   4. postvoid residual.

3. How much urine normally remains in the bladder after voiding?
   1. 50 ml or less
   2. 100 ml or less
   3. 200 ml or less
   4. 250 ml or less

4. The patient has reflex incontinence. What serious reaction may occur in this patient if the bladder becomes overdistended?
   1. stress incontinence.
   2. orthostatic hypotension.
   3. autonomic dysreflexia.
   4. tachycardia.

5. When a person voids inappropriately because of an inability to get to the toilet, this is called:
   1. urge incontinence.
   2. functional incontinence.
   3. reflex incontinence.
   4. stress incontinence.

6. Stimuli that may encourage voiding include:
   1. decreasing the fluid intake to less than 2000 ml/day.
   2. drinking caffeine and cola drinks.
   3. pressing down on the abdomen.
   4. pouring warm water over the perineum, and drinking water while on the toilet.

7. The patient who is incontinent of urine is at risk for:
   1. urinary tract infection and urinary calculi (stones).
   2. upper respiratory infection and pelvic infection.
   3. bradycardia and thrombophlebitis.
   4. diarrhea and skin breakdown.

8. The treatment for fecal neurogenic incontinence is to:
   1. cleanse the colon, usually with enemas and suppositories.
   2. treat the underlying medical condition.
   3. schedule toileting based on the patient's usual time of defecation.
   4. teach pelvic muscle exercises and biofeedback.

9. A patient has blood and mucus in his stool. This type of fecal incontinence is:
   1. neurogenic.
   2. symptomatic.
   3. anorectal.
   4. overflow.

10. Causes of overflow fecal incontinence include:
    1. nerve damage that causes weak pelvic muscles.
    2. colon or rectal disease.
    3. loss of anal reflexes in patients with dementia.
    4. constipation in which the rectum is constantly distended.

11. A patient with fecal incontinence may need laxatives to:
    1. relieve constipation.
    2. establish bowel control.
    3. improve the loss of anal sphincter tone.
    4. reverse the loss of the anal reflex.

12. What is a common reason for urethral obstruction in males?
    1. Vasoconstriction
    2. Hypertension
    3. Kidney obstruction
    4. Prostate enlargement

13. Which of the following diagnostic procedures is used to determine whether the patient is emptying the bladder completely?
    1. Postvoid residual
    2. Imaging procedures
    3. Cystometry
    4. Urodynamic testing

14. A patient is scheduled for a cystoscopy and he asks the nurse what this test is. The nurse answers that cystoscopy:
    1. evaluates the neuromuscular function of the bladder.
    2. may be ordered to create images of the urinary structures.
    3. uses a scope inserted through the urethra to visualize the urethra and bladder.
    4. detects involuntary passage of urine when abdominal pressure increases.

15. The patient has just been prescribed an antidepressant for treatment of urge incontinence. She asks the nurse why an antidepressant is prescribed for this. The nurse answers that it:
    1. improves sphincter tone.
    2. reduces overactive bladder contractions.
    3. relaxes the internal sphincter.
    4. causes bladder contraction.

PART III: CHALLENGE YOURSELF!

M. Getting Ready for NCLEX.

Choose the most appropriate answer or select all that apply.

1. The first step in the medical management of fecal overflow incontinence is to:
   1. treat the underlying medical condition.
   2. teach pelvic muscle exercises and biofeedback.
   3. cleanse the colon, often with enemas and suppositories.
   4. schedule toileting based on the patient's usual time of defecation.

2. The patient has fecal incontinence. What does the nurse provide for the patient in order to prevent constipation? Select all that apply.
   1. Protein
   2. Fiber
   3. Carbohydrates
   4. Potassium
   5. Fluids

Nursing Care Plan.

Read the following situation and answer questions 3-5. For more information, refer to Nursing Care Plan, The Patient with Stress Incontinence, p. 364 in your textbook.

An 80-year-old resident in a long-term care facility complains of having trouble "holding my urine." She is unable to control urine if she strains, coughs, or laughs. She is the mother of five children, all born at home. She reports no other complaints except for arthritis in her hips and knees and hypertension. Fear of losing control of her urine has caused her to avoid leaving her room except for meals. She is wearing perineal pads to keep her dry. Physical Examination: Height 5' 3". Weight 179 lbs. Heart and breath sounds normal.

3. Which symptoms are indicative of stress incontinence in this patient?

4. What are factors that have contributed to her stress incontinence?

5. What are the most important nursing interventions to improve her urinary control? Select all that apply.
   1. Instruct her how to do Kegel perineal exercises.
   2. Inspect the perineal area and buttocks, reporting signs of irritation.
   3. Advise to empty her bladder every 2 hours while awake.
   4. Decrease fluid intake.
   5. Discourage coffee, tea, and alcohol.

Loss, Death, and End-of-Life Care

 Go to http://evolve.elsevier.com/Linton/medsurg/ for additional activities and exercises.

NCLEX CATEGORIES:

Safe and Effective Care Environment:
Coordinated Care

Health Promotion and Maintenance

Psychosocial Integrity

Physiological Integrity: Basic Care and Comfort, Physiological Adaptation

OBJECTIVES

1. Describe beliefs and practices related to death and dying.
2. Describe responses of patients and their families to terminal illness and death.
3. Identify nursing diagnoses that are appropriate for the terminally ill.
4. Identify nursing goals that are appropriate for the terminally ill.
5. Identify nursing interventions to meet the needs of terminally ill and dying patients.
6. Discuss the needs of the terminally ill patient's significant others.
7. Discuss the ways nurses can intervene to meet the needs of the terminally ill patient's significant others.
8. Explore the responses of the nurse who works with the terminally ill.
9. Explore the needs of the nurse who works with terminally ill patients.
10. Identify issues related to caring for the dying patient, including advance directives, do-not-resuscitate decisions, brain death, organ donations, and pronouncement of death.

PART I: MASTERING THE BASICS

A. Beliefs About Death.
Which of the following are common beliefs about death for a 68-year-old person? Select all that apply.
1. Seldom thinks about death.
2. Death is temporary and reversible.
3. Afraid of prolonged death.
4. Faces death of family members and peers.
5. Sees death as inevitable.
6. Examines death as it relates to various meanings, such as freedom from discomfort.
7. Own death can be avoided.
8. Afraid of prolonged health problems.

B. Key Terms.
Match the physical manifestations of approaching death in the numbered column with the most appropriate term in the lettered column.

1. _____   Breathing is rapid and deep with periods of apnea.

2. _____   Breathing becomes irregular, gradually slowing down to terminal gasps.

3. _____   Grunting and noisy tachypnea.

A. Death rattle
B. Cheyne-Stokes breathing
C. "Guppy breathing"

C. Grieving Process.

Match the definition or description in the numbered column with the most appropriate stage of grieving in the lettered column. Answers may be used more than once.

1. _____ Patient or family members may become outraged with situations.
2. _____ Peaceful acknowledgment of the loss.
3. _____ Patient realizes the loss is final and the situation cannot be altered.
4. _____ Patient refuses to acknowledge the loss.
5. _____ Patient wishes for more time or wishes to avoid the loss.
6. _____ Patient expresses feelings that the loss is occurring as a punishment for past actions and may try to negotiate with a higher power for more time.
7. _____ Protects the patient and family from the reality of the loss.

A. Depression
B. Anger
C. Denial
D. Acceptance
E. Bargaining

D. Beliefs About Death.

Match the belief about death in the numbered column with the most appropriate age group in the lettered column. Answers may be used more than once.

1. _____ Sees death as inevitable.
2. _____ Faces death of parents and family members.
3. _____ Examines death as it relates to various meanings, such as freedom from discomfort.
4. _____ Sees death as future event.
5. _____ Faces death of peers.
6. _____ May experience death anxiety.

A. Young adulthood
B. Middle adulthood
C. Older adulthood

E. Fears of Dying.

Which of the following are related to the fear of meaninglessness? Select all that apply.

1. Assure patient that medication will be given promptly, as needed.
2. Express worth of dying person's life.
3. Simple presence of person to provide support and comfort.
4. Holding hands, touching, and listening.
5. Provide consistent pain control.
6. Dying person reviews his or her life.
7. Prayers, thoughts, and feelings provide comfort.

F. Key Terms.

Match the definition in the numbered column with the most appropriate term in the lettered column.

1. _____ The body's cooling after death
2. _____ Discoloration in the skin after death
3. _____ Stiffening of the body after death

A. Rigor mortis
B. Livor mortis
C. Algor mortis

PART II: PUTTING IT ALL TOGETHER

G. Multiple Choice/Multiple Response.

Choose the most appropriate answer or select all that apply.

1. Which change occurs preceding death?
   1. Blood pressure rises.
   2. Breathing sounds are quiet.
   3. Pulse slows.
   4. Extremities turn red.

2. Which of the following are associated with the death rattle? Select all that apply.
   1. Suffocation
   2. Mouth breathing
   3. Tightness in the chest
   4. Noisy respirations
   5. Accumulation of mucus
   6. Wet-sounding respirations

3. In what parts of the body is livor mortis generally most obvious?
   1. Skin of extremities
   2. Fingers and toes
   3. Face and chest
   4. Back and buttocks

4. Which cultural group values stoicism at death?
   1. Greeks
   2. Mexicans
   3. Vietnamese
   4. Swedes

5. What is the last sense to remain intact during the death process?
   1. Vision
   2. Smell
   3. Hearing
   4. Touch

6. Where does the sense of touch decrease first in a dying person?
   1. Face
   2. Abdomen
   3. Arms
   4. Legs

7. Why does the patient who is dying appear to stare?
   1. The blink reflex is lost gradually.
   2. Vision is blurred.
   3. There is decreased lubrication of the eye.
   4. Decreased circulation to the eye occurs progressively.

8. Which body function ceases first in the dying person?
   1. Heartbeat
   2. Respiration
   3. Brain function
   4. Kidney function

9. Which of the following are criteria to determine death? Select all that apply.
   1. Unresponsiveness to external stimuli that would usually be painful
   2. Complete absence of spontaneous breathing
   3. Total lack of reflexes
   4. A flat EEG for 8 hours

10. Which criterion must be present for brain death to be pronounced and life support disconnected by the physician?
    1. All brain function must cease.
    2. Coma or unresponsiveness must be present.
    3. Absence of all brain stem reflexes must be noted.
    4. Apnea must be present.

11. What causes livor mortis after death?
    1. Skin loses elasticity and breaks down easily.
    2. There is a breakdown of red blood cells.
    3. Chemical changes prevent muscle relaxation.
    4. Circulation decreases and the body cools.

12. Which religious group believes that the body should not be shrouded until sacraments have been performed?
    1. Muslims
    2. Orthodox Jews
    3. Protestants
    4. Roman Catholics

13. The durable power of attorney for health care can be used only if the physician certifies in writing that the person is:
    1. incapable of making decisions.
    2. brain dead.
    3. unresponsive or in a coma.
    4. lacking reflexes.

14. The Patient Self-Determination Act requires that institutions must inform patients about:
    1. rules and regulations about CPR.
    2. the right to have an autopsy.
    3. the right to initiate advance directives.
    4. rules and regulations about the delivery of hospice care.

PART III: CHALLENGE YOURSELF!

H. Getting Ready for NCLEX.

Choose the most appropriate answer or select all that apply.

1. Place sequential order (from 1-5) the Kübler-Ross stages of grieving.
    A. _____   Acceptance
    B. _____   Depression
    C. _____   Bargaining
    D. _____   Denial
    E. _____   Anger

2. Place in sequential order (from 1-3) the Rando stages of grieving.
    A. _____   Confrontation
    B. _____   Avoidance
    C. _____   Accommodation

3. Which are physical manifestations of approaching death? Select all that apply.
    1. Decreased pain and touch perception
    2. Involuntary blinking of the eyes
    3. Eyelids remain open
    4. Cold, clammy skin
    5. Jaw is clenched
    6. Swallowing is difficult
    7. Gag reflex is stimulated
    8. Drop in blood pressure

The Patient with Cancer

 Go to http://evolve.elsevier.com/Linton/medsurg/ for additional activities and exercises.

NCLEX CATEGORIES:

Safe and Effective Care Environment:
Coordinated Care, Safety and Infection Control

Health Promotion and Maintenance

Psychosocial Integrity

Physiological Integrity: Basic Care and Comfort, Pharmacological Therapies, Reduction of Risk Potential, Physiological Adaptation

OBJECTIVES

1. Explain the differences between benign and malignant tumors.
2. List the most common sites of cancer in men and women.
3. Describe measures to reduce the risk of cancer.
4. Define terms used to name and classify cancer.
5. List nursing responsibilities in the care of patients having diagnostic tests to detect possible cancer.
6. Explain the nursing care of patients undergoing each type of cancer therapy: surgery, radiation, chemotherapy, and biotherapy.
7. Assist in developing a nursing care plan for the terminally ill patient with cancer and the patient's family.

PART I: MASTERING THE BASICS

A. Key Terms.
Match the definition in the numbered column with the most appropriate term in the lettered column.

1. _____ Tending to progress in virulence; has the characteristics of becoming increasingly undifferentiated, invading surrounding tissues, and colonizing distant sites

2. _____ Cancer-causing agent

3. _____ The use of radiation in the treatment of cancer and other diseases

4. _____ Process by which cancer spreads to distant sites

5. _____ Drugs used to treat cancer, including hematopoietic growth factors, biologic response modifiers, and monoclonal antibodies

6. _____ An agent that inhibits the maturation or reproduction of malignant cells

7. _____ Tumor; may be benign or malignant

8. _____ Use of chemicals to treat illness

9. _____ Not malignant

A. Radiotherapy
B. Benign
C. Chemotherapy
D. Metastasis
E. Neoplasm
F. Malignant
G. Antineoplastic
H. Carcinogen
I. Biotherapy

B. Radiation Therapy.

Which of the following normal cells are most sensitive to radiation? Select all that apply.

1. Nail beds
2. Digestive and urinary tract linings
3. Respiratory tract lining
4. Skin
5. Lymph tissue
6. Ovaries
7. Kidneys
8. Lungs
9. Testes
10. Hair follicle
11. Bone marrow

C. Drug Therapy.

Of the following drugs, which types of antineoplastic drugs are frequently used in chemotherapy? Select all that apply.

1. Diuretics
2. Bronchodilators
3. Hormones
4. Mitotic inhibitors
5. Narcotics
6. Alkylating agents
7. Antithyroid drugs
8. Antiemetics
9. Sedatives
10. Antihypertensives
11. Antitumor antibiotics
12. Hypnotics
13. Biologic response modifiers

D. Drug Therapy.

Which of the following are major systemic side effects of antineoplastic drugs? Select all that apply.

1. Dry mouth
2. Bone marrow suppression
3. Urinary retention
4. Sedation
5. Nausea and vomiting
6. Constipation
7. Dizziness
8. Alopecia
9. Electrolyte imbalance
10. Tachycardia

E. Warning Signs of Cancer.

Which of the following are warning signs of cancer? Select all that apply.

1. Nausea and vomiting
2. Nagging cough and hoarseness
3. Change in bowel or bladder habits
4. Heart palpitations and tachycardia
5. Sores that do not heal
6. Dyspnea and trouble breathing
7. Change in warts or moles

F. Stages of Tumors.

Match the definition in the numbered column with the most appropriate stage in the lettered column.

1. _____ There is limited spread of the cancer in the local area, usually to nearby lymph nodes.

2. _____ The malignant cells are confined to the tissue of origin; there is no invasion of other tissues.

3. _____ The cancer has metastasized to distant parts of the body.

4. _____ The tumor is larger or has spread from the site of origin into nearby tissues, or both; regional lymph nodes are likely to be involved.

A. Stage I
B. Stage II
C. Stage III
D. Stage IV

G. Drug Therapy.

Match the side effect in the numbered column with the most appropriate drug in the lettered column.

1. _____ Pulmonary inflammation and fibrosis

2. _____ Neurotoxicity resulting in numbness and tingling of extremities

3. _____ Toxic effects on the heart that may lead to heart failure

4. _____ Hypersensitivity

A. Vincristine (Oncovin)
B. Doxorubicin (Adriamycin)
C. Bleomycin (Blenoxane)
D. Paclitaxel (Taxol)

PART II: PUTTING IT ALL TOGETHER

H. Multiple-Choice Questions.
Choose the most appropriate answer.

1. What is the second most common cause of death in the United States?
   1. Heart disease
   2. Cancer
   3. Accident
   4. Stroke

2. What is the effect on cells and tissue when DNA of a normal cell is exposed to a carcinogen and irreversible changes occur in the DNA?
   1. The cell appears abnormal but continues to function normally.
   2. The cell is in a latent period before increased growth forms tumors.
   3. A tumor develops.
   4. Transformed cells relocate to remote sites.

3. A patient whose primary tumor has grown and spread to regional lymph nodes but not to distant sites is staged:
   1. T1, N2, M1.
   2. T2, N1, M0.
   3. T0, N3, M1.
   4. T4, N0, M0.

4. A patient has cancer that has been staged T1, N0, M0. The nurse would interpret this information as:
   1. minimal size and extension of tumor.
   2. no sign of tumor.
   3. malignancy in epithelial tissue but not in basement membrane.
   4. progressively increasing size and extension.

5. A treatment likely to be curative when tumors are confined in one area is:
   1. radiotherapy.
   2. chemotherapy.
   3. immunotherapy.
   4. surgery.

6. Radiation has immediate and delayed effects on cells; the immediate effect is:
   1. cell death.
   2. alteration of DNA, which impairs cell's ability to reproduce.
   3. interruption of the clotting cascade.
   4. cell starvation.

7. Which side effect occurs in patients undergoing radiotherapy and also in patients taking antineoplastic drugs?
   1. Phlebitis at infusion site
   2. Erythema and peeling of skin
   3. Alopecia
   4. Cardiomyopathy

8. The highest rate of death from prostate, colon, and breast cancer occurs among:
   1. Caucasians.
   2. Latinos.
   3. Native Americans.
   4. African-Americans.

9. What is the most dangerous side effect of antineoplastic drugs?
   1. Alopecia
   2. Nausea and vomiting
   3. Electrolyte imbalance
   4. Bone marrow suppression

10. A drug that boosts the body's natural defenses to combat malignant cells is:
    1. vincristine.
    2. interferon.
    3. doxorubicin (Adriamycin).
    4. paclitaxel (Taxol).

11. Invasive procedures are minimized in patients with:
    1. leukopenia.
    2. thrombocytopenia.
    3. anemia.
    4. agranulocytosis.

12. Compromised host precautions may be needed for patients with:
    1. leukopenia.
    2. thrombocytopenia.
    3. anemia.
    4. weight loss.

13. Which of the following tumors is malignant?
    1. Fibroma
    2. Lipoma
    3. Melanoma
    4. Myoma

14. Which diagnostic procedure is used to detect cancers of the central nervous system, spinal column, neck bones, and joints?
    1. Magnetic resonance imaging (MRI)
    2. Computed tomography (CT)
    3. Positron emission tomography (PET)
    4. Contrast radiographs

PART III: CHALLENGE YOURSELF!

I.   Getting Ready for NCLEX.

Choose the most appropriate answer or select all that apply.

1. A patient experiences erythema and peeling of skin while receiving radiation therapy. Which of the following are appropriate nursing interventions for this patient? Select all that apply.
   1. Increase fluid intake.
   2. Use lotions.
   3. Watch for excessive bruising and bleeding.
   4. Report fever.
   5. Keep skin moist.
   6. Wear cotton clothing.

2. The outcome criterion, a patient's completion of essential activities without dyspnea or tachycardia, is related to patients with:
   1. alopecia.
   2. loss of a body part.
   3. anemia.
   4. denial.

3. The priority care for patients experiencing neurotoxicity from antineoplastic drugs is to:
   1. monitor for edema.
   2. protect the patient from infection.
   3. protect extremities from injury.
   4. assess skin turgor.

4. What is appropriate teaching for the patient who is having external radiation therapy?
   1. "The treatment may be painful for the first 5 minutes, but the pain will subside."
   2. "You will be radioactive as long as the machine is turned on."
   3. "Skin markings made by the radiologist are used to mark areas that will not be irradiated."
   4. "Skin over the area being treated may become discolored and irritated."

5. Which of the following are characteristics of malignant tumors? Select all that apply.
   1. Usually slow growth rate
   2. Invade surrounding tissue
   3. Cells closely resemble those of tissue of origin
   4. Recurrence is common after removal
   5. Metastasis frequently occurs
   6. Little tissue destruction

6. Which of the following are common oncologic emergencies? Select all that apply.
   1. Superior vena cava syndrome
   2. Pulmonary edema
   3. Hypertension
   4. Hypercalcemia
   5. Syndrome of inappropriate antidiuretic hormone (SIADH)
   6. Spinal cord compression
   7. Disseminated intravascular coagulation

Nursing Care Plan.

Read the following situation and answer questions 7-10. For more information, refer to Nursing Care Plan, The Patient with Cancer, p. 411 in your textbook.

A 63-year-old man recently diagnosed with lung cancer is being treated with radiotherapy and chemotherapy. He states he is fatigued and weak since starting his therapy. He has had mild nausea, anorexia, and occasional diarrhea. He complains of a dry mouth and is having some dysphagia. The skin over the area being radiated is tender. He is married, is the father of three grown children, and is an insurance salesman. He smoked one pack of cigarettes a day for 30 years, having quit smoking 10 years ago. He continues to work part time.

7. Which patient teaching points will the nurse emphasize with this patient, regarding his radiotherapy? Select all that apply.
   1. Do not wash off skin markings.
   2. Do not apply lotion to irritated skin.
   3. Advise him to avoid crowds and people with infection.
   4. Eat small, frequent meals.
   5. Do frequent, gentle mouth care.

8. Anzemet is ordered for the nausea and vomiting he experiences while undergoing chemotherapy. What are the main side effects of this drug? Select all that apply.
   1. Abdominal pain
   2. Dizziness
   3. Headache
   4. Bradycardia

9. This patient has a stage II tumor. What is the meaning of the stage II classification?
    1. Malignant cells are confined to the tissue of origin.
    2. The cancer has metastasized to distant parts of the body.
    3. The tumor is larger and has spread from the site of origin into nearby tissues.
    4. There is limited spread of the cancer in the local area, usually to nearby lymph nodes.

10. This patient develops signs of bone marrow suppression as a result of his chemotherapy. What is the priority nursing intervention?
    1. Avoid exposure to sun and harsh chemicals.
    2. Use a soft toothbrush.
    3. Schedule activities to prevent overtiring.
    4. Protect from injury.

The Patient with an Ostomy

 Go to http://evolve.elsevier.com/Linton/medsurg/ for additional activities and exercises.

NCLEX CATEGORIES:

Safe and Effective Care Environment: Safety and Infection Control

Health Promotion and Maintenance

Psychosocial Integrity

Physiological Integrity: Basic Care and Comfort, Reduction of Risk Potential, Physiological Adaptation

OBJECTIVES

1. List the indications for ostomy surgery to divert urine or feces.
2. Describe nursing interventions to prepare the patient for ostomy surgery.
3. Explain the types of procedures used for fecal diversion.
4. Assist in developing a nursing process to plan care for the patient with each of the following types of fecal diversion: ileostomy, continent ileostomy, ileoanal reservoir, and colostomy.
5. Explain the types of procedures done for urinary diversion.
6. Assist in developing a nursing care plan for the patient with each of the following types of urinary diversion: ureterostomy, ileal conduit, and continent internal reservoir.
7. Discuss content to be included in teaching patients to learn to live with ostomies.

PART I: MASTERING THE BASICS

A. Key Terms.

Match the definition in the numbered column with the most appropriate term in the lettered column.

1. _____ Opening created to drain contents of an organ
2. _____ Surgically created opening in the kidney to drain urine
3. _____ Surgically created opening into the urinary bladder
4. _____ Surgical procedure that creates an opening into a body structure
5. _____ Capable of controlling natural impulses; in relation to an ostomy, able to retain feces or urine
6. _____ Surgically created opening in the ureter
7. _____ Downward displacement
8. _____ Communication or connection between two organs or parts of organs
9. _____ Surgically created opening in the ileum
10. _____ Surgically created opening in the colon

A. Anastomosis
B. Colostomy
C. Continent
D. Ileostomy
E. Nephrostomy
F. Ostomy
G. Prolapse
H. Stoma
I. Ureterostomy
J. Vesicostomy

B. Application of Ostomy Pouch.

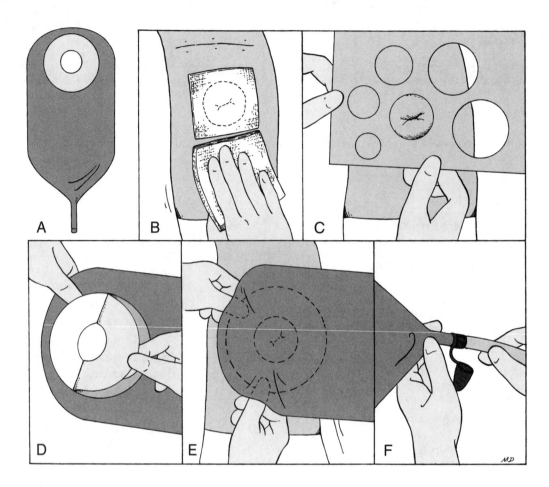

1. Match the steps in the numbered column below with the corresponding correct letters (A-F, showing stages of application) in the figure above (Figure 26-7, textbook p. 439).

    1. _____   Gently press into place with the pouch drain pointed toward the floor.
    2. _____   Remove the backing from the adhesive of the new pouch.
    3. _____   Connect the drain to the tubing or close the drain, if appropriate.
    4. _____   Gather supplies.
    5. _____   Use a stoma template to measure the size of the stoma.
    6. _____   Wash hands and put on gloves.
    7. _____   Remove the old pouch and clean the area around the stoma.
    8. _____   Cut an opening the same size as the stoma into the skin barrier and adhesive.
    9. _____   Place a gauze square over the stoma to absorb the drainage.
    10. _____   Place the opening in the new pouch over the stoma.
    11. _____   Secure the tubing to the sheets or according to agency policy.

2. Why is sizing the ostomy pouch so important during the first 6–8 weeks postoperatively?

3. If edema occurs after the first week postoperatively, this most likely indicates:
    1. improperly fitting collection device.
    2. infection.
    3. capillary hemorrhage.
    4. poor circulation.

C. Colostomy Types.

1. Use the figure below (Figure 26-5, textbook p. 433). Label each type of colostomy (A–D) and indicate the type of drainage passed by each (E–G).

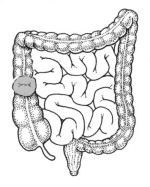

1. _____

_____

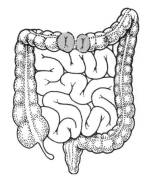

2. _____

_____

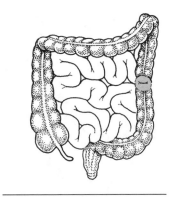

3. _____

_____

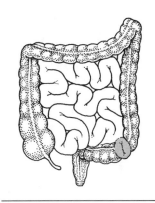

4. _____

_____

<table>
<tr><td>A. Descending colostomy</td><td>E. Passes liquid to semisolid stool</td></tr>
<tr><td>B. Ascending colostomy</td><td>F. Passes softly formed stool</td></tr>
<tr><td>C. Transverse colostomy</td><td>G. Passes liquid material</td></tr>
<tr><td>D. Sigmoid colostomy</td><td></td></tr>
</table>

2. What are the two main long-term complications of colostomies?

1. _____

2. _____

3. What type of medication can be inserted into a colostomy stoma to stimulate evacuation?
   1. Laxative liquid
   2. Hyperosmolar laxative
   3. Rectal suppository
   4. Nystatin

D. Types of Urinary Diversions.

1. Using the figure below, label the types of urinary diversion procedures (A–E) using the following terms.

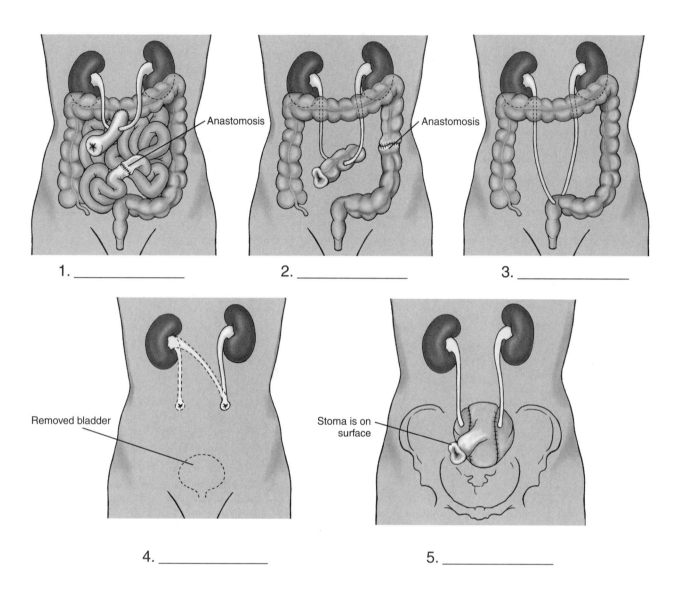

1. _____

2. _____

3. _____

4. _____

5. _____

    A. Continent internal ileal reservoir
    B. Colon (sigmoid) conduit
    C. Ureterosigmoidostomy
    D. Ileal conduit
    E. Cutaneous ureterostomy

2. What are two serious consequences of urinary tract infections following ureterostomy? Select two that apply.
    1. Stenosis
    2. Hemorrhage
    3. Kidney damage
    4. Septicemia

3. What is the treatment for yeast infections around the ureterostomy stoma?
   1. Nystatin powder
   2. Antibiotic ointment
   3. Steroid ointment
   4. Soap and water

4. If odor is a problem with ureterostomy, the pouch can be soaked for 20–30 minutes in:
   1. 50% alcohol.
   2. normal saline.
   3. vinegar water.
   4. baking soda and water.

PART II: PUTTING IT ALL TOGETHER

E. Multiple Choice/Multiple Response.

Choose the most appropriate answer or select all that apply.

1. A colostomy is performed by bringing a loop of the intestine through the wall of the:
   1. bladder.
   2. rectum.
   3. abdomen.
   4. stomach.

2. Which complication of colostomy involves the narrowing of the abdominal opening around the base of the stoma?
   1. Prolapse
   2. Stenosis
   3. Obstruction
   4. Evisceration

3. What is the result of the loss of bicarbonate in ileostomy drainage?
   1. Hypokalemia
   2. Hypercalcemia
   3. Metabolic acidosis
   4. Fluid volume excess

4. The nurse notices that the patient's ileal conduit stoma has turned black. The nurse notifies the physician immediately, because it may mean that:
   1. ureteral obstruction has occurred.
   2. circulation is impaired.
   3. wound infection is present.
   4. prolapse has occurred.

5. After bowel resection for the ileal conduit procedure, the nurse should expect:
   1. necrosis of the wound.
   2. temporary ileus.
   3. gray-black stoma.
   4. ureteral calculi.

6. The Kock pouch is made with a section of:
   1. sigmoid colon.
   2. jejunum.
   3. ileum.
   4. ascending colon.

7. Which foods tend to produce thicker stools?
   1. Milk and cottage cheese
   2. Fresh fruits
   3. Green, leafy vegetables
   4. Pasta and boiled rice

8. Why is a nasogastric tube placed in a patient with bowel obstruction?
   1. Dilate the digestive tract
   2. Decompress the bowel
   3. Provide method of feeding
   4. Improve peristalsis

9. What is a complication of colostomy irrigation?
   1. Obstruction
   2. Diarrhea
   3. Infection
   4. Perforated bowel

10. A patient with an ileoanal reservoir is prescribed metronidazole (Flagyl), and asks the nurse why this drug is prescribed. The nurse answers that Flagyl is given to treat:
    1. pain.
    2. bleeding.
    3. inflammation.
    4. fluid volume deficit.

11. A patient with a colostomy is experiencing weakness when the colostomy is irrigated. Which manifestation requires the nurse to contact the physician?
    1. Prolapse
    2. Perforated bowel
    3. Diarrhea
    4. Red stoma

12. Which of the following is a sign of bowel obstruction?
    1. Bloody stools
    2. Fever
    3. Abdominal distention
    4. Hypotension

13. Which of the following is a major long-term complication caused by coughing in a patient with a colostomy?
    1. Prolapse
    2. Stenosis
    3. Obstruction
    4. Inflammation

14. Which is a complication of ureterostomy?
    1. Obstruction
    2. Perforation
    3. Hydronephrosis
    4. Prolapse

15. Which drug is used to treat a rash around the stoma of a patient with an ureterostomy?
    1. Tetracycline
    2. Neosporin
    3. Benadryl
    4. Nystatin

16. Which group has the highest rate of colon and rectal cancers that are commonly treated with ostomies?
    1. Asians
    2. African-Americans
    3. Caucasians
    4. Native Americans

17. Which type of patient with a colostomy should be given a two-piece appliance that allows frequent pouch changes without skin trauma?
    1. Jewish
    2. Native American
    3. Asian
    4. Muslim

18. Following ileostomy surgery, the stoma is inspected for bleeding and:
    1. edema.
    2. rough edges.
    3. temperature.
    4. color.

19. Following ileostomy surgery, what should the nurse examine when checking the base of the stoma? Select all that apply.
    1. Purulent drainage
    2. Redness
    3. Amount of drainage present
    4. Skin breakdown

20. When does ileostomy drainage occur after surgery?
    1. First 6 hours
    2. 10–12 hours
    3. 24–48 hours
    4. After 72 hours

21. Postoperative ileostomy patients may experience electrolyte imbalances due to:
    1. passage of liquid stool.
    2. bleeding around the stoma.
    3. poor circulation.
    4. infection.

22. What are factors that contribute to a prolapsed stoma in a colostomy? Select all that apply.
    1. Increased abdominal pressure
    2. Coughing
    3. Poor blood supply
    4. Peristomal hernia
    5. Poorly attached stoma
    6. Abdominal opening that is too small

PART III: CHALLENGE YOURSELF!

F. Getting Ready for NCLEX.

Choose the most appropriate answer or select all that apply.

1. If the color of the stoma is pale or blue following ileostomy surgery, what should the nurse do? Select all that apply.
    1. Cleanse skin around stoma with soap and water.
    2. Apply a protective skin barrier before replacing the pouch.
    3. Notify the physician.
    4. Check the pouch hourly to detect leakage.

2. What does a small amount of bleeding around the base of a new stoma indicate?
    1. Infection
    2. Tissue injury
    3. Adequate blood supply
    4. Poor circulation

3. A postoperative ileostomy patient becomes confused. What is the nursing intervention for this mental status change?
    1. Check the pouch hourly.
    2. Watch for neuromuscular status weakness.
    3. Measure tissue turgor.
    4. Monitor serum electrolytes.

4. Which foods should patients with continent ileostomies avoid initially? Select all that apply.
   1. Pasta
   2. Coffee
   3. Berries
   4. Nuts
   5. Boiled rice
   6. Fresh fruit

5. A nurse notices that the patient's colostomy is not draining properly. What is the appropriate nursing action to take?
   1. Place a gloved finger in the stoma to dilate it.
   2. Use a larger catheter to irrigate.
   3. Inform the physician.
   4. Push the catheter in 3 inches.

6. The nurse is taking care of a patient with an ileostomy. The nurse is watching for signs of small bowel obstruction. To reduce the risk of obstruction, what is the appropriate diet for this patient?
   1. Low fiber
   2. Low cholesterol
   3. Soft, bland foods
   4. High residue

7. A patient with an ileostomy one week postoperatively has a pulse of 120 bpm, respirations 28/min, temperature of 101° F, and a rigid abdomen. The nurse suspects that this patient has which complication?
   1. Obstruction
   2. Peritonitis
   3. Inflammation
   4. Evisceration of the site

Nursing Care Plan.
Read the following situation and answer questions 8-9. For more information, refer to Nursing Care Plan, Providing Nursing Care for the Patient with a Colostomy, p. 434 in your textbook.

A 47-year-old Asian-American patient had a bowel resection and permanent colostomy in the descending colon to remove a malignant tumor. He is 3 days post-surgery. He reports adequate pain control with IV morphine. He has had no nausea and vomiting but has a nasogastric tube attached to low suction. He is NPO and is receiving IV fluids at 150 ml per hour.

8. How often does the nurse check his pouch to detect leakage?

9. A physician orders 1000 ml of D_5W to infuse over 8 hours. The drop factor is 15 drops per 1 ml. The nurse sets the flow rate at how many drops per minute? (Round to the nearest tenth).

Neurologic Disorders

Go to http://evolve.elsevier.com/Linton/medsurg/ for additional activities and exercises.

NCLEX CATEGORIES:

Safe and Effective Care Environment: Safety and Infection Control

Health Promotion and Maintenance

Psychosocial Integrity

Physiological Integrity: Pharmacological Therapies, Reduction of Risk Potential, Physiological Adaptation

OBJECTIVES

1. Identify common neurologic changes in the older person and the implications of these for nursing care.
2. Describe the diagnostic tests and procedures used to evaluate neurologic dysfunction and the nursing responsibilities associated with each.
3. Identify the uses, side effects, and nursing interventions associated with common drug therapies used in patients with neurologic disorders.
4. Describe the signs and symptoms associated with increased intracranial pressure (ICP) and the medical therapies used in treatment.
5. List the components of the nursing assessment of the patient with a neurologic disorder.
6. Describe the pathophysiologic condition, signs and symptoms, complications, and medical or surgical treatment for patients with selected neurologic disorders.
7. Assist in developing a nursing care plan for the patient with a neurologic disorder.

PART I: MASTERING THE BASICS

A. Key Terms.
Match the definition in the numbered column with the most appropriate term in the lettered column.

1. _____ Abnormal extension of the upper extremities with extension of the lower extremities
2. _____ Weakness on one side of the body
3. _____ Abnormal flexion of the upper extremities with extension of the lower extremities
4. _____ Pain in a nerve or along the course of a nerve
5. _____ Inflammation of brain tissue
6. _____ Effects on the autonomic nervous system
7. _____ Affecting the same side
8. _____ Paralysis on one side of the body
9. _____ Affecting the opposite side
10. _____ Within the skull

A. Dysautonomia
B. Contralateral
C. Decerebrate posturing
D. Decorticate posturing
E. Encephalitis
F. Hemiparesis
G. Hemiplegia
H. Intracranial
I. Ipsilateral
J. Neuralgia

B. Key Terms. Neurotransmitters.

Which of the following are neurotransmitters? Select all that apply.

1. Acetylcholine
2. Thyroxine
3. Epinephrine
4. Norepinephrine
5. Insulin
6. Myosin

C. Age-Related Changes.

Which of the following are possible neurologic changes associated with normal aging? Select all that apply.

1. Nerve cells increase in number.
2. Brain weight is reduced.
3. The size of ventricles is reduced.
4. Increased plaques and tangled fibers are found in nerve tissue.
5. Pupillary response to light is slower.
6. Pupil of the eye is larger.
7. Reaction time increases.

D. Pupillary Evaluation.

Which of the following are normal characteristics of pupils that are noted in pupillary evaluation? Select all that apply.

1. Size: 6 mm
2. Shape: Round
3. Reactivity: React quickly to light

E. Key Terms. Levels of Consciousness.

Complete the statements in the numbered column with the most appropriate term in the lettered column. Some terms may be used more than once, and some terms may not be used.

1. Decreased responsiveness accompanied by lack of spontaneous motor activity is _____.

2. A patient who cannot be aroused even by powerful stimuli is _____.

3. The most accurate and reliable indicator of neurologic status is the _____.

4. Excessive drowsiness is _____.

5. If a patient is stuporous but can be aroused, the patient is _____.

6. Unnatural drowsiness or sleepiness is _____.

A. Agitation
B. Level of consciousness
C. Combativeness
D. Somnolence
E. Neuromuscular response
F. Lethargy
G. Comatose
H. Pupillary evaluation
I. Semicomatose
J. Stupor

F. Common Neurologic Disorders.

1. Complete the statements in the numbered column with the most appropriate term in the lettered column.

   1. _____ Inflammation of the coverings of the brain and spinal cord caused by either viral or bacterial organisms
   2. _____ Inflammation of brain tissue usually caused by a virus
   3. _____ A rapidly progressing disease that affects the motor component of the peripheral nervous system
   4. _____ A progressive degenerative disorder that results in an eventual loss of coordination and control over involuntary motor movement
   5. _____ A chronic, progressive disease in which the amount of acetylcholine available at the neuromuscular junction is reduced
   6. _____ A degenerative neurologic disease that is also known as *Lou Gehrig's disease*
   7. _____ A chronic, progressive, degenerative disease attacking the myelin sheath, disrupting motor pathways of the CNS

   A. Meningitis
   B. Parkinson disease
   C. Guillain-Barré syndrome
   D. Encephalitis
   E. Multiple sclerosis (MS)
   F. Amyolateral sclerosis (ALS)
   G. Myasthenia gravis

2. Match the definition in the numbered column with the most appropriate neurologic disease in the lettered column. Some diseases may be used more than once, and some diseases may not be used.

1. _____ A disease characterized by intense pain along nerve lines in the face
2. _____ Acute paralysis of the seventh cranial nerve
3. _____ Paralysis associated with a loss in motor coordination caused by cerebral damage
4. _____ Progressive muscle weakness, fatigue, pain, and respiratory problems years after the initial infection, illness, and recovery

A. Cerebral palsy
B. Bell's palsy
C. Postpolio syndrome
D. Trigeminal neuralgia

G. Autonomic Nervous System.
Which responses are controlled by the parasympathetic nervous system? Select all that apply.
1. Bronchial dilation
2. Pupil constriction
3. Increased gut peristalsis and tone in lumen
4. Pupil dilation
5. Bronchial constriction
6. Decreased gut peristalsis and tone in lumen
7. Increased rate and force of cardiac contractions
8. Flight-or-fight response
9. Mediates rest response

H. Brain Dysfunctions.
Which of the following dysfunctions are related to the cerebellum? Select all that apply.
1. Loss of steady gait
2. Dysfunction occurring on the same side as the offending lesion
3. Motor dysfunction on the opposite side from the lesion
4. Loss of steady, balanced posture

I. Diagnostic Procedures.
Match the intervention or description in the numbered column with the appropriate diagnostic test in the lettered column. Some diagnostic tests may be used more than once.

1. _____ A shampoo is done before the test, and medications, such as anticonvulsants and stimulants, are withheld 24–48 hours before the test.
2. _____ Tell the patient to expect to lie still on a stretcher while the dye is injected and radiographs of the head are taken.
3. _____ A cannula is usually inserted into the femoral artery, and a catheter is advanced to the carotid or vertebral arteries.
4. _____ Needle electrodes are placed on several points over a nerve and muscles supplied by the nerve.
5. _____ Have the patient void before the procedure to reduce discomfort from the position.
6. _____ Inform the radiologist about any allergies to iodine, shellfish, or contrast media.
7. _____ Patient must remain on one side in a knee-to-chest position.
8. _____ Because air, blood, bone, tissue, and CSF have varying densities, they appear in various shades of gray in this test.
9. _____ A contrast dye is injected, followed by a series of radiographs.

A. Lumbar puncture
B. CT scan
C. Cerebral angiography
D. Electromyography (EMG)
E. Electroencephalogram (EEG)

J. Key Terms. Brain Surgery.
Match the definition or description in the numbered column with the most appropriate term in the lettered column.

1. _____ Surgery that requires opening the skull
2. _____ Excision of a segment of the skull
3. _____ Procedure done to repair a skull defect

A. Cranioplasty
B. Craniotomy
C. Craniectomy

K. Key Terms. Head Trauma.

Match the definition in the numbered column with the most appropriate term in the lettered column.

1. _____ Head trauma in which there is no visible injury to the skull or brain

2. _____ Head trauma in which there is actual bruising and bleeding in the brain tissue

3. _____ A collection of blood, usually clotted, which may be classified as subdural or epidural

A. Contusion(s)
B. Hematoma
C. Concussion

L. Key Terms. Scalp Injuries.

Which of the following are common scalp injuries? Select all that apply.

1. Lacerations
2. Fissures
3. Contusions
4. Abrasions
5. Hematomas
6. Tumors

M. Clinical Manifestations of Parkinson Syndrome.

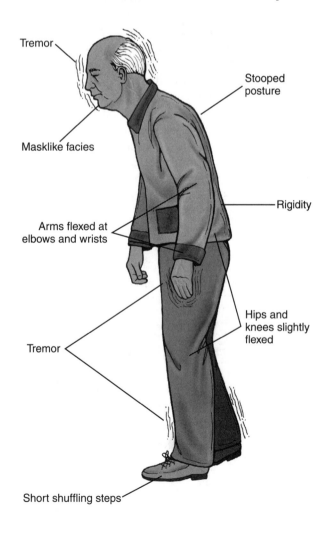

Tremor
Stooped posture
Masklike facies
Rigidity
Arms flexed at elbows and wrists
Hips and knees slightly flexed
Tremor
Short shuffling steps

1. Refer to the figure. Match the description of symptoms of Parkinson disease in the numbered column with the most appropriate term in the lettered column. Some terms may be used more than once, and some may not be used.

1. _____ Trembling, shaking type of movement usually seen in upper extremities
2. _____ Stiffness
3. _____ Extremely slow movements
4. _____ Movement of thumb against fingertips

A. Bradykinesia
B. Tremor
C. Bradycardia
D. Rigidity
E. Pill-rolling
F. Dementia

2. What are the three major symptoms (major triad) of Parkinson syndrome? Select all that apply.
1. Aching
2. Monotone voice
3. Tremors at rest
4. Rigidity
5. Slumped posture
6. Bradykinesia

3. What is characteristic of the tremors of a patient with Parkinson syndrome?

4. What are the two main goals for the patient with Parkinson disease?

N. Drug Therapy.
Match the uses of drugs in the numbered column with names of drugs used for MS in the lettered column.

1. _____ Antiinflammatory drug used during period of exacerbation

2. _____ Antiinflammatory drug used to encourage remission

3. _____ Drug used to decrease the frequency of recurrent neurologic episodes in relapsing-remitting MS

4. _____ Drug used to treat the spasticity experienced by MS patients

A. Betaseron (interferon beta-1b)
B. Prednisone
C. Baclofen
D. ACTH

O. Divisions of Trigeminal Nerve (Figure 27-20, p. 485).

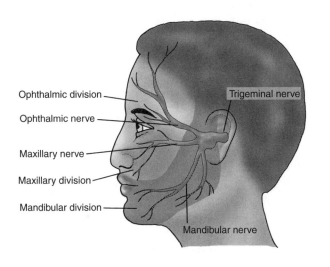

1. What disease is characterized by intense pain along one of the three branches of the trigeminal nerve?

2. What is the main focus of nursing care for the patient with trigeminal neuralgia?

3. What other problems does this patient have due to nerve involvement? Select all that apply.
   1. Imbalanced nutrition
   2. Social isolation
   3. Increased ICP
   4. Hypertension
   5. Ineffective tissue perfusion

PART II: PUTTING IT ALL TOGETHER

P. Multiple Choice/Multiple Response.

Choose the most appropriate answer or select all that apply.

1. To minimize headache following a lumbar puncture, what should be increased?
   1. Calcium
   2. Fluid intake
   3. Potassium
   4. Ambulation

2. The family should be advised that a craniotomy can take as long as:
   1. 2 hours.
   2. 6 hours.
   3. 12 hours.
   4. 24 hours.

3. As ICP increases and perfusion is reduced, oxygen delivery to cerebral tissue is:
   1. increased.
   2. bypassed.
   3. reduced.
   4. stopped.

4. A patient with increased ICP has a "blown pupil." Which of the following describes this condition?
   1. Dilated
   2. Pinpoint
   3. Reacts to light
   4. Unequal to the other pupil

5. The pupils may become dilated and fixed as ICP rises due to pressure on the:
   1. oculomotor nerve.
   2. cerebellum.
   3. hypothalamus.
   4. optic nerve.

6. Which neurons transmit information toward the central nervous system (CNS)?
   1. Sensory
   2. Motor
   3. Efferent
   4. Axon

7. A type of headache in which the pain is usually unilateral and has a warning is called:
   1. cluster.
   2. migraine.
   3. tension.
   4. sinus.

8. A patient is having frequent seizure activity. As a result, which of the following are used excessively by the large number of hyperactive neurons? Select all that apply.
   1. Calcium
   2. Potassium
   3. Oxygen
   4. Glucose
   5. Sodium
   6. Acetylcholine

9. What is used in the initial management of bacterial meningitis?
   1. Corticosteroids
   2. Antihistamines
   3. Anticholinergics
   4. Antimicrobials

10. What is the priority common source of anxiety for many patients with Guillain-Barré syndrome?
    1. Communication
    2. Self-esteem
    3. Circulation
    4. Elimination

11. In order to reduce the symptoms of Parkinson disease, what is L-dopa converted to as it crosses the blood-brain barrier?
    1. Epinephrine
    2. Dopamine
    3. Norepinephrine
    4. Acetylcholine

12. Which cranial nerve is tested by asking the patient to swallow on command?
    1. Vagus (CN X)
    2. Trigeminal (CN V)
    3. Facial (CN VII)
    4. Glossopharyngeal (CN IX)

13. In a patient with myasthenia gravis, what does rapid improvement of muscle strength after administration of edrophonium chloride (Tensilon) indicate?
    1. Hypertensive crisis
    2. Adrenergic crisis
    3. Myasthenic crisis
    4. Cholinergic crisis

14. Which priority measures are indicated for patients with increased ICP? Select all that apply.
    1. Raise the head of the bed 90 degrees.
    2. Increase fluids and monitor carefully.
    3. Monitor for changes in level of consciousness.
    4. Check pupillary reactivity.

15. Which drugs are commonly used in the treatment of patients with increased ICP? Select all that apply.
    1. Hyperosmolar agents (mannitol)
    2. Corticosteroids
    3. Diuretics (furosemide)
    4. Antihypertensives
    5. Barbiturates

16. Which are characteristics of reflexes in the older patient? Select all that apply.
    1. Jerky
    2. Tremors present
    3. Slower
    4. Remain intact

17. What physical therapy programs are most helpful for patients with Parkinson disease? Select all that apply.
    1. Crutch walking
    2. Massage
    3. Cold compresses
    4. Exercise
    5. Gait retraining

18. What are ways to improve mobility for a patient with Parkinson disease? Select all that apply.
    1. Scoot to the edge of a chair before trying to stand.
    2. March in place before starting to walk.
    3. Use cotton sheets to make it easier to move in and out of bed.
    4. Practice lifting the foot as if to step over an object on the floor to initiate walking.

PART III: CHALLENGE YOURSELF!

Q. Getting Ready for NCLEX.

Choose the most appropriate answer or select all that apply.

1. A nurse is caring for a patient with amyolateral sclerosis. What is the priority patient problem?
   1. Impaired physical mobility
   2. Ineffective airway clearance
   3. Impaired verbal communication
   4. Decreased cardiac output

2. What is the priority cause of nutritional problems in patients with amyolateral sclerosis?
   1. Oropharyngeal muscle weakness
   2. Paralysis of respiratory muscles
   3. Dysphagia
   4. Progressive illness of patient

3. Match the nursing diagnosis for patients with meningitis in the numbered column with the "related to" statement in the lettered column.

   1. _____ Ineffective cerebral tissue perfusion
   2. _____ Ineffective breathing pattern
   3. _____ Acute pain
   4. _____ Risk for injury
   5. _____ Deficient fluid volume
   6. _____ Risk for disuse syndrome

   A. Confusion, seizures, restlessness
   B. Irritation of the meninges
   C. Bedrest
   D. Increased ICP
   E. Vomiting and fever
   F. Depression of the respiratory center

Nursing Care Plan.

Read the following situation and answer questions 4-7. (For more information, refer to Nursing Care Plan, Nursing Care of a Patient with a Head Injury, p. 468 in your textbook.)

A 27-year-old man was injured in a motorcycle accident 3 days ago. He is now alert and oriented to person and place but not to time.

4. What is the most reliable indicator of mental status in this patient?
   1. Blood pressure
   2. Pulse
   3. Level of consciousness
   4. Pupil equality

5. What is a late sign of increased ICP due to pressure on the third cranial nerve?
   1. Jerky tracking of eyes
   2. Altered motor function
   3. Dilated pupils
   4. Hemiparesis

6. How high should this patient's bed be raised to prevent increased ICP?
   1. 15 degrees
   2. 30 degrees
   3. 45 degrees
   4. 90 degrees

7. What nursing measures are likely to be the most helpful in the management of seizures for this patient? Select all that apply.
   1. Keep the patient flat on his back.
   2. Remove any objects that could cause harm.
   3. Call a medical emergency if a generalized tonic-clonic seizure lasts more than 4 minutes.
   4. Hold the patient down so that he is not thrashing.
   5. Place a padded tongue blade between his teeth.

Cerebrovascular Accident

chapter

28

 Go to http://evolve.elsevier.com/Linton/medsurg/ for additional activities and exercises.

NCLEX CATEGORIES:

Safe and Effective Care Environment: Safety and Infection Control

Health Promotion and Maintenance

Psychosocial Integrity

Physiological Integrity: Pharmacological Therapies, Reduction of Risk Potential, Physiological Adaptation

OBJECTIVES

1. Discuss the risk factors for cerebrovascular accident (CVA).
2. Identify two major types of CVA.
3. Describe the pathophysiology, signs and symptoms, and medical treatment for each type of CVA.
4. Describe the neurologic deficits that may result from CVA.
5. Explain the tests and procedures used to diagnose a CVA, and nursing responsibilities for patients undergoing those tests and procedures.
6. List data to be included in the nursing assessment of the CVA patient.
7. Assist in developing a nursing process for a CVA patient during the acute and rehabilitation phases.
8. Specify criteria used to evaluate the outcomes of nursing care for the CVA patient.
9. Identify resources for the CVA patient and family.
10. Discuss criteria used to identify patients eligible for treatment with recombinant tissue plasminogen activator (rt-PA).

PART I: MASTERING THE BASICS

A. Key Terms.
Match the definition in the numbered column with the most appropriate term in the lettered column.

1. _____ Inability to speak clearly because of neurologic damage that impairs normal muscle control
2. _____ Drooping of the upper eyelid
3. _____ Difficulty speaking, reading, and writing
4. _____ Double vision
5. _____ The inability to understand words or the inability to respond with words, or both
6. _____ Loss of half the field of vision; loss is on the side opposite the brain lesion
7. _____ Partial inability to initiate coordinated voluntary motor acts
8. _____ Ability to speak clearly but without meaning
9. _____ Difficulty swallowing
10. _____ Paralysis of one side of the body

A. Hemiplegia
B. Nonfluent aphasia
C. Dyspraxia
D. Dysarthria
E. Ptosis
F. Homonymous hemianopsia
G. Expressive aphasia
H. Aphasia
I. Dysphagia
J. Diplopia

B. Key Terms.

Match the definition or description in the numbered column with the most appropriate term in the lettered column. Some terms may be used more than once, and some terms may not be used.

1. _____ An important warning condition for a possible later stroke

2. _____ A buildup of fatty deposits in the blood vessels

3. _____ The common name for cerebrovascular accident

4. _____ A temporary neurologic deficit caused by impairment of cerebral blood flow

5. _____ A "swooshing" noise in a clogged carotid artery that can be auscultated in diagnosing a TIA

6. _____ Opening an obstructed blood vessel and removing the plaque

A. Bruit
B. Transient ischemic attack (TIA)
C. Angioplasty
D. Stroke
E. Endarterectomy
F. Atherosclerosis

C. Central Nervous System.

Match the definition or description in the numbered column with the most appropriate term in the lettered column. Some terms may be used more than once.

1. _____ The part of the brain that controls the left side of the body

2. _____ The part of the brain that controls the right side of the body

3. _____ The part of the brain that controls vital basic functions, including respiration, heart rate, and consciousness

4. _____ The part of the brain that coordinates movement, balance, and posture

5. _____ The circulatory system in the cerebrum

6. _____ The part of the brain that includes the midbrain, pons, and medulla

A. Cerebellum
B. Brainstem
C. Cerebrovascular system
D. Right hemisphere
E. Left hemisphere

D. Control Zones of the Brain (Figure 28-1, p. 491).

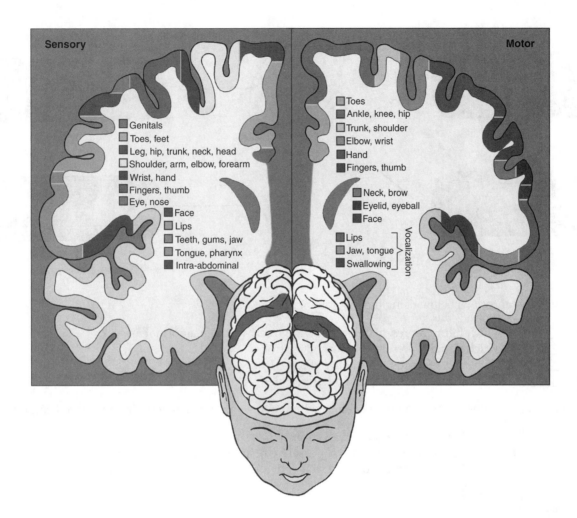

1. Which part of the brain receives and interprets sensory information?
   1. Frontal lobe
   2. Parietal lobe
   3. Occipital lobe
   4. Temporal lobe

2. Which part of the cerebrum initiates motor activity for various parts of the body?
   1. Frontal lobe
   2. Parietal lobe
   3. Occipital lobe
   4. Temporal lobe

3. Which part of the brain controls balance, coordination, and posture?
   1. Frontal lobe
   2. Cerebellum
   3. Thalamus
   4. Cerebrum

E. Types of Stroke (Figure 28-4, p. 498).

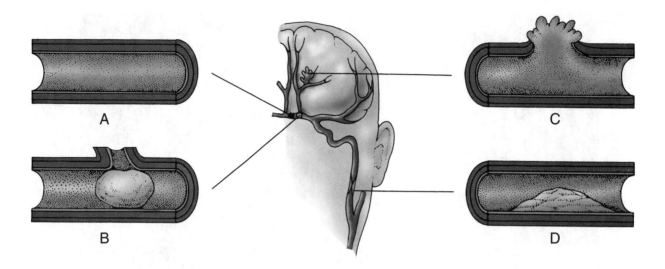

1. Answer the questions below using the diagram above.

    1. _____ Which figure represents blood flowing freely through a normal artery?
    2. _____ Which figure represents a thrombotic stroke?
    3. _____ Which figure represents a hemorrhagic stroke?
    4. _____ Which figure represents an embolic stroke?

2. Match the definition in the numbered column with the most appropriate term in the lettered column.

    1. _____ Caused by cerebral arterial wall rupture
    2. _____ Caused by obstruction of blood vessel by plaque, blood clot, or both
    3. _____ Caused by obstruction forming in blood vessel of the brain

    A. Thrombotic stroke
    B. Embolic stroke
    C. Hemorrhagic stroke

PART II: PUTTING IT ALL TOGETHER

F. Multiple Choice/Multiple Response.
Choose the most appropriate answer or select all that apply.

1. One of the most important needs of the acute stroke patient is to be turned and repositioned at least every:
    1. 2 hours.
    2. 4 hours.
    3. 8 hours.
    4. 12 hours.

2. Turning and repositioning the stroke patient will reduce the incidence of:
    1. hypertension.
    2. skin breakdown.
    3. headache.
    4. cerebral edema.

3. A warning condition for a possible later stroke is:
    1. TIA.
    2. paralysis.
    3. hemorrhage.
    4. cyanosis.

4. Which diagnostic test shows narrowing of cerebral blood vessels?
   1. CT scan
   2. MRI
   3. EEG
   4. Angiography

5. Which of the following are possible causes of constipation in the patient with a stroke? Select all that apply.
   1. Infection
   2. Cerebral edema
   3. Immobility
   4. Dehydration
   5. Drug therapy

6. The main focus of the rehabilitation phase following a stroke is to:
   1. cure the disease process.
   2. assist the patient into remission.
   3. prevent another stroke from occurring.
   4. return the patient to the highest functional level possible.

7. The most frequent cause of death following a stroke is:
   1. kidney failure.
   2. pneumonia.
   3. seizure.
   4. heart attack.

8. What (approximate) percentage of individuals who experience a TIA will have a stroke within 5 years?
   1. 10%
   2. 20%
   3. 30%
   4. 40%

9. What is a priority problem immediately following a stroke?
   1. Oxygenation
   2. Hydration
   3. Nutrition
   4. Thermoregulation

10. What is a common sensory-perceptual problem in a patient with a stroke?
    1. Weakness
    2. Paralysis
    3. Diplopia
    4. Dysphagia

11. A patient who does not feel pressure or pain due to lost sensation following a stroke is at risk for:
    1. aphasia.
    2. paralysis.
    3. injury.
    4. infection.

12. A patient experiencing an acute stroke should receive a thrombolytic drug within:
    1. 90 minutes.
    2. 2 hours.
    3. 3 hours.
    4. 6 hours.

13. Which term is used to describe speech impaired to the point that the person has almost no ability to communicate?
    1. Global aphasia
    2. Expressive aphasia
    3. Receptive aphasia
    4. Nonfluent aphasia

14. Which of the following are signs of a stroke? Select all that apply.
    1. Sudden, severe headache with no known cause
    2. Sudden trouble seeing
    3. Tremors of extremities at rest
    4. Rigidity of movement
    5. Sudden trouble speaking
    6. Numbness or weakness of the face, arm, or leg

15. According to the NIH Stroke Scale, which variables are assessed in a patient who has had a CVA? Select all that apply.
    1. Level of consciousness
    2. Visual field testing
    3. Motor function of arms
    4. Best language (describe a picture)
    5. Blood pressure
    6. Sensory comparison side to side
    7. Temperature
    8. Pupillary reaction

PART III: CHALLENGE YOURSELF!

G. Getting Ready for NCLEX.

Choose the most appropriate answer or select all that apply.

1. Which factors create problems related to physical mobility for a patient with a stroke? Select all that apply.
    1. Edema
    2. Dyspraxia
    3. Hypertension
    4. Visual field disturbances
    5. Hemiplegia

2. Match the uses of drugs in the numbered column with the drugs used for treatment of stroke in the lettered column.

    1. _____ Used to treat cerebral edema
    2. _____ Used to treat hemorrhagic stoke by dilating and preventing spasms in cerebral blood vessels
    3. _____ Used to reduce intracranial pressure by reducing cerebral inflammation
    4. _____ Used to prevent strokes caused by thrombi
    5. _____ Used to dissolve clots that cause acute ischemic stroke
    6. _____ Used to treat seizures, if seizures are present with stroke
    7. _____ Used to destroy thrombi

    A. Anticonvulsants, such as phenytoin and phenobarbital
    B. Platelet aggregation inhibitors, such as aspirin
    C. Hyperosmotic agents, such as mannitol
    D. Streptokinase
    E. Calcium channel blockers, such as nimodipine
    F. Tissue plasminogen activator (t-PA), and recombinant tissue plasminogen activator (rt-PA)
    G. Corticosteroids

3. According to *Healthy People 2010*, what is the role of the nurse in stroke prevention and treatment? Select all that apply.
    1. Spread the word about risk factors for and warning signs of stroke.
    2. Participate in stroke and blood pressure screenings.
    3. Engage in and promote physical activity.
    4. Assist patients to locate anti-smoking campaigns.
    5. Encourage yearly eye exams.
    6. Help patients obtain treatment for depression following a stroke.

4. Match the nursing diagnosis for the patient with a stroke in the numbered column with the most appropriate "related to" statement in the lettered column.

    1. _____ Risk for injury
    2. _____ Deficient fluid volume
    3. _____ Anxiety
    4. _____ Imbalanced nutrition: less than body requirements
    5. _____ Interrupted family processes
    6. _____ Impaired verbal communication
    7. _____ Impaired physical mobility

    A. Dysphagia, inability to feed self
    B. Loss of function, fear of disability
    C. Inadequate intake, dysphagia
    D. Weakness, paralysis, impaired balance
    E. Paralysis
    F. Anticipated need for assistance after discharge
    G. Aphasia

5. The initial assessment of a patient suspected of having an acute stroke is directed at determining the type and extent of stroke. According to the Cincinnati Pre-hospital Stroke Scale, what is an abnormal finding when the patient is asked to show teeth or smile? Fill in the blank.

    _____

6. The nurse is monitoring a newly admitted patient with a possible stroke. What is an abnormal finding when the patient is asked to close both eyes and hold both arms straight out for 10 seconds? Fill in the blank.

    _____

7. When administering the Cincinnati Prehospital Stroke Scale, what are abnormal findings that may indicate the patient is having a stroke, when the patient is asked to repeat a simple phrase, such as "You can't teach an old dog new tricks"? Select all that apply.
   1. Uses correct words, but speaks slowly
   2. Slurs words together
   3. Uses the wrong words
   4. Speaks with a lisp
   5. Unable to speak

8. Diminished or lost sensation in body parts occurs in many stroke patients. The patient who does not feel pressure or pain is susceptible to:
   1. injury.
   2. infection.
   3. pneumonia.
   4. dyspnea.

9. In the acute phase following a stroke, if the patient has homonymous hemianopsia, the environment is arranged so that the important items are available on the:
   1. unaffected side.
   2. affected side.
   3. left side.
   4. right side.

Spinal Cord Injury

 Go to http://evolve.elsevier.com/Linton/medsurg/ for additional activities and exercises.

NCLEX CATEGORIES:

Safe and Effective Care Environment: Safety and Infection Control

Health Promotion and Maintenance

Psychosocial Integrity

Physiological Integrity: Basic Care and Comfort, Reduction of Risk Potential, Physiological Adaptation

OBJECTIVES

1. Explain the impact of spinal cord injury.
2. Describe the diagnostic tests used to evaluate spinal cord injuries and related nursing responsibilities.
3. Explain the physical effects of spinal cord injury.
4. Describe the medical and surgical treatment during the acute phase of spinal cord injury.
5. List the data to be included in the nursing assessment of the patient with a spinal cord injury.
6. Identify nursing diagnoses, goals, interventions, and outcome criteria for the patient with a spinal cord injury.
7. Describe the nursing care for the patient undergoing a laminectomy.
8. State the goals of rehabilitation for the patient with spinal cord injury.

PART I: MASTERING THE BASICS

A. Key Terms.
Match the definition in the numbered column with the most appropriate term in the lettered column.

1. _____ Loss of motor and sensory function in all four extremities due to damage to the spinal cord

2. _____ Soft, in relation to muscle; lacking tone

3. _____ Abnormally exaggerated response of the autonomic nervous system to a stimulus

4. _____ Loss of motor and sensory function due to damage to the spinal cord that spares the upper extremities but, depending on the level of the damage, affects the trunk, pelvis, and lower extremities

5. _____ Increased muscle tone characterized by sudden, involuntary muscle spasms

6. _____ Area of skin supplied by sensory nerve fibers from a single posterior spinal root

7. _____ Surrounded with a sheath

A. Paraplegia
B. Myelinated
C. Tetraplegia; quadriplegia
D. Dermatome
E. Flaccid
F. Spasticity
G. Autonomic dysreflexia

B. Key Terms.

Match the statements in the numbered column with the most appropriate term in the lettered column. Some terms may be used more than once.

1. _____ Removal of all or part of the posterior arch of the vertebra

2. _____ The placement of a piece of donor bone, commonly taken from the hip, into the area between the involved vertebrae

3. _____ Used to determine sensory loss

4. _____ The surgical procedure done to alleviate compression of the spinal cord or nerves

A. Dermatome chart
B. Spinal fusion
C. Laminectomy

C. Spinal Cord Injury

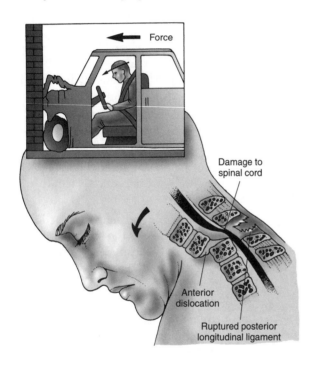

1. Where do most spinal injuries occur? Select the two most common locations.
   1. _____ Cervical
   2. _____ Thoracic
   3. _____ Lumbar
   4. _____ Sacral

2. What is the greatest priority in the acute phase of a spinal cord injury?
   1. Keep a patent airway.
   2. Prevent further cord injury.
   3. Preserve cord function.
   4. Immobilize the patient.

3. During the acute phase, what procedure may be done to decrease pressure on the spinal cord?
   1. Placement of halo device
   2. Decompressive laminectomy
   3. Placement of Crutchfield tongs
   4. Lumbar puncture

4. Explain why the traditional head-tilt–chin-lift method of opening the airway is inappropriate in spinal cord–injured patients.

PART II: PUTTING IT ALL TOGETHER

D. Multiple Choice/Multiple Response.

Choose the most appropriate answer or select all that apply.

1. The halo device is used to provide immobilization and alignment of the:
   1. cervical vertebrae.
   2. thoracic vertebrae.
   3. lumbar vertebrae.
   4. sacral vertebrae.

2. Prompt intervention following autonomic dysreflexia (AD) must be directed toward severe:
   1. hypertension.
   2. hypotension.
   3. infection.
   4. lung compromise.

3. Patients with skull tongs are maintained on:
   1. bedrest with ambulation three times a day.
   2. isolation precautions.
   3. high-roughage diets.
   4. strict bedrest.

4. Following an ileus, the patient will be given oral fluids and food when:
   1. the swallow reflex returns.
   2. the patient is no longer anorexic.
   3. bladder continence returns.
   4. peristalsis returns.

5. Using the "Grading Scale for Muscle Strength," (Table 29-4) the nurse would score a finding of full active range of motion against gravity and resistance as:
   1. 1.
   2. 2.
   3. 3.
   4. 5.

6. Which type of spinal cord injury will result in a loss of motor control below the waist?
   1. C4
   2. C7
   3. T4
   4. T10

7. Which action is indicated in the management of spasticity in the spinal cord–injured patient?
   1. Increase tactile stimuli.
   2. Administer antihypertensive medications.
   3. Perform passive ROM exercises at least four times a day.
   4. Turn and reposition the patient at least every 4 hours.

8. Which procedure is a visualization of the spinal cord and vertebrae through the injection of a radiopaque dye directly into the subarachnoid space of the spinal cord?
   1. Myelography
   2. Electromyography
   3. Lumbar puncture
   4. Electroencephalography

9. Injuries at or above C5 may result in instant death because the:
   1. innervation to the phrenic nerve is interrupted.
   2. sympathetic innervation to the heart is blocked.
   3. sensory nerves to the brain are interrupted.
   4. saphenous nerve can no longer transmit impulses.

10. The spinal cord–injured patient may have difficulty maintaining body temperature within a normal range because the:
    1. hypothalamus can no longer regulate temperature.
    2. regulatory mechanisms of vasoconstriction and sweating are lost.
    3. peripheral nerves to the skin are interrupted.
    4. skin is not able to lose heat through evaporation.

11. At the scene of an accident involving a patient with spinal cord injury, emergency personnel will apply a hard cervical collar around the patient's neck to immobilize the:
    1. skull.
    2. spinal column.
    3. brain.
    4. upper part of the body.

12. Which type of traction is applied to a fiberglass jacket and is used to immobilize and align the cervical vertebrae and relieve compression of nerve roots?
    1. Philadelphia collar
    2. Gardner-Wells tongs
    3. Crutchfield tongs
    4. Halo ring

13. Which condition is an exaggerated sympathetic response to stimuli, such as bladder distention, that produces severe hypertension with the potential for seizures and stroke?
    1. Spinal cord injury
    2. Autonomic dysreflexia
    3. Meningitis
    4. Amyotrophic lateral sclerosis

14. As spinal shock begins to subside and reflex activity returns, the patient with a spinal cord injury is at risk for:
    1. respiratory arrest.
    2. autonomic dysreflexia.
    3. ileus.
    4. coma.

15. Which statements are true about spinal shock? Select all that apply.
    1. Reflex activity below the level of the injury temporarily ceases
    2. Immediate, transient response to injury
    3. Paralysis is flaccid during this time
    4. Exaggerated response of the autonomic nervous system in patients whose injury is at or above the T6 level
    5. Resolution of spinal shock occurs when spastic, involuntary movement of extremities ceases

16. What is the reason why most spinal cord–injured patients can maintain bowel function?
    1. Most spinal cord injuries occur above the T6 level.
    2. Peristalsis is interrupted by most spinal cord injuries, but responds to fecal mass.
    3. The bowel musculature has its own neural center that responds to fecal distention.
    4. The bowel function is not affected by spinal cord injuries.

17. Which are factors that contribute to problems with the integumentary system of the spinal cord–injured patient? Select all that apply.
    1. Immobility
    2. Loss of sensation
    3. Impaired temperature regulation
    4. Spastic activity
    5. Interrupted vasomotor tone of the vascular system

18. What are the main reasons a patient with spinal cord injury may experience ineffective individual coping? Select all that apply.
    1. Disturbed sensory perception
    2. Feeding self-care deficit
    3. Overwhelming losses
    4. Limited potential for recovered function

19. What are the main reasons a spinal cord–injured patient is at risk for injury? Select all that apply.
    1. Involuntary muscle spasms
    2. Lack of motor function
    3. Lack of sensory function
    4. Involvement of intercostal muscles
    5. Orthostatic hypotension

PART III: CHALLENGE YOURSELF!

E. Getting Ready for NCLEX.

Choose the most appropriate answer or select all that apply.

1. The nurse is taking care of a patient who is maintained in cervical traction while on a conventional bed. Which is the best method for changing positions of this patient?
    1. Assisted ambulation
    2. Range-of-motion exercises
    3. "Log-rolling"
    4. Grasping the muscles

2. When the spinal cord–injured patient has spasticity, to what is nursing management directed? Select all that apply.
    1. Prevention of infection
    2. Prevention of muscle atrophy
    3. Prevention of contracture
    4. Prevention of dyspnea

3. During the time of flaccid paralysis, the nurse must be diligent in performing:
   1. active range-of-motion exercises.
   2. passive range-of-motion exercises.
   3. coughing and deep-breathing exercises.
   4. early ambulation.

4. The nurse is caring for a postlaminectomy patient. Which finding is reported to the physician?
   1. WBC of $7,000/mm^3$
   2. Blood pressure 125/80 mm Hg
   3. Clear drainage from incision site
   4. Respirations of 18/min

5. When the nurse is taking care of a postoperative laminectomy patient, what nursing interventions are implemented to promote tissue perfusion? Select all that apply.
   1. Apply pneumatic stockings
   2. Assist the patient with ROM exercises
   3. Administer analgesics for pain relief
   4. Follow strict hand hygiene technique
   5. Auscultate breath sounds

6. Which are characteristics the spinal cord–injured patient may feel during the initial acute phase of adaptation? Select all that apply.
   1. Rage
   2. Depression
   3. Verbal abuse
   4. Shock
   5. Disbelief
   6. Denial

7. After the period of reaction for the spinal cord–injured patient subsides, the nurse should focus interventions related to altered self-concept on patient:
   1. independence and control.
   2. protection from harm.
   3. expression of anger and bargaining.
   4. reassurance of body image.

8. Which are safety measures the nurse should take while caring for a spinal cord–injured patient who is experiencing spastic paralysis? Select all that apply.
   1. Secure the patient with a protective strap across the chest.
   2. Avoid stimulation of the spastic extremity.
   3. Grasp the muscle when performing range-of-motion exercises or positioning the patient.
   4. Support joints above and below the affected muscle group with palms of hands.

9. The patient with spinal cord injury is at risk for injury. What nursing measures will help prevent venous thromboembolism in this patient? Select all that apply.
   1. Pressure stockings
   2. Sequential compression devices when patient is up walking
   3. Administer injections above the level of paralysis.
   4. Use of the incentive spirometer.
   5. Apply firm pressure to the diaphragm when assisting with breathing exercises.

10. The patient with spinal cord injury is experiencing a sudden pounding headache, facial flushing, and increased blood pressure. What is the priority nursing action to take for this patient?
    1. Check the indwelling catheter for occlusion.
    2. Remove any fecal impaction.
    3. Raise the patient's head to a 45-degree angle.
    4. Perform passive range-of-motion exercises.

11. Which are health promotion considerations to teach a spinal cord–injured patient who is being discharged from the hospital? Select all that apply.
    1. Bathe in tepid water with mild soap; dry thoroughly.
    2. Wear cotton undergarments.
    3. Eat a balanced diet, with high amounts of potassium and calcium.
    4. When in bed, turn at least every 2 hours.
    5. Sit up in a chair at least twice a day.

Acute Respiratory Disorders

 Go to http://evolve.elsevier.com/Linton/medsurg/ for additional activities and exercises.

NCLEX CATEGORIES:

Safe and Effective Care Environment: Safety and Infection Control

Health Promotion and Maintenance

Psychosocial Integrity

Physiological Integrity: Pharmacological Therapies, Reduction of Risk Potential, Physiological Adaptation

OBJECTIVES

1. Identify data to be collected in the nursing assessment of the patient with a respiratory disorder.
2. Identify the nursing implications of age-related changes in the respiratory system.
3. Describe diagnostic tests or procedures for respiratory disorders and nursing interventions.
4. Explain nursing care of patients receiving therapeutic treatments for respiratory disorders.
5. For selected respiratory disorders, describe the pathophysiology, signs and symptoms, complications, diagnostic measures, and medical treatment.
6. Assist in developing a nursing care plan for the patient who has an acute respiratory disorder.

PART I: MASTERING THE BASICS

A. Key Terms.

Match the definition in the numbered column with the most appropriate term in the lettered column.

1. _____ Dry, rattling sound caused by partial bronchial obstruction

2. _____ Rapid respiratory rate

3. _____ Presence of air in the pleural cavity that causes the lung on the affected side to collapse

4. _____ Temporary cessation of breathing

5. _____ Low oxygen level in body tissues

6. _____ Movement of air into and out of the lungs

7. _____ Rales; abnormal lung sounds heard on auscultation

8. _____ Difficulty breathing when lying down

9. _____ Accumulation of blood in the pleural space

10. _____ Low level of oxygen in the blood

11. _____ Blood flow through blood vessels of tissue

12. _____ Collapsed lung or part of a lung

13. _____ Difficulty breathing

14. _____ Excess carbon dioxide in the blood

A. Atelectasis
B. Crackles
C. Dyspnea
D. Hemothorax
E. Hypercapnia
F. Hypoxemia
G. Hypoxia
H. Orthopnea
I. Pneumothorax
J. Rhonchus
K. Tachypnea
L. Tissue perfusion
M. Ventilation
N. Apnea

B. Lower Respiratory Tract.

1. Using the figure below (Figure 30-1B, textbook p. 542) label the structures (A–I).

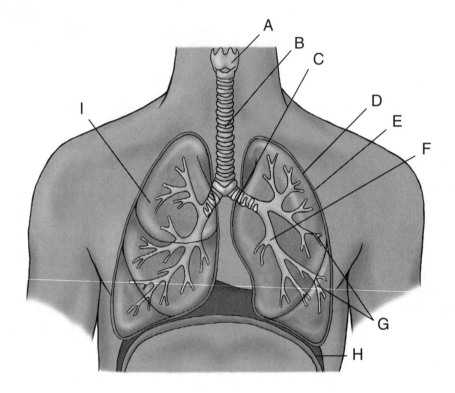

A. _____		F. _____	
B. _____		G. _____	
C. _____		H. _____	
D. _____		I. _____	
E. _____			

2. How many lobes are in the right and left lungs?

   Right lung _____ Left lung _____

3. Which characteristics of the right bronchus explain why foreign bodies from the trachea are more likely to enter the right bronchus than the left bronchus? Select all that apply.
   1. The right bronchus is longer.
   2. The right bronchus is wider.
   3. The right bronchus is straighter vertically.
   4. The right bronchus has a greater horizontal slant.

C. Age-Related Changes.

1. Which of the following are age-related changes that occur in the pharynx and the larynx? Select all that apply.
   1. Loss of elasticity of laryngeal muscles
   2. Louder voice
   3. Thickening of the vocal cords
   4. Muscle atrophy
   5. Gravelly voice

2. Which of the following are age-related changes in the respiratory system? Select all that apply.
   1. Increased lung elasticity
   2. Enlargement of bronchioles
   3. Decreased number of functioning alveoli
   4. Rib cage becomes more rigid
   5. Diaphragm widens
   6. Atrophy of respiratory muscles

3. Which of the following age-related respiratory system changes cause the older adult to be more susceptible to lung infections? Select all that apply.
   1. Decreased work of breathing
   2. Less effective cough
   3. Relaxed chest movement
   4. Diaphragm flattens
   5. Decreased ability to inhale and exhale

D. Diagnostic Procedures.

Match the description of the diagnostic tests and procedures in the numbered column with the most appropriate term in the lettered column. Answers may be used more than once.

1. _____ Detects pulmonary embolism and other obstructive conditions
2. _____ Used to visualize abnormalities in the respiratory system
3. _____ Aspiration of pleural fluid so that it can be examined for pathogens
4. _____ Measures culture and sensitivity of sputum
5. _____ Detects alterations in oxygenation status, including alkalosis or acidosis
6. _____ Distinguishes malignant from benign cells and evaluates effectiveness of cancer treatment
7. _____ Must remain NPO until gag reflex returns
8. _____ Report dyspnea and asymmetric chest movement following procedure
9. _____ Assure patient that radiation dose is small and that isotope is quickly eliminated
10. _____ Apply pressure at the puncture site for 5–10 minutes
11. _____ Collect the specimen early in the morning before breakfast

A. Ventilation-perfusion scan (lung scan)
B. Fiberoptic bronchoscopy
C. Sputum analysis examination
D. Arterial blood gas analysis
E. Thoracentesis
F. Positive emission tomography (PET) scan

E. Types of Breathing Patterns.

Match the descriptions of breathing patterns in the numbered columns with the most appropriate term in the lettered column. Some terms may be used more than once.

1. _____ Respiratory rate faster than 20 breaths/minute
2. _____ Periodic deep breaths (more than 3 sighs per minute)
3. _____ Regular deep breaths, faster than 20 breaths per minute
4. _____ Regular even breaths, 12–20 breaths per minute
5. _____ Varying, irregular breaths with sudden periods of apnea
6. _____ Breaths progressively deeper, becoming more shallow, followed by periods of apnea
7. _____ Gradual rise in end-expiratory level with each successive breath
8. _____ Associated with severe brain pathology
9. _____ Causes include fever and pain
10. _____ Associated with emphysema
11. _____ Related to the use of sedatives and narcotics
12. _____ Related to metabolic acidosis, diabetic ketoacidosis, and renal failure

A. Normal
B. Tachypnea
C. Bradypnea
D. Sighing respirations
E. Cheyne-Stokes respirations, apnea
F. Kussmaul's respirations (with hyperventilation)
G. Biot's respirations
H. Obstructive breathing

F. Rib Fractures.

List one nursing goal, three outcome criteria, and five nursing interventions for the following nursing diagnosis for the patient with fractured ribs.

Nursing Diagnosis

Ineffective breathing pattern related to pain that occurs with ventilation

Nursing Goal

1. _____

Outcome Criteria

1. _____
2. _____
3. _____

Nursing Interventions

1. _____
2. _____
3. _____
4. _____
5. _____

G. Pulmonary Embolus.

Which of the following are signs and symptoms of pulmonary embolus (PE)? Select all that apply.

1. Fever and tachycardia
2. Skin cool and dry
3. Sudden chest pain
4. Cough and hemoptysis
5. Spontaneous onset of chest wall tenderness

H. Artificial Airways.

Match the definition or description in the numbered column with the most appropriate term in the lettered column.

1. _____ Tube used with a surgically created opening through the neck into the trachea
2. _____ Curved tube used to maintain an airway temporarily
3. _____ Soft rubber tube inserted through the nose and extended to the base of the tongue
4. _____ Long tube inserted through the mouth or nose into the trachea

A. Endotracheal tube
B. Nasal airway
C. Tracheostomy tube
D. Oral airway

I. Drug Therapy.

Match the definition or description in the numbered column with the most appropriate term in the lettered column.

1. _____ Suppress cough reflex
2. _____ Dry up nasal secretions
3. _____ Relax smooth muscle in the bronchial airways and blood vessels
4. _____ Kill or inhibit growth of bacteria, viruses, or fungi
5. _____ Reduce frequency of acute asthma attacks (not used to stop them after they've started)
6. _____ Inhibit allergic response; prevent asthmatic attacks
7. _____ Cause constriction of nasal blood vessels and reduce swelling of mucous membranes
8. _____ Antiinflammatory drugs used to treat asthma
9. _____ Thin respiratory secretions so that they are more readily mobilized and can be coughed up
10. _____ Dissolve clots and used to treat pulmonary emboli
11. _____ Reduce thickness of mucus and used to treat bronchitis and asthma

A. Decongestants
B. Antitussives
C. Expectorants
D. Antihistamines
E. Mast cell stabilizers
F. Bronchodilators
G. Corticosteroids
H. Leukotriene inhibitors
I. Mucolytics
J. Antimicrobials
K. Thrombolytics

J. Thoracic Surgery.

Match the definition or description in the numbered column with the most appropriate term in the lettered column.

1. _____ Surgical incision of the chest wall
2. _____ Removal of entire lung
3. _____ Stripping of the membrane that covers the visceral pleura
4. _____ Performed by inserting an endoscope through a small thoracic incision
5. _____ Removal of ribs
6. _____ Preset amount of oxygenated air delivered during each ventilator breath
7. _____ Collapsed alveoli

A. Tidal volume
B. Thoracotomy
C. Pneumonectomy
D. Thoracoplasty
E. Atelectasis
F. Decortication of lung
G. Thoracoscopy

K. Bronchioles and Alveoli.

Label the structures in the figure below. Refer to Figure 30-2 in your textbook, p. 543.

A. _____
B. _____
C. _____
D. _____
E. _____

PART II: PUTTING IT ALL TOGETHER

L. Multiple Choice/Multiple Response.

Choose the most appropriate answer.

1. Who is at risk for having aspiration pneumonia?
    1. Chronically ill patients
    2. Patients with tube feedings
    3. Immunosuppressed patients
    4. Smokers

2. For a patient with influenza, which type of drugs must be started within 24–48 hours after the onset of symptoms and continued for 10 days?
    1. Antimicrobials
    2. Antifungals
    3. Antivirals
    4. Corticosteroids

3. Which type of influenza vaccine is recommended for adults over the age of 50 and all health care workers?
    1. Live vaccine (FluMist)
    2. Inactivated vaccine
    3. First-generation antiviral
    4. Second-generation antiviral

4. What is a common reason for thoracic surgery?
    1. Emphysema
    2. Pneumonia
    3. Asthma
    4. Chest injury

5. Which of the following conditions indicates a medical emergency?
    1. Pneumothorax
    2. Acute bronchitis
    3. Pleurisy
    4. Pneumonia

6. Which abnormal breath sound is due to fluid accumulation in the alveoli and does not clear with coughing?
    1. Wheezes
    2. Rhonchi
    3. Fine crackles
    4. Coarse crackles

7. Chest physiotherapy should be performed:
    1. eight times each day.
    2. after meals.
    3. before meals.
    4. at bedtime.

8. The technique of positioning the patient to facilitate gravitational movement of respiratory secretions toward the bronchi and trachea for expectoration is:
    1. postural drainage.
    2. chest percussion.
    3. chest vibration.
    4. clapping.

9. If excessive secretions that the patient cannot expectorate accumulate in the oral or nasal airway, what may be required?
    1. Spirometry
    2. A lung scan
    3. An MRI
    4. Suctioning

10. What are risks associated with using intermittent positive-pressure breathing (IPPB) treatments?
    1. Atelectasis
    2. Respiratory alkalosis
    3. Contamination of fluid reservoir
    4. Bronchospasm

11. With simple oxygen masks for patients, flow rates from the flowmeter should be adjusted to:
    1. 1–6 liters/min.
    2. 6–10 liters/min.
    3. 10–12 liters/min.
    4. 15–20 liters/min.

12. Ventilators are most commonly required for patients with:
    1. oxygen toxicity.
    2. tachycardia.
    3. hypoxemia.
    4. hyperventilation.

13. The preset amount of oxygenated air delivered during each ventilator breath is called the:
    1. vital capacity.
    2. nebulizing dose.
    3. tidal volume.
    4. respiratory rate.

14. The total number of breaths delivered per minute with mechanical ventilation is called the:
    1. oxygen level setting.
    2. tidal volume setting.
    3. pressure setting.
    4. respiratory rate setting.

15. What is prescribed to keep the pressure in the lungs above the atmospheric pressure at the end of expiration?
    1. The oxygen level setting
    2. The tidal volume setting
    3. Positive end-expiratory pressure (PEEP)
    4. Negative inspiratory pressure

16. Which factor interferes with accurate measurement of the pulse oximeter?
    1. Hypotension
    2. Hyperthermia
    3. Vasodilation
    4. Heart rate

17. Which group of people abstains from using tobacco?
    1. Greek Orthodox
    2. Protestants
    3. Mormons
    4. Orthodox Jews

18. Which herb is often taken to decrease the duration and severity of a cold?
    1. Ginkgo
    2. Ginseng
    3. Kava kava
    4. Echinacea

PART III: CHALLENGE YOURSELF!

M. Getting Ready for NCLEX.

Choose the most appropriate answer or select all that apply.

1. To prevent the spread of germs from person to person, a priority "respiratory etiquette" health promotion behavior which nurses should teach is:
    1. a common cold from a viral cause does not require antimicrobial therapy.
    2. cover your mouth and nose when coughing or sneezing.
    3. wash your hands with soap and warm water for at least 20 seconds.
    4. adequate nutrition is available to reduce susceptibility to infectious organisms.

2. The primary nursing diagnosis for the patient who has fractured ribs is Ineffective breathing pattern related to:
    1. increased sputum production.
    2. ineffective cough.
    3. pain.
    4. atelectasis.

3. The patient with a pulmonary embolism is going home from the hospital with a prescription for Coumadin, following a week of heparin therapy in the hospital. What are the key teaching points for discharge teaching? Select all that apply.
    1. Use a soft toothbrush.
    2. Avoid constricting clothing.
    3. Place a pillow under both knees when sitting.
    4. Be sure to attend clinic follow-up appointments for monitoring of partial thromboplastin time (PTT).

Nursing Care Plan.

Read the following situation and answer questions 4-6. For more information, refer to Nursing Care Plan, The Patient with Pneumonia, p. 572 in your textbook.

A 78-year-old woman is admitted to the hospital with pneumonia. Nursing diagnoses include Ineffective airway clearance, Impaired gas exchange, Activity intolerance, and Imbalanced nutrition: less than body requirements. Her vital signs are: temperature, 103.5° F; pulse, 98; respiration, 28; blood pressure, 160/94. Lung sounds clear to auscultation. She states she has "shortness of breath."

4. Which nursing diagnosis should the nurse plan to address first?

5. Does this patient exhibit any signs of hypoxemia?

6. What nursing action is indicated regarding this patient's temperature?

Chronic Respiratory Disorders

 Go to http://evolve.elsevier.com/Linton/medsurg/ for additional activities and exercises.

NCLEX CATEGORIES:

Safe and Effective Care Environment: Safety and Infection Control

Health Promotion and Maintenance

Psychosocial Integrity

Physiological Integrity: Pharmacological Therapies, Reduction of Risk Potential, Physiological Adaptation

OBJECTIVES

1. Identify examples of chronic inflammatory, obstructive, and restrictive pulmonary diseases.
2. Explain the relationship between cigarette smoking and chronic respiratory disorders.
3. For selected chronic respiratory disorders, describe the pathophysiology, signs and symptoms, complications, diagnostic measures, and medical treatment.
4. Assist in developing a nursing care plan for the patient who has a chronic respiratory disorder.

PART I: MASTERING THE BASICS

A. Key Terms.

Match the definition in the numbered column with the most appropriate term in the lettered column.

1. _____ One of many occupational diseases caused by inhalation of particles of industrial substances

2. _____ Permanent dilation of a portion of the bronchi or bronchioles

3. _____ A collection of inflammatory cells commonly surrounded by fibrotic tissue that represents a chronic inflammatory response to infectious or noninfectious agents

4. _____ A condition characterized by episodes of bronchospasm that causes wheezing and dyspnea; reactive airway disease

5. _____ A disorder characterized by loss of lung elasticity with trapping of air, retained carbon dioxide, and dyspnea

6. _____ Inflammation of the lung

7. _____ Right-sided heart failure secondary to pulmonary disease

8. _____ Placement of a radiation source in the body to treat a malignancy

9. _____ Bronchial inflammation

10. _____ Interstitial fibrosis caused by inhalation of asbestos fibers

A. Granuloma
B. Asthma
C. Brachytherapy
D. Pneumoconiosis
E. Asbestosis
F. Bronchiectasis
G. Pneumonitis
H. Bronchitis
I. Emphysema
J. Cor pulmonale

B. COPD.

1. Which varying combinations of conditions make up chronic obstructive pulmonary disease (COPD)? Select all that apply.
   1. Asthma
   2. Right-sided heart failure
   3. Pneumonia
   4. Chronic bronchitis
   5. Emphysema

2. Which are goals of medical treatment for COPD? Select all that apply.
    1. Attain symptom relief.
    2. Slow disease progression.
    3. Improve exercise tolerance.
    4. Prevent and treat complications.

C. Impaired Gas Exchange.

What are signs and symptoms of impending respiratory failure to watch for with patients experiencing impaired gas exchange? Select all that apply.
    1. Easy bruising
    2. Tachypnea
    3. Deep respirations
    4. Diaphoresis
    5. Bradycardia
    6. Loss of consciousness

D. Hypoxemia.

Explain why the red blood cell count is typically elevated in patients with chronic hypoxemia.

E. Oxygen Therapy.

In the treatment of COPD, the initial flow of oxygen is usually 1–3 liters/min. Why are high levels of oxygen not administered to COPD patients?

F. Tuberculosis.

Which of the following are reasons for the rise in the incidence of tuberculosis in the United States since 1986? Select all that apply.
    1. Development of drug-resistant strains
    2. Increased population of people with HIV
    3. Increased cigarette smoking population
    4. Increased irritating substances in the environment

G. Diagnostic Tests for Tuberculosis.

Which diagnostic tests are done to confirm the diagnosis of tuberculosis? Select all that apply.
    1. Fiberoptic bronchoscopy
    2. Sputum cultures
    3. Acid-fast smears of body fluids
    4. Tuberculin skin tests
    5. Auscultation of the lungs
    6. Pulmonary function tests
    7. Chest radiographs

H. Occupational Lung Disease.

Which of the following are examples of offending substances that may lead to occupational lung diseases? Select all that apply.
    1. Bacteria
    2. Fungi
    3. Dust
    4. Chlorine
    5. Asbestos
    6. Coal dust
    7. Viruses

I. Pulmonary Disorders.

1. Match the signs and symptoms in the numbered column with their respective conditions in the lettered column.

    1. _____ Productive cough, exertional dyspnea, and wheezing
    2. _____ Cough, night sweats, chest pain and tightness, fatigue, and anorexia
    3. _____ Dyspnea on exertion; may display use of accessory muscles of respiration; barrel chest

    A. Emphysema
    B. Chronic bronchitis
    C. Tuberculosis

2. Which of the following are increased by cigarette smoking? Select all that apply.
    1. Emphysema
    2. Cardiovascular disease
    3. Renal disease
    4. Esophageal reflux
    5. Chronic bronchitis

J. Nursing Diagnoses/COPD.

Match the nursing diagnosis for the patient with COPD in the numbered column with the "related to" statement in the lettered column.

1. _____ Impaired gas exchange

2. _____ Ineffective airway clearance

3. _____ Anxiety

4. _____ Altered nutrition: less than body requirements

5. _____ Risk for infection

6. _____ Activity intolerance

7. _____ Decreased cardiac output

A. Decreased ciliary action, increased secretions, weak cough
B. Alveolar destruction, bronchospasm, air trapping
C. Anorexia, dyspnea
D. Right-sided heart failure
E. Increased secretions, weak cough
F. Inability to meet oxygen needs
G. Hypoxemia

PART II: PUTTING IT ALL TOGETHER

K. Multiple Choice/Multiple Response.

Choose the most appropriate answer or select all that apply.

1. What are the three major airway characteristics of a patient with asthma? Select all that apply.
   1. Inflammation
   2. Obstruction
   3. Edema
   4. Hyperresponsiveness
   5. Bronchodilation

2. Why does the opening of the airways decrease in size in patients with asthma? Select all that apply.
   1. Contracted smooth muscle
   2. Redness
   3. Loss of elasticity
   4. Inflammation

3. A serious complication of bronchoconstriction is:
   1. hypoxemia.
   2. hypotension.
   3. drowsiness.
   4. bradycardia.

4. According to the NIH 2007 Guidelines, which are the four major components of medical treatment for asthma? Select all that apply.
   1. Assess and monitor asthma severity and control
   2. Education for partnership in care
   3. Control of environmental factors
   4. Medications
   5. Eliminate risk factors

5. The best position for patients with bronchial asthma is:
   1. supine.
   2. prone.
   3. side-lying.
   4. Fowler's.

6. Arterial blood gas findings that should be reported to the physician if they occur in patients with impaired gas exchange include:
   1. PaO_2 decreases, pH increases.
   2. PaO_2 increases, pH increases.
   3. PaO_2 decreases, $PaCO_2$ increases.
   4. PaO_2 increases, $PaCO_2$ increases.

7. A nasal cannula is preferred over a face mask because the mask may increase the patient's feeling of:
   1. insecurity.
   2. safety.
   3. suffocation.
   4. self-esteem.

8. In patients with emphysema, which causes patients to use accessory muscles for breathing? Select all that apply.
   1. Lungs are often hyperinflated
   2. The diaphragm is flattened
   3. Pursed-lip breathing
   4. Hyperventilation

9. The most serious complications of COPD are respiratory failure and:
   1. kidney failure.
   2. heart failure.
   3. brain hemorrhage.
   4. hypovolemic shock.

10. The term *blue bloater* is used to describe patients with:
    1. advanced emphysema.
    2. pneumonia.
    3. adult respiratory distress syndrome.
    4. advanced chronic bronchitis.

11. The term *pink puffer* is used to describe some patients with emphysema who have normal skin color due to:
    1. normal arterial blood gases.
    2. unlabored respirations.
    3. barrel-chest formation.
    4. normal body temperature.

12. What is the most reliable diagnostic test for COPD?
    1. Chest radiograph
    2. Magnetic resonance imaging (MRI)
    3. Pulmonary function test
    4. Complete blood count (CBC)

13. Drugs that are ordered to decrease airway resistance and the work of breathing for patients with COPD are called:
    1. vasoconstrictors.
    2. diuretics.
    3. calcium channel blockers.
    4. bronchodilators.

14. The preferred route of administration of bronchodilator drugs for patients with COPD is by:
    1. mouth.
    2. inhalation.
    3. intramuscular injection.
    4. intravenous injection.

15. During the physical examination of patients with COPD, the nurse observes the neck for:
    1. edema.
    2. distended veins.
    3. enlarged lymph nodes.
    4. cyanosis.

16. What is the recommended daily fluid intake to help thin secretions in patients with impaired gas exchange?
    1. 600–800 ml
    2. 1000–1500 ml
    3. 2500–3000 ml
    4. 4000–5000 ml

17. Which of the following contributes to increased feelings of restlessness and anxiety in the asthma patient?
    1. Decreased arterial oxygen
    2. Increased arterial carbon dioxide
    3. Increased heart rate
    4. Increased respiratory rate

18. During the physical examination of patients with COPD, the thorax is inspected for the classic:
    1. pink color.
    2. blue tinge.
    3. pulmonary edema.
    4. barrel-chest shape.

19. Which are signs and symptoms of airway obstruction in the patient with COPD? Select all that apply.
    1. Headache
    2. Tachycardia
    3. Abnormal breath sounds
    4. Dyspnea
    5. Dizziness

20. Why are patients with COPD encouraged to drink extra fluids each day?
    1. Decrease body temperature
    2. Increase circulation
    3. Liquefy secretions
    4. Prevent kidney stones

21. The work of breathing is increased with COPD, which in turn increases the patient's:
    1. caloric requirements.
    2. requirements for calcium.
    3. requirements for sodium.
    4. dietary roughage requirements.

22. The recommended diet for the patient who is dyspneic is a soft diet with:
    1. low salt.
    2. low protein.
    3. low calories.
    4. frequent, small meals.

23. If the COPD patient becomes excessively dyspneic or develops tachycardia during activity, the patient should:
    1. increase the activity slowly.
    2. stop the activity.
    3. sit down briefly and then resume activity.
    4. drink a full glass of water.

24. The nurse monitors the patient with chronic bronchitis and emphysema for which of the following signs of heart failure? Select all that apply.
    1. Bradycardia
    2. Tachycardia
    3. Increasing dyspnea
    4. Dehydration
    5. Dependent edema

25. A persistent, productive cough with bloody sputum (hemoptysis) is a common symptom of:
    1. emphysema.
    2. cystic fibrosis.
    3. sinusitis.
    4. tuberculosis.

26. The most common preventive drug therapy for tuberculosis is:
    1. prednisone.
    2. isoniazid.
    3. gamma globulin.
    4. aminophylline.

27. The patient who is thought to have active tuberculosis is isolated at first. Which of the following is *not* necessary related to the care of the patient?
    1. Good hand hygiene
    2. Wearing masks
    3. Wearing gowns
    4. Standard Precautions

PART III: CHALLENGE YOURSELF!

L. Getting Ready for NCLEX.

Choose the most appropriate answer or select all that apply.

1. Which of the following problems develop when status asthmaticus is not treated? Select all that apply.
    1. Pneumothorax
    2. Acidosis
    3. Right-sided heart failure
    4. Renal failure
    5. Liver failure

2. Which complications occur when severe, persistent bronchospasm is not treated? Select all that apply.
    1. Constriction of bronchial smooth muscle
    2. Thickening of airway tissues
    3. Air trapping in the alveoli
    4. Hypoinflation of the lungs

3. What is the treatment for a patient with a positive TB skin test, a negative chest radiograph, and who is at risk for tuberculosis? Select all that apply.
    1. Treat prophylactically to prevent development of active tuberculosis.
    2. Repeat the chest radiograph in 6 months.
    3. No treatment is needed.
    4. Take isoniazid for 9–12 months.

4. Which are contributing factors to and appropriate nursing interventions for a patient with active tuberculosis who is experiencing social isolation? Select all that apply.
    1. Good hand hygiene by patient and health care providers.
    2. Wear particulate masks (disposable respirators) during contact with the patient.
    3. Wear gowns during all contact with the patient.
    4. Explain to the patient that isolation is temporary to protect others from infection.
    5. Encourage the patient to express feelings about the diagnosis and isolation.

5. Which foods must be avoided by patients who are taking isoniazid?
    1. Aged cheese
    2. Dairy products
    3. Grapefruit
    4. Bananas

Nursing Care Plan.

Refer to Nursing Care Plan, The Patient with Chronic Obstructive Pulmonary Disease, p. 592 in the textbook, and answer questions 6-12.

6. What signs and symptoms of COPD does this patient exhibit? Select all that apply.
    1. Fatigue
    2. Orthopnea
    3. Productive cough
    4. Clear sputum
    5. Normal respiratory rate
    6. Bluish skin color
    7. Pursed-lip breathing
    8. Barrel-shaped thorax

7. Why does the nurse monitor this patient for peripheral edema?

8. Which signs of heart failure would the nurse be monitoring? Select all that apply.
   1. Increasing dyspnea
   2. Increasing urine output
   3. Bradycardia
   4. Dependent edema

9. What are the most serious complications of COPD? Select all that apply.
   1. Renal failure
   2. Liver failure
   3. Respiratory failure
   4. Heart failure

10. Which of the following are characteristics of emphysema? Select all that apply.
    1. Elastic recoil decreases.
    2. Lungs becomes hypoinflated.
    3. Respiratory bronchiole walls break down.
    4. Alveolar walls enlarge and break down.
    5. Ruptured blebs cause the lung to collapse.

11. What is the priority nursing diagnosis for this patient?

12. What tasks for this patient could be assigned to unlicensed assistive personnel? Select all that apply.
    1. Monitor vital signs and arterial blood gases.
    2. Assist to comfortable high-Fowler's position in bed.
    3. Observe respiratory status before and after use of bronchodilator.
    4. Encourage 2500–3000 ml of fluid daily.
    5. Provide comfort measures.
    6. Identify stressors in addition to hypoxemia.
    7. Provide pleasant environment for meals.
    8. Monitor sputum color and body temperature.
    9. Monitor for signs of heart failure, especially peripheral edema.
    10. Assist with oral hygiene.

Hematologic Disorders

 Go to http://evolve.elsevier.com/Linton/medsurg/ for additional activities and exercises.

NCLEX CATEGORIES:

Safe and Effective Care Environment: Safety and Infection Control

Health Promotion and Maintenance

Psychosocial Integrity

Physiological Integrity: Pharmacological Therapies, Reduction of Risk Potential, Physiological Adaptation

OBJECTIVES

1. List the components of the hematologic system and describe their role in oxygenation and hemostasis.
2. Identify data to be collected when assessing a patient with a disorder of the hematologic system.
3. Describe tests and procedures used to diagnose disorders of the hematologic system and nursing considerations for each.
4. Describe nursing care for patients undergoing common therapeutic measures for disorders of the hematologic system.
5. Describe the pathophysiology, signs and symptoms, medical diagnosis, and medical treatment for selected disorders of the hematologic system.
6. Assist in planning nursing care for a patient with a disorder of the hematologic system.

PART I: MASTERING THE BASICS

A. Key Terms.
Match the definition in the numbered column with the most appropriate term in the lettered column.

1. _____ Person with type AB-positive blood who can receive transfusions with any type of blood because all the common antigens (A, B, and Rh) are present in the blood

2. _____ A purplish skin lesion resulting from blood leaking outside the blood vessels

3. _____ A reduction in the number of red blood cells or in the quantity of hemoglobin

4. _____ A small (1–3 mm) red or reddish-purple spot on the skin resulting from blood capillaries breaking and leaking small amounts of blood into the tissues

5. _____ A primary function of the hematologic system

6. _____ Person with type O-negative blood who can donate blood to anyone because none of the common antigens are present in the blood

7. _____ Changes in blood pressure and pulse as person moves from lying to sitting to standing positions

8. _____ Red or reddish-purple skin lesion 3 mm or more in size that results from blood leaking outside of the blood vessels

9. _____ Control of bleeding

A. Anemia
B. Oxygenation
C. Ecchymosis
D. Orthostatic vital sign changes
E. Petechia
F. Purpura
G. Universal donor
H. Universal recipient
I. Hemostasis

B. Anemia and Coagulation Disorders.

Match the descriptions in the numbered column with the appropriate type of anemia or coagulation disorder in the lettered column. Answers may be used more than once.

1. _____ Results from complete failure of bone marrow

2. _____ Occurs when a person does not absorb vitamin B$_{12}$ from the stomach

3. _____ A genetic disease carried on a recessive gene

4. _____ Results from diet low in iron or inability of the body to absorb enough iron from GI tract

5. _____ Causes include cancer chemotherapy and radiation

6. _____ Secondary disorder to another pathologic process, such as sepsis, shock, burns, or obstetric complications

7. _____ Hypercoagulable state with thrombosis and hemorrhage

8. _____ Genetic disease in which a person lacks blood-clotting factors normally found in the plasma

9. _____ May be caused by drugs (such as streptomycin and chloramphenicol) and exposure to toxic chemicals and radiation

10. _____ Symptoms include weakness, sore tongue, and numbness of hands or feet

11. _____ Misshapen red blood cells become fragile and rupture easily

A. Thrombocytopenia
B. Disseminated intravascular coagulation (DIC)
C. Hemophilia
D. Pernicious anemia
E. Sickle cell anemia
F. Iron deficiency anemia
G. Aplastic anemia

C. Anemia.

Which of the following are ways the body compensates when a person is anemic with chronic blood loss? Select all that apply.

1. Increased heart rate
2. Decreased respiratory rate
3. Blood redistributed toward the skin
4. Increased production of erythropoietin

D. Thrombocytopenia.

Which of the following are signs and symptoms of thrombocytopenia? Select all that apply.

1. Petechiae
2. Gingival bleeding
3. Fever
4. Orthostatic hypotension
5. Epistaxis
6. Purpura

E. Drug Therapy.

Match the drug action and the appropriate nursing intervention in the numbered column with the name of the drug(s) in the lettered column. Answers may be used more than once.

1. _____ Replaces iron

2. _____ Stimulates the bone marrow to produce red blood cells

3. _____ Intramuscular injection; must be given every month for the rest of the person's life, if the patient has pernicious anemia

4. _____ May be given by intravenous or subcutaneous injection; patient is usually treated three times per week until the hematocrit is 30–33

A. Vitamin B$_{12}$
B. Ferrous sulfate
C. Epoietin alfa
D. Iron dextran

PART II: PUTTING IT ALL TOGETHER

F. Multiple Choice/Multiple Response.

Choose the most appropriate answer or select all that apply.

1. A condition in which there are too many blood cells is called:
   1. pernicious anemia.
   2. aplastic anemia.
   3. hemolytic anemia.
   4. polycythemia vera.

2. The treatment for autoimmune hemolytic anemia is:
   1. vitamin B$_{12}$ injections.
   2. a ferrous sulfate and high-iron diet.
   3. an iron dextran and high-carbohydrate diet.
   4. corticosteroids and blood transfusions.

3. The treatment for aplastic anemia is:
   1. vitamin B_{12} injections.
   2. a ferrous sulfate and high-iron diet.
   3. an iron dextran and high-carbohydrate diet.
   4. transfusions, antibiotics, and corticosteroids.

4. Treatment for sickle cell crisis includes:
   1. a ferrous sulfate and high-iron diet.
   2. an iron dextran and high-carbohydrate diet.
   3. aggressive intravenous hydration and IV morphine.
   4. corticosteroids and platelet transfusions.

5. For each unit of packed RBCs transfused, the patient's hemoglobin should increase approximately:
   1. 10 g/dl.
   2. 5 g/dl.
   3. 3 g/dl.
   4. 1 g/dl.

6. Red or reddish-purple spots 3 mm or larger that are the result of blood vessels breaking are:
   1. petechiae.
   2. purpura.
   3. ecchymoses.
   4. nodes.

7. Patients with low red blood cell counts may have:
   1. bradycardia.
   2. hypotension.
   3. bleeding problems.
   4. tachycardia.

8. The patient is receiving packed red blood cells, because of a low hematocrit and hemoglobin. Which are symptoms of low hematocrit and hemoglobin? Select all that apply.
   1. Shortness of breath
   2. Bradycardia
   3. Decreased blood pressure
   4. Chest pain
   5. Fatigue
   6. Lightheadedness

9. Once blood is picked up from the blood bank, the transfusion should be started within:
   1. 5 minutes.
   2. 20 minutes.
   3. 30 minutes.
   4. 2 hours.

10. Platelets are generally administered when a patient's platelet count drops below:
    1. 10,000/mm^3.
    2. 15,000/mm^3.
    3. 20,000/mm^3.
    4. 300,000/mm^3.

11. If platelets are ordered before a procedure such as a lumbar puncture or endoscopy to prevent postprocedure bleeding, the platelets should be administered:
    1. 1 week before the procedure.
    2. 1 day before the procedure.
    3. 6 hours before the procedure.
    4. immediately before the procedure.

12. The treatment for hemophilia is:
    1. plasma and cryoprecipitate transfusions.
    2. red blood cell transfusions and antibiotics.
    3. white blood cell transfusions and potassium.
    4. platelet and anticoagulant transfusions.

13. Symptoms of thrombocytopenia include:
    1. fatigue and pallor.
    2. petechiae and purpura.
    3. nausea and vomiting.
    4. tachycardia and palpitations.

14. Treatment for thrombocytopenia in cancer patients receiving chemotherapy or radiation therapy includes:
    1. red blood cell transfusions and iron.
    2. white blood cell transfusions and antibiotics.
    3. platelet transfusions.
    4. cryoprecipitate transfusions and anticonvulsants.

15. The condition in which a person has too few platelets circulating in the blood is called:
    1. leukemia.
    2. anemia.
    3. lymphoma.
    4. thrombocytopenia.

16. Four types of blood transfusion reactions include hemolytic, circulatory overload, febrile, and:
    1. thrombocytopenic.
    2. anaphylactic.
    3. anemic.
    4. leukopenic.

17. Feverfew, garlic, and ginkgo are herbs that affect:
    1. wound healing.
    2. blood clotting.
    3. resistance to infection.
    4. kidney function.

18. What is the role of the spleen related to the hematologic system?
    1. Produces platelets
    2. Manufactures clotting factors
    3. Removes old blood cells from circulation
    4. Synthesizes vitamins

19. How many liters of blood circulating through the body does a healthy adult have?
    1. 2 liters
    2. 6 liters
    3. 10 liters
    4. 24 liters

20. What is the most common site for a bone marrow biopsy?
    1. Posterior iliac crest
    2. Sternum
    3. Femur
    4. Tibia

21. What is a term used to describe the series of events that occur in the process of blood clotting?
    1. Anticoagulation
    2. Hemostasis
    3. Hemolysis
    4. Coagulation cascade

22. Which of the following are antigens found on the cell membranes of red blood cells? Select all that apply.
    1. A antigens
    2. B antigens
    3. AB antigens
    4. O antigens
    5. Rhesus (Rh) antigens
    6. pH antigens

23. Which of the following are types of blood transfusion reactions? Select all that apply.
    1. Hemolytic
    2. Anaphylactic
    3. Febrile
    4. Circulatory overload
    5. Anemic

PART III: CHALLENGE YOURSELF!

G. Getting Ready for NCLEX.

Choose the most appropriate answer or select all that apply.

1. Which of the following bone marrow sites produce the majority of red blood cells and platelets? Select all that apply.
   1. Humerus
   2. Sternum
   3. Pelvis

2. Which of the following functions of the liver are related to hematologic functions? Select all that apply.
   1. Manufactures red blood cells
   2. Manufactures clotting factors
   3. Clears old and damaged red blood cells from the circulation
   4. Stores glucose in the form of glycogen
   5. Aids in phagocytosis of bacteria

3. Which of the following are nursing actions for the patient at risk for injury from low red blood cell counts? Select all that apply.
   1. Allow for rest between periods of activity.
   2. Elevate the patient's head on pillows to reduce shortness of breath.
   3. Administer analgesics as prescribed.
   4. Decrease daily fluid intake.
   5. Increase food intake of iron.

4. Which of the following are nursing actions for the patient at risk for injury from bleeding? Select all that apply.
   1. Avoid intramuscular injections.
   2. Use a soft-bristled toothbrush.
   3. Avoid foods high in vitamin D.
   4. Avoid the use of suppositories.

5. Which of the following foods are high in iron content? Select all that apply.
   1. Fish
   2. Dark green vegetables
   3. Red meats
   4. Beans
   5. Pasta
   6. Rice

6. The nurse is collecting data from a patient with a hematologic disorder. What characteristics may be indicative of an underlying hematologic disorder? Select all that apply.
   1. Kussmaul's respirations
   2. Easy bruising
   3. Elevated temperature
   4. Chronic fatigue
   5. Periods of unusually long bleeding
   6. Hypertension

7. Which of the following manifestations might indicate a hematologic problem in a patient? Select all that apply.
   1. Severe headache
   2. High fever
   3. Changes in vision
   4. Epistaxis
   5. Heart palpitations
   6. Chest pain
   7. Joint pain
   8. Kidney pain
   9. Cold intolerance
   10. Fatigue
   11. Dyspnea
   12. Bradypnea

8. The patient with anemia has been prescribed ferrous sulfate. Which are nursing actions related to administration of this drug? Select all that apply.
   1. Have the patient take the drug with milk.
   2. Encourage the patient to take the drug with food.
   3. Tell the patient to drink through a straw, if the ferrous sulfate is given in liquid form.
   4. Explain that stools may turn black.
   5. Avoid taking with foods containing tyramine.

9. Which of the following are related to administering iron dextran to a patient with anemia? Select all that apply.
   1. Monitor the patient for hypersensitivity reactions.
   2. Test dose before starting treatment.
   3. Give intramuscular injections only in the lower outer quadrant of the buttock.
   4. Use the Z-track technique when giving an intramuscular injection.
   5. Inject the medication slowly.
   6. Massage the area.

10. If a patient with anemia is orthostatic and tilt-positive, which should be increased?
    1. Carbohydrates
    2. Fiber
    3. Fluids
    4. Vitamins

Nursing Care Plan.
Refer to the Nursing Care Plan, The Patient in Sickle Cell Crisis, p. 620 in the textbook, and answer questions 11-21.

11. What data has been collected about this patient that indicates sickle cell crisis?

12. What patient problem should the nurse address first when the patient is admitted to the emergency department?
    1. Acute pain
    2. Risk for injury related to orthostatic hypotension
    3. Risk for fluid volume deficit
    4. Anxiety related to hospitalization

13. What changes in the heart occur as the patient's body tries to compensate for persistently low red blood cell counts?

14. Which of the following are signs and symptoms related to stressors that can trigger a sickle cell crisis? Select all that apply.
    1. Infection
    2. Dehydration
    3. Overexertion
    4. Edema
    5. Hot weather changes
    6. Smoking
    7. High-fat diet

15. What causes the pain in sickle cell anemia?

16. What are probable causes of the fever this patient has?

17. How long do sickle cell crises typically last?

18. What is commonly prescribed for pain relief during a sickle cell crisis?

19. Why is aggressive IV hydration indicated during sickle cell crisis?

20. Why should the nurse pay special attention to the temperature of this patient?

21. What is a common fear in patients with sickle cell crisis?

Immunologic Disorders

Go to http://evolve.elsevier.com/Linton/medsurg/ for additional activities and exercises.

NCLEX CATEGORIES:

Safe and Effective Care Environment: Safety and Infection Control

Health Promotion and Maintenance

Psychosocial Integrity

Physiological Integrity: Pharmacological Therapies, Reduction of Risk Potential, Physiological Adaptation

OBJECTIVES

1. List the components of the immune system and describe their role in innate immunity, acquired immunity, and tolerance.
2. List the data to be collected when assessing a patient with a disorder of the immune system.
3. Describe the tests and procedures used to diagnose disorders of the immune system and nursing considerations for each.
4. Describe the nursing care for patients undergoing common therapeutic measures for disorders of the immune system.
5. Describe the pathophysiology, signs and symptoms, medical diagnosis, and medical treatment for selected disorders of the immune system.
6. Assist in developing a nursing care plan for a patient with a disorder of the immune system.

PART I: MASTERING THE BASICS

A. Key Terms.
Match the definition or description in the numbered column with the most appropriate term in the lettered column.

1. _____ Resistance to or protection from a disease

2. _____ Certain white blood cells (neutrophils, monocytes, and macrophages) that engulf and destroy invading pathogens, dead cells, and cellular debris

3. _____ Class of fatty acids that regulates vasodilation, temperature elevation, white blood cell activation, and other physiologic processes

4. _____ Freely circulating Y-shaped antigen-binding protein produced by B lymphocytes and plasma cells

5. _____ Disease-causing microorganism

6. _____ A substance, usually a protein, that is capable of stimulating a response from the immune system

7. _____ Defensive system that is operational at all times, consisting of anatomic and physiologic barriers, the inflammatory response, and the ability of certain cells to phagocytose invaders

8. _____ Defensive response by T_C cells aimed at intracellular defects such as viruses and cancer

9. _____ Antibody-mediated or cell-mediated response that is specific to a particular pathogen and is activated when needed

10. _____ Defensive response by B cells assisted by T_H cells, aimed at invading microorganisms such as bacteria

11. _____ Membrane-bound, Y-shaped binding protein produced by B lymphocytes; called *antibody* when released from the cell membrane

12. _____ Actions taken to help protect patients with low white blood cell counts from infection

13. _____   Cancer of the white blood cells in
which the bone marrow produces too
many immature white blood cells

A. Acquired immunity
B. Antibody
C. Antibody-mediated immunity
D. Antigen
E. Cell-mediated immunity
F. Compromised host precautions
G. Eicosanoid
H. Immunity
I. Immunoglobulin
J. Innate immunity
K. Leukemia
L. Pathogen
M. Phagocytes

B. Immune System.

Match the organ in the numbered column with its function in the lettered column.

1. _____   Lymph nodes
2. _____   Bone marrow
3. _____   Spleen
4. _____   Thymus

A. Participate(s) in the maturation of T
lymphocytes
B. Act(s) as filter to remove microorganisms from
the lymph fluid before it returns to the blood
C. Filter(s) and destroy(s) microorganisms in the
blood
D. Produce(s) white blood cells

C. White Blood Cells.

Match the type of white blood cell in the numbered column with its function in the lettered column.

1. _____   Basophils
2. _____   B lymphocytes
3. _____   Neutrophils
4. _____   Monocytes
5. _____   Eosinophils
6. _____   Mast cells
7. _____   T lymphocytes

A. Called *macrophages* when they enter tissue;
powerful phagocytes
B. Initiate inflammatory response; circulate in
blood and release histamine

C. Fight bacterial infections; most numerous type
of the white blood cells
D. Combat parasitic infections; associated with
allergies
E. Manufacture immunoglobulins and stimulate
the production of antibodies
F. Store histamine; located in body tissues
G. Secrete cytokines, facilitating body's immune
system

D. Immunity.

*Match the definition or description in the numbered
column with the most appropriate term in the lettered
column. Some terms may be used more than once.*

1. _____   Process of ingesting and digesting
invading pathogens, dead cells, and
cellular debris
2. _____   Process of self-recognition that occurs
as part of normal neonatal growth
and development
3. _____   Response initiated when IgM immunoglobulins on the surface of B lymphocytes detect a foreign antigen
4. _____   System activated only when needed
in response to a specific antigen;
can be antibody-mediated or cell-
mediated
5. _____   Response aimed at intracellular
defects caused by viruses and cancer;
responsible for delayed hypersensitivity reactions and transplant organ
tissue rejection
6. _____   System that consists of anatomic and
physiologic barriers, inflammatory
response, and action of phagocytic
cells
7. _____   Defense systems present at birth
8. _____   Defense systems specific to a particular pathogen
9. _____   Immunity responsible for delayed
hypersensitivity reactions
10. _____   Immunity aimed at invading microorganisms such as bacteria

A. Acquired immunity
B. Innate immunity
C. Tolerance
D. Phagocytosis
E. Antibody-mediated immunity
F. Cell-mediated immunity

E. Lines of Defense.
Match the description of the body's first lines of defense in the numbered column with the most appropriate anatomic and physiologic barriers in the lettered column. Answers may be used more than once.

1. _____ Acidic: inhibits growth of organisms

2. _____ Secretes lysozyme, an antimicrobial enzyme

3. _____ Contains antibody IgA and phagocytes

4. _____ Acts as protective covering and secretes substances that inhibit growth of pathogens

A. Skin
B. Sweat glands
C. GI and GU mucosae
D. Respiratory and gastrointestinal secretions

F. Immunity.
Which of the following are related to active acquired antibody immunity? Select all that apply.

1. Occurs when a person produces his or her own antibodies in response to a pathogen
2. Occurs when a person receives a vaccination
3. Permanent type of immunity
4. Occurs when an antibody produced by a person is transferred to another person
5. Immunity lasts only 1–2 months after antibodies have been received
6. Occurs when a person has an infection and produces his or her own antibodies
7. Immunity obtained from gamma globulin injections given to people exposed to hepatitis

G. Systemic Lupus Erythematosus.
Which of the following are symptoms of systemic lupus erythematosus (SLE)? Select all that apply.

1. Characteristic rash
2. Easy bruising
3. Photosensitivity with exposure to sunlight
4. Arthritis
5. Proteinuria
6. Petechiae
7. Hematologic disorder, such as leukopenia

H. Shift to the Right.
List two conditions that may cause a "shift to the right" on a CBC.

1. _____

   _____

2. _____

   _____

I. Diagnostic Procedures.
Match the diagnostic test in the numbered column with the disease or disorder it is used to diagnose in the lettered column. Answers may be used more than once.

1. _____ Antinuclear antibody test

2. _____ Bone marrow biopsy

3. _____ Lymphangiography

4. _____ Liver-spleen scan

5. _____ Skin tests

A. Hodgkin's disease
B. Hypersensitivities
C. Leukemia
D. SLE

J. Bone Marrow Transplants.

Which of the following are indications for bone marrow transplant? Select all that apply.
1. Thrombocytopenia
2. High doses of chemotherapy
3. High doses of radiation therapy
4. Hypersensitivity reaction
5. Aplastic anemia

K. Bone Marrow Transplants.

1. Which of the following are descriptions of an allogenic bone marrow transplant? Select all that apply.
   1. Requires a matched donor
   2. Procedure in which a patient's own bone marrow is returned to the patient
   3. Best option for patients with a solid tumor that has not metastasized to the bone marrow, such as patients with breast cancer or lymphoma
   4. Type of transplant that has been done the longest
   5. Used to restore bone marrow function in patients with leukemia

2. Which of the following describe peripheral blood stem cell transplants? Select all that apply.
   1. Newest type of transplant, which is becoming the most common type
   2. Procedure in which a patient's own bone marrow is harvested before chemotherapy and radiation therapy
   3. Following harvesting of stem cells through apheresis, the patient is treated with chemotherapy and radiation therapy
   4. Procedure in which colony-stimulating factors are administered to the patient to stimulate the bone marrow to produce white blood cells
   5. Procedure that reduces the duration of neutropenia

L. Complications.

Which of the following are major complications of bone marrow and peripheral blood stem cell transplants? Select all that apply.
1. Hemorrhage
2. Infection
3. Shock
4. Thrombocytopenia
5. Graft-versus-host disease

M. Neutropenia.

Which are causes of neutropenia? Select all that apply.
1. Decreased bone marrow production
2. Chemotherapy
3. Hypersensitivity reactions
4. Radiation therapy
5. Autoimmune reactions

N. Leukemia.

Explain why a patient with leukemia may have signs of anemia, such as fatigue, paleness, tachycardia, and tachypnea.

O. Nursing Diagnoses/Leukemia.

Which are common nursing diagnoses for patients with acute leukemia? Select all that apply.
1. Risk for injury
2. Risk for acute confusion
3. Impaired oral mucous membrane
4. Urinary retention
5. Imbalanced nutrition
6. Fatigue

P. Immune System Disorders.

Match the definition or description in the numbered column with the appropriate immune system disorder in the lettered column.

1. _____ Cancer of the white blood cells
2. _____ Cancer of the lymph system staged as low-, intermediate-, or high-grade
3. _____ Cancer of the lymph system characterized by the presence of Reed-Sternberg cells in the lymph nodes
4. _____ Cancer of the plasma cells in the bone marrow
5. _____ Autoimmune disease that affects multiple organs

A. SLE
B. Hodgkin's disease
C. Leukemia
D. Non-Hodgkin's lymphoma
E. Multiple myeloma

Q. Hypersensitivity.

Which are antigens that may cause an immediate hypersensitivity reaction? Select all that apply.
1. Insect stings
2. Pollen
3. Organ transplant cells; transplanted graft rejection
4. Blood transfusion cells; mismatched blood transfusion
5. Dust

R. Compromised Host Precautions.

Which are nursing actions indicated for a patient on compromised host precautions? Select all that apply.
1. Hand hygiene: All persons entering the patient's room must wash their hands.
2. Staff use of masks: Masks are required.
3. Dietary concerns: Serve only cooked or canned foods.
4. Patient's use of masks: Patient should wear a clean mask while in his or her room.
5. Scheduling of patient appointments: Plan follow-up appointment at clinic in one week.

S. Lymphatic System.

Using the figure below (Figure 33-1, textbook p. 627), label the parts of the lymphatic system.

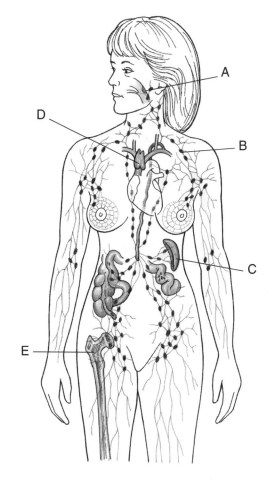

A. _____

B. _____

C. _____

D. _____

E. _____

PART II: PUTTING IT ALL TOGETHER

T. Multiple Choice/Multiple Response.

Choose the most appropriate answer or select all that apply.

1. The body's defense network against infection is the:
    1. cardiovascular system.
    2. respiratory system.
    3. immune system.
    4. circulatory system.

2. Which filters microorganisms from the lymph fluid before it is returned to the bloodstream?
    1. Thymus
    2. Bone marrow
    3. Spleen
    4. Lymph node

3. The body's first line of defense is:
    1. skin and inflammation.
    2. phagocytosis and kidney.
    3. blood vessels and kidney.
    4. skin and mucous membranes.

4. Which is responsible for delayed hypersensitivity reactions and rejection of transplanted tissue?
    1. Humoral immunity
    2. Interferon immunity
    3. Cell-mediated immunity
    4. Antibody-mediated immunity

5. The most numerous white blood cells are the:
    1. neutrophils.
    2. basophils.
    3. lymphocytes.
    4. eosinophils.

6. A class of fatty acids that regulates vasodilation, temperature elevation, white blood cell activation, and other immune processes includes:
    1. cytokines.
    2. eicosanoids.
    3. lymphocytes.
    4. neutrophils.

7. Substances that make the antigen more recognizable to neutrophils, monocytes, and macrophages are:
    1. eicosanoids.
    2. eosinophils.
    3. antibodies.
    4. cytokines.

8. When there is a breakdown of tolerance, what types of diseases occur?
    1. Autoimmune
    2. Viral
    3. Bacterial
    4. Cancers

9. Which are examples of autoimmune disorders? Select all that apply.
    1. Rheumatoid arthritis
    2. SLE
    3. Graves' disease
    4. Leukemia
    5. Type 1 diabetes mellitus

10. The body's ability to determine self from non-self is called:
    1. tolerance.
    2. phagocytosis.
    3. immunity.
    4. inflammation.

11. A "shift to the left" on a CBC indicates that more than 60% of white blood cells are:
    1. lymphocytes.
    2. basophils.
    3. eosinophils.
    4. neutrophils.

12. A blood test that detects antibodies present in the blood that may indicate autoimmune disorders is:
    1. complete blood count (CBC).
    2. Western blot test.
    3. antinuclear antibody test.
    4. T cell counts.

13. Which diagnostic procedure is done to detect and identify microorganisms in blood?
    1. Western blot
    2. Viral load
    3. Complete blood count (CBC)
    4. Blood culture

14. The function of colony-stimulating factors (CSFs) is to stimulate the:
    1. bone marrow to produce more blood cells.
    2. heart to increase the force of contraction.
    3. kidney to promote the reabsorption of water.
    4. bronchi of the lung to dilate.

15. A condition that puts a patient at increased risk of infection is:
    1. anemia.
    2. thrombocytopenia.
    3. eosinophilia.
    4. neutropenia.

16. A cancer of the white blood cells in which the bone marrow produces too many immature WBCs is:
    1. Hodgkin's disease.
    2. non-Hodgkin's lymphoma.
    3. leukemia.
    4. multiple myeloma.

17. The reason pus may not be seen even though infection is present in a patient with leukemia is that patients with leukemia do not have normal:
    1. platelets.
    2. red blood cells.
    3. white blood cells.
    4. cytokines.

18. When a patient's absolute neutrophil count falls below 1000/mm^3, what precautions are instituted?
    1. Enteric precautions
    2. Droplet precautions
    3. Compromised host precautions
    4. Transmission-based precautions

19. What minimizes the chance of the recipient's immune system attacking the transplanted organ?
    1. Administration of steroids
    2. Tissue matching of donor to recipient
    3. Administration of antibiotics
    4. Administration of platelets

20. Exaggerated immune responses that are uncomfortable and potentially harmful are:
    1. hypersensitivity reactions.
    2. bacterial lung infections.
    3. tachycardic reactions.
    4. peripheral neuropathy reactions.

PART III: CHALLENGE YOURSELF!

U. Getting Ready for NCLEX.

Choose the most appropriate answer or select all that apply.

1. What is the priority nursing diagnosis for a patient with acute leukemia?
   1. Fatigue
   2. Imbalanced nutrition
   3. Risk for injury
   4. Ineffective self health management

2. Which change in vital signs may indicate sepsis, a common complication of leukemia?
   1. Tachycardia
   2. Dyspnea
   3. Hypertension
   4. Decreased temperature

3. A common finding in patients with leukemia is a hematocrit below 30 g/dl and hemoglobin below 10 g/dl, indicating the condition of:
   1. anemia.
   2. thrombocytopenia.
   3. leukopenia.
   4. sepsis.

4. What presents the greatest risk to patients with leukemia?
   1. Hemorrhage
   2. Anemia
   3. Infection
   4. Fatigue

5. A patient with leukemia has been placed on compromised host precautions. Which nursing actions are indicated for this patient? Select all that apply.
   1. Keep invasive procedures to a minimum.
   2. Careful attention to aseptic technique must be maintained.
   3. Designate a particular thermometer and sphygmomanometer to use exclusively when caring for this patient.
   4. Encourage the patient to shower daily, using bar soap.
   5. Minimize waiting times in waiting rooms when scheduling follow-up appointments.
   6. Instruct the patient not to handle flowers and plants.
   7. Humidifiers may be used, as long as they have containers of water.

Human Immunodeficiency Virus and Acquired Immunodeficiency Syndrome

 Go to http://evolve.elsevier.com/Linton/medsurg/ for additional activities and exercises.

NCLEX CATEGORIES:

Safe and Effective Care Environment: Safety and Infection Control

Health Promotion and Maintenance

Psychosocial Integrity

Physiological Integrity: Basic Care and Comfort, Pharmacological Therapies, Reduction of Risk Potential, Physiological Adaptation

OBJECTIVES

1. Describe the history of human immuno-deficiency virus and acquired immuno-deficiency syndrome.
2. Explain the pathophysiology and etiology of HIV infection.
3. List risk factors associated with human immunodeficiency virus infection.
4. Identify complications associated with human immunodeficiency virus infection.
5. Identify criteria for diagnosis of acquired immunodeficiency syndrome.
6. Name the major human immunodeficiency vi-rus drugs, indications, side effects, and nursing considerations.
7. Describe appropriate nursing care and patient teaching of the HIV and AIDS patient.

PART I: MASTERING THE BASICS

A. Key Terms.

Match the definition or description in the numbered column with the most appropriate term in the lettered column.

1. _____ Medication that interferes with the maturation of viral particles.

2. _____ Disease that is now viewed less as a fatal illness than as a manageable chronic condition.

3. _____ Medication regimen or a combination of drugs that is recommended when the viral load reaches certain levels.

4. _____ Retrovirus that causes AIDS.

A. AIDS (acquired immunodeficiency syndrome)
B. HAART (highly active antiretroviral therapy)
C. HIV (human immunodeficiency virus)
D. Protease inhibitor

B. Signs and Symptoms.

Which are common signs and symptoms of HIV infec-tion? Select all that apply.

1. Heart palpitations
2. Abdominal pain
3. Fever
4. Night sweats
5. Swollen lymph nodes

C. Major Complications.

Which of the following are major complications of HIV infection? Select all that apply.

1. Hemorrhage
2. Opportunistic infections
3. Weight loss
4. Edema
5. Dementia
6. Malnutrition

D. Wasting Syndrome.

Which factors contribute to the wasting syndrome experienced by patients with HIV infection? Select all that apply.

1. Liver disorder
2. Kidney failure
3. Malabsorption of nutrients
4. Reduced food intake

E. Cancers with HIV Infection.

List four types of cancers that may occur in 40% of patients with HIV infection.

1. _____

2. _____

3. _____

4. _____

F. Transmission of HIV.

How is HIV transmitted? Select all that apply.

1. Saliva
2. Breast milk
3. Semen
4. Urine
5. Blood
6. Vaginal fluids
7. Tears
8. Sweat

G. Opportunistic Infections.

Match the description in the numbered column with the opportunistic infection complication in the lettered column. Answers may be used more than once.

1. _____ People become infected by ingesting contaminated, undercooked meats or vegetables.
2. _____ Main symptom is severe, persistent, watery diarrhea.
3. _____ Second leading cause of death among AIDS patients.
4. _____ Occurs in about 80% of HIV patients.
5. _____ Mainly transmitted by blood and body fluids through unprotected sex.
6. _____ Infection starts with primary outbreak, then latency and possible reactivation later.
7. _____ Fungal infection with symptom of thrush.

8. _____ Symptoms include shortness of breath upon exertion, fever, and a nonproductive cough.

A. Candidiasis
B. *Pneumocystis jiroveci* pneumonia
C. Herpes simplex
D. Cytomegalovirus
E. Toxoplasmosis
F. Cryptosporidiosis

H. Oncologic Conditions.

Match the description in the numbered column with the oncological condition in the lettered column. Answers may be used more than once.

1. _____ Appears as a macular, painless, non-pruritic skin lesion
2. _____ Hypoxia may occur when respiratory system is affected
3. _____ A fever for more than 2 weeks is a symptom
4. _____ Avoiding unprotected sex is the only means of prevention
5. _____ Diagnosis by CT scan and lumbar puncture

A. Kaposi sarcoma
B. Lymphoma

I. Drug Therapy.

Match the description in the numbered column with the correct drug(s) used to treat patients with HIV infection in the lettered column. Answers may be used more than once, and some may not be used.

1. _____ Used in patients with HIV to slow the replication and progression of the virus by interfering with HIV replication inside the CD4 cell.
2. _____ Used in patients with HIV to slow the replication and progression of HIV by blocking an enzyme so that the infected cell cannot produce any more HIV proteins.

A. Nucleoside reverse transcriptase inhibitors (NRTIs) (AZT, Retrovir)
B. Protease inhibitors (Invirase, Norvir)
C. Non-nucleoside reverse transcriptase inhibitors (NNRTIs) (Viramune)

J. Explain why patients with HIV infection are at increased risk for cancer.

K. Diagnostic Bloodwork.

List four types of diagnostic bloodwork that may aid in the diagnosis of HIV infection. Select all that apply.

1. ELISA
2. Western blot
3. PTT
4. T cell count
5. Viral load count
6. Lipid profile

PART II: PUTTING IT ALL TOGETHER

L. Multiple Choice/Multiple Response.

Choose the most appropriate answer or select all that apply.

1. What is the leading cause of death in people with AIDS?
    1. Kaposi sarcoma
    2. Malnutrition
    3. Pneumonia
    4. Encephalopathy

2. About how long after infection does the body produce enough antibodies to be detected by standard HIV testing?
    1. 2–3 days
    2. 1 week
    3. 12 weeks
    4. 6 months

3. Which substances remain at high levels throughout the course of HIV infection?
    1. HIV antibodies
    2. CD8 cells
    3. CD4 cells
    4. Red blood cells

4. Antiviral medications are given to patients with HIV infection to:
    1. prevent viral replication and destroy infected cells.
    2. destroy viral cells that are infected.
    3. slow viral replication and progression.
    4. destroy bacteria and prevent infection.

5. Which test for HIV infection is the most reliable diagnostic test?
    1. ELISA
    2. Western Blot
    3. CD4 count
    4. CD8 count

6. How many newly diagnosed HIV infections occur annually in the United States?
    1. 20,000
    2. 40,000
    3. 100,000
    4. 540,000

7. Which drug is used to treat opportunistic fungal infections in people with HIV infection?
    1. AZT
    2. Retrovir
    3. Amphotericin B
    4. Bactrim

8. Which opportunistic infection is treated with Bactrim and Pentamidine?
    1. *Pneumocystis jiroveci* pneumonia
    2. Candidiasis
    3. Histoplasmosis
    4. Cytomegalovirus

9. What is the usual combination of drugs for HIV patients who are started on the medication regimen called HAART?
    1. Antimicrobials and protease inhibitor
    2. NRTIs and protease inhibitor
    3. NRTIs and NNRTIs
    4. Antimycotics and NNRTIs

10. What is the most serious problem with HAART therapy?
    1. Resistance
    2. Hypolipidemia
    3. Renal failure
    4. Infection

11. What type of cells does HIV gradually destroy that are essential for resisting pathogens?
    1. Neutrophils
    2. T4 cells
    3. B cells
    4. Eosinophils

12. HIV is passed from person to person primarily through:
    1. air droplet contact.
    2. hand-to-mouth contact.
    3. exposure to bodily fluids.
    4. mouth-to-mouth contact.

13. The leading cause of death in people with AIDS is:
    1. herpes zoster.
    2. dermatitis.
    3. pneumonia.
    4. Kaposi sarcoma.

14. For many women, one of the first symptoms of HIV infection is:
    1. vaginal candidiasis.
    2. burning on urination.
    3. menstrual irregularities.
    4. hemorrhoids.

15. A type of skin cancer that has dramatically increased as a result of AIDS is:
    1. *Pneumocystis jiroveci* pneumonia.
    2. melanoma.
    3. Kaposi sarcoma
    4. venereal warts.

16. The medical treatment of HIV infection includes the use of zidovudine (AZT, Retrovir), which is given to:
    1. cure AIDS.
    2. prevent transmission to sexual partners.
    3. treat the secondary infections of AIDS.
    4. slow the progress of AIDS.

17. Drugs such as clindamycin, Pentamidine, and Bactrim are used to:
    1. prevent or treat opportunistic infections.
    2. slow the progress of AIDS.
    3. decrease the dermatitis associated with AIDS.
    4. increase T4 lymphocytes.

18. The risk of transmission of HIV increases with:
    1. donating blood.
    2. unprotected sex.
    3. hugging and kissing.
    4. using restrooms.

19. The transmission of HIV can occur through:
    1. saliva.
    2. sweat.
    3. urine.
    4. blood.

20. The patient with AIDS is at high risk for opportunistic infections because of:
    1. altered skin integrity.
    2. increased HIV antibodies.
    3. decreased CD4 cells.
    4. fatigue.

21. Patients with AIDS may have disturbed thought processes due to:
    1. anxiety.
    2. dementia.
    3. anemia.
    4. brain damage.

22. As the number of CD4 cell counts decreases, the patient becomes increasingly susceptible to:
    1. myelosuppression.
    2. anemia.
    3. tuberculosis.
    4. opportunistic infections.

23. Which tissue can be infected by HIV?
    1. Pancreas
    2. Stomach
    3. Kidney
    4. Lymph nodes

24. Which of the following diagnostic tools are included in the examination of patients with HIV? Select all that apply.
    1. CD4 count
    2. HIV viral load
    3. CBC
    4. Lipid profile
    5. Electrolyte screen
    6. BUN
    7. Toxoplasmosis antibody titers

PART III: CHALLENGE YOURSELF!

M. Getting Ready for NCLEX.

Choose the most appropriate answer or select all that apply.

1. Which of the following are teaching points for patients with toxoplasmosis? Select all that apply.
   1. Avoid dark green vegetables
   2. Avoid undercooked raw meats
   3. Practice good hand hygiene
   4. Prevent dehydration
   5. Avoid cat litterboxes
   6. Avoid ingestion of potentially contaminated water

2. Which are common side effects of HAART therapy? Select all that apply.
   1. Decreased triglycerides
   2. Increased cholesterol
   3. Nausea and vomiting
   4. Peripheral neuropathy

3. Which are nutrition teaching points for the patient with HIV? Select all that apply.
   1. Thoroughly cook meats and poultry.
   2. Thaw frozen foods at room temperature.
   3. Eat small, frequent meals high in lactose.
   4. Eat meals low in fat.

4. Which are common nursing diagnoses for patients with HIV infection? Select all that apply.
   1. Risk for aspiration
   2. Anxiety
   3. Risk for injury
   4. Fluid volume excess
   5. Imbalanced nutrition
   6. Urinary stress incontinence
   7. Impaired oral mucous membranes

5. What is one of the major reasons for noncompliance among patients receiving HAART therapy?
   1. Muscle weakness
   2. Nightmares
   3. Gastrointestinal upset
   4. Hypersensitivity reactions

6. Which of the following are signs and symptoms during the later stages of AIDS? Select all that apply.
   1. Fever
   2. Hypertension
   3. Confusion
   4. Weight loss
   5. Night sweats
   6. Swollen lymph nodes

7. The best way to prevent transmission of HIV is to:
   1. use condoms during all sexual contact.
   2. wash hands thoroughly following contact with HIV-positive people.
   3. avoid risky behaviors.
   4. get plenty of rest and eat a nutritious diet.

8. Which are therapeutic communication techniques that the nurse can use to show support for patients with HIV infection? Select all that apply.
   1. Be reassuring.
   2. Be positive.
   3. Be accepting.
   4. Be sensitive.
   5. Be courteous.

Nursing Care Plan.

Refer to Nursing Care Plan, The Patient with HIV Infection, p. 659 in the textbook, and answer questions 9-10.

9. What is the priority nursing diagnosis for this patient with HIV infection?

10. Which nursing interventions for this patient could be assigned to unlicensed assistive personnel? Select all that apply.
    1. Advise patient of the kinds of side- and adverse effects that she might experience.
    2. Explain the importance of continuing the drugs under medical supervision.
    3. Discuss ways to conserve energy.
    4. Assist patient with ambulation.
    5. Weigh weekly.
    6. Assist with oral hygiene.

Cardiac Disorders

 Go to http://evolve.elsevier.com/Linton/medsurg/ for additional activities and exercises.

NCLEX CATEGORIES:

Safe and Effective Care Environment: Safety and Infection Control

Health Promotion and Maintenance

Psychosocial Integrity

Physiological Integrity: Basic Care and Comfort, Pharmacological Therapies, Reduction of Risk Potential, Physiological Adaptation

OBJECTIVES

1. Label the major parts of the heart.
2. Describe the flow of blood through the heart and coronary vessels.
3. Name the elements of the heart's conduction system.
4. State the order in which normal impulses are conducted through the heart.
5. Explain the nursing considerations for patients having procedures to detect or evaluate cardiac disorders.
6. Identify nursing implications for common therapeutic measures, including drug, diet, or oxygen therapy; pacemakers and cardioverters; cardiac surgery; and cardiopulmonary resuscitation.
7. Explain the pathophysiology, risk factors, signs and symptoms, complications, and treatment for selected cardiac disorders.
8. List the data to be obtained in assessing the patient with a cardiac disorder.
9. Assist in developing nursing care plans for patients with cardiac disorders.

PART I: MASTERING THE BASICS

A. Key Terms.

Match the definition or description in the numbered column with the most appropriate term in the lettered column.

1. _____ Slow heart rate, usually defined as fewer than 60 beats per minute (bpm)

2. _____ Rapid heart rate, usually defined as greater than 100 bpm

3. _____ Abnormal thickening and hardening of the arterial walls caused by fat and fibrin deposits

4. _____ Obstruction of a blood vessel with a blood clot transported through the bloodstream

5. _____ A sound heard on auscultation of the heart that usually indicates turbulent blood flow across heart valves

6. _____ Abnormal thickening, hardening, and loss of elasticity of the arterial walls

7. _____ The amount of blood in a ventricle at the end of diastole; the pressure generated at the end of diastole

8. _____ Disturbance of rhythm; arrhythmia

9. _____ Study of the movement of blood and the forces that affect it

10. _____ A heartbeat that is strong, rapid, or irregular enough that the person is aware of it

11. _____ Fainting

12. _____ The amount of resistance the ventricles must overcome to eject the blood volume

13. _____ Backward flow

14. _____ Death of myocardial tissue caused by prolonged lack of blood and oxygen supply

15. _____ Passage of blood through the vessels of an organ

A. Murmur
B. Thromboembolism
C. Hemodynamics
D. Regurgitation
E. Syncope
F. Atherosclerosis
G. Bradycardia
H. Perfusion
I. Preload
J. Myocardial infarction
K. Palpitation
L. Tachycardia
M. Afterload
N. Arteriosclerosis
O. Dysrhythmia

B. Cardiac Function.
Match the definition or description in the numbered column with the most appropriate term in the lettered column.

1. _____ The delivery of a synchronized electric shock to the myocardium to restore normal sinus rhythm

2. _____ Place where electrical impulse is initiated in heart

3. _____ Terminal ends of bundle branches that cause ventricles to contract

4. _____ The amount of blood (measured in liters) ejected by each ventricle per minute

5. _____ Adaptations made by the heart and circulation to maintain normal cardiac output

6. _____ The ability of a cell to generate an impulse without external stimulation

7. _____ The ability of cardiac muscle to shorten and contract

8. _____ Enlargement of existing cells, resulting in increased size of an organ or tissue

9. _____ A wall that divides a body cavity

10. _____ Termination of fibrillation, usually by electric shock

11. _____ Contraction phase of the cardiac cycle

12. _____ The ability of the cell to transmit electrical impulses rapidly and efficiently to distant regions of the heart

13. _____ Formation of a blood clot

14. _____ Relaxation phase of the cardiac cycle

A. Cardiac output
B. Systole
C. Conductivity
D. SA node
E. Compensation
F. Defibrillation
G. Contractility
H. Cardioversion
I. Diastole
J. Hypertrophy
K. Purkinje fibers
L. Thrombosis
M. Septum
N. Automaticity

C. Cardiac Innervation.
Which of the following are increased by the sympathetic nervous system? Select all that apply.
1. Amount of blood in the ventricles
2. Heart rate
3. Force of contractions
4. Speed of conduction through the AV node

D. Preload and Afterload.

1. Which are factors that increase preload? Select all that apply.
   1. Dehydration
   2. Hemorrhage
   3. Increased venous return to the heart
   4. Overhydration
   5. Venous vasodilation

2. Which are factors that increase afterload? Select all that apply.
   1. Vasodilation
   2. Hypertension
   3. Vasoconstriction
   4. Aortic stenosis

E. Age-Related Changes.

Which are age-related changes in the heart? Select all that apply.

1. Decreased density of heart muscle connective tissue
2. Decreased elasticity of myocardium
3. Increased cardiac contractility
4. Valves may thicken and stiffen
5. Emptying of chambers may be incomplete
6. Increased number of pacemaker cells in the SA node
7. Increased number of nerve fibers in ventricles
8. Cardiac response to stress is slower

F. Diagnostic Blood Tests.

Match the characteristic of laboratory tests in the numbered column with the appropriate test in the lettered column.

1. _____ Indicates the body's ability to defend itself against infection and inflammation; elevated with acute myocardial infarction (AMI)
2. _____ Indicates damage to myocardial cells
3. _____ Protein found in cardiac muscle
4. _____ Determination of body's ability to maintain acid-base balance

A. Myoglobin
B. Arterial blood gas
C. Creatine phosphokinase (CPK)
D. WBC

G. Heart Chambers.

Match the characteristic in the numbered column with the appropriate heart chamber in the lettered column. Some terms may be used more than once.

1. _____ Contains the highest pressure in the heart
2. _____ Receives blood through the tricuspid valve
3. _____ Cone-shaped, has the thickest muscle mass of the four chambers
4. _____ Receives blood saturated with oxygen from the four pulmonary veins
5. _____ Receives blood from the inferior and superior vena cava

A. Right atrium (RA)
B. Right ventricle (RV)
C. Left atrium (LA)
D. Left ventricle (LV)

H. Diagnostic Procedures.

Match the definition or description in the numbered column with the appropriate diagnostic test or procedure in the lettered column. Some answers may be used more than once.

1. _____ An ambulatory ECG that provides continuous monitoring
2. _____ A transducer used to pick up sound waves and convert them to electrical impulses
3. _____ A high-resolution, three-dimensional image of the heart; cardiac tissue is imaged without lung or bone interference
4. _____ An exercise tolerance test that is a recording of an individual's cardiovascular response during a measured exercise challenge
5. _____ Study of electrical activity of the heart
6. _____ A procedure in which a catheter is advanced into the heart chambers or coronary arteries under fluoroscopy
7. _____ Test that may determine pressures in the RA, RV, and pulmonary artery
8. _____ Electrodes placed on the surface of the skin pick up the electrical impulses of the heart
9. _____ The patient ambulates on a treadmill or a stationary bicycle while connected to a monitor
10. _____ Heart ultrasound that is a visualization and recording of the size, shape, position, and behavior of the heart's internal structures
11. _____ Noninvasive measurement of oxygen saturation
12. _____ Use of catheters with multiple electrodes inserted through the femoral vein to record the heart's electrical activity
13. _____ Fast form of imaging technology that allows for high-quality images of the heart as it contracts and relaxes

A. Stress test
B. Cardiac catheterization
C. Electrocardiogram (ECG)
D. Echocardiogram
E. Electrophysiology study (EPS)
F. MRI
G. Holter monitor
H. Pulse oximetry
I. Ultrafast computed tomography (electron-beam CT)

I. Complications of Coronary Artery Disease.

Match the description of complications of coronary artery disease (CAD) in the numbered column with the most appropriate term in the lettered column. Some terms may not be used.

1. _____ Disturbances in heart rhythm
2. _____ When the injured left ventricle is unable to meet the body's circulatory demands
3. _____ The most frequent cause of death after an AMI; marked by hypotension and decreasing alertness
4. _____ When clots form in the injured heart chambers, they may break loose and travel to the lung
5. _____ A fatal complication in which weakened areas of the ventricular wall bulge and burst

A. Ventricular aneurysm/rupture
B. Mitral stenosis
C. Dysrhythmias
D. Hemorrhage
E. Cardiogenic shock
F. Thromboembolism
G. Heart failure

J. Mitral Stenosis.

Complete the statement in the numbered column with the most appropriate term in the lettered column. Some terms may not be used.

1. _____ The leading cause of mitral stenosis
2. _____ The chamber of the heart that dilates to accommodate the amount of blood not ejected in patients with mitral stenosis

3. _____ When collecting data for the assessment of the patient with mitral stenosis, the nurse takes the vital signs and auscultates for _____.

A. Heart murmur
B. Rheumatic heart disease
C. Left ventricle
D. Left atrium
E. Right ventricle

K. Drug Therapy.

1. Match the drug classification in the numbered column with its use and action in the lettered column.

1. _____ Diuretics
2. _____ Antianginals
3. _____ Antiplatelets
4. _____ Cardiac glycosides
5. _____ Thrombolytics

A. Increase cardiac output
B. Dissolve clots
C. Prevent strokes
D. Decrease fluid retention
E. Relieve pain

2. Match the drug used for cardiac disorders in the numbered column with its classification in the lettered column. Some terms may not be used.

1. _____ Nitroglycerin
2. _____ Aspirin, dipyridamole (Persantine), and clopidogrel (Plavix)
3. _____ Heparin and warfarin (Coumadin)
4. _____ Morphine and meperidine hydrochloride (Demerol)
5. _____ Furosemide (Lasix) and hydrochlorothiazide (Esidrix, HCTZ, and Oretic)
6. _____ Streptokinase, sotalol hydrochloride (Betapace), and tissue plasminogen activator
7. _____ Digoxin (Lanoxin) and digitoxin

A. Anticholinergics
B. Antianginals
C. Analgesics
D. Antiplatelet agents
E. Antidysrhythmics
F. Diuretics
G. Fibrinolytics (antithrombolytics)
H. Anticoagulants
I. Cardiac glycosides
J. ACE inhibitors

L. Drug Therapy.

Match the use(s) of AMI drug therapy in the numbered column with the specific drug in the lettered column. Some drugs may be used more than once, and some may not be used.

1. _____ Used for chest pain
2. _____ Administered through an IV or into the coronary arteries to dissolve thrombi
3. _____ Following the administration of antithrombolytics, this drug is administered to prevent further clot formation
4. _____ Administered for ventricular tachy-cardia
5. _____ Increases myocardial contractility and decreases the heart rate

A. Furosemide (Lasix)
B. Streptokinase
C. Digitalis
D. Morphine sulfate
E. Atropine sulfate
F. Lidocaine
G. Heparin

M. ECG.

Match the ECG change in the numbered column with the feature of AMI in the lettered column.

1. _____ The T wave is inverted.
2. _____ There is ST segment elevation.
3. _____ A significant Q wave is present; the Q wave is greater than one-third the height of the R wave.

A. Ischemia
B. Infarction
C. Injury

N. Heart Failure.

For the following signs and symptoms of heart failure (HF), indicate whether they are indicative of (A) right-sided or (B) left-sided failure.

1. _____ Dependent edema
2. _____ Decreasing BP readings
3. _____ Increased central venous pressure
4. _____ Anxious, pale, and tachycardic
5. _____ Jugular vein distention
6. _____ Abdominal engorgement
7. _____ Crackles, wheezes, dyspnea, and cough
8. _____ Pulmonary edema
9. _____ Decreased urinary output

O. Drug Therapy.

Match the actions of drugs used to treat heart failure in the numbered column with the drug or drug classification in the lettered column. Some answers may be used more than once, and some answers may not be used.

1. _____ Improve(s) pump function by increasing contractility and decreasing heart rate
2. _____ Decrease(s) circulating fluid volume and decrease(s) preload
3. _____ Decrease(s) anxiety, dilate(s) the vasculature, and reduce(s) myocardial consumption in the acute stage

A. Heparin
B. Morphine
C. Diuretics
D. Streptokinase
E. Cardiac glycosides or inotropic agents such as digoxin

P. Heart Failure.

Match the nursing diagnosis for the patient with heart failure in the numbered column with the "related to" statement in the lettered column.

1. _____ Fluid volume excess
2. _____ Impaired gas exchange
3. _____ Anxiety
4. _____ Decreased cardiac output
5. _____ Activity intolerance

A. Inability to perform activities
B. Decreased pulmonary perfusion
C. Mechanical failure
D. Ineffective cardiac pumping
E. Edema and inability to breathe

Q. Heart Circulation.
In the Figure 35-2 (p. 665) below, label the parts (A–M) of the heart.

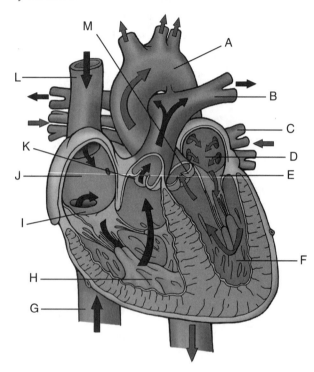

A. _____
B. _____
C. _____
D. _____
E. _____
F. _____
G. _____
H. _____
I. _____
J. _____
K. _____
L. _____
M. _____

R. Conduction System.
In the Figure 35-4 below (p. 667), label the parts (A–E) of the conduction system of the heart.

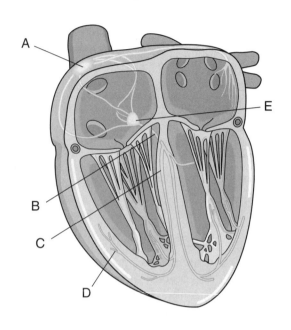

A. _____
B. _____
C. _____
D. _____
E. _____

PART II: PUTTING IT ALL TOGETHER

S. Multiple Choice/Multiple Response.
Choose the most appropriate answer or select all that apply.

1. The pressure is highest in which heart chamber?
   1. Right atrium
   2. Left atrium
   3. Right ventricle
   4. Left ventricle

2. The first branches of the systemic circulation are the:
   1. subclavian arteries.
   2. coronary arteries.
   3. carotid arteries.
   4. brachial arteries.

3. The ventricles contract when the electrical impulse reaches the:
   1. SA node.
   2. AV node.
   3. Purkinje fibers.
   4. bundle of His.

4. Stroke volume, the amount of blood ejected with each ventricular contraction, depends on myocardial:
   1. contractility.
   2. excitability.
   3. conductivity.
   4. automaticity.

5. If the valves of the heart do not close properly, the patient is said to have:
   1. infarction.
   2. murmur.
   3. necrosis.
   4. tachycardia.

6. Which are ways to increase oxygen supply to the myocardium? Select all that apply.
   1. Administer supplemental oxygen.
   2. Increase the rate of myocardial contraction.
   3. Coronary artery vasodilation.
   4. Increase antiplatelet activity.

7. Which of the following is more likely to occur in older adults as the cardiovascular system adapts more slowly to changes in position?
   1. Tachycardia
   2. Bradycardia
   3. Postural hypotension
   4. Headache

8. A noninvasive measure of cardiac output is:
   1. cardiac catheterization.
   2. pulse pressure.
   3. angioplasty.
   4. blood gas measurement.

9. A normal ECG finding is documented as a normal:
   1. tachycardia.
   2. sinus rhythm.
   3. bradycardia.
   4. ventricular gallop.

10. The patient is taking a stress test. Which of the following symptoms require that the stress test be stopped immediately? Select all that apply.
    1. Angina
    2. Increased heart rate
    3. Diaphoresis
    4. Slower respirations
    5. Falling blood pressure

11. The normal cardiac output is:
    1. 1–3 liters/min.
    2. 4–8 liters/min.
    3. 10–13 liters/min.
    4. 15–20 liters/hour.

12. Patients with AMI often exhibit:
    1. respiratory acidosis.
    2. respiratory alkalosis.
    3. elevated cholesterol levels.
    4. decreased WBC count.

13. What type of diet is generally recommended for cardiac patients?
    1. Low-fat, high-calcium
    2. Low-fat, high-fiber
    3. Low-sodium, low-protein
    4. High-sodium, low-potassium

14. If fluid retention accompanies the cardiac problem, the physician may order restriction of:
    1. potassium.
    2. sodium.
    3. fat.
    4. calcium.

15. The purpose of temporary and permanent pacemakers is to improve cardiac output and tissue perfusion by restoring regular:
    1. blood volume.
    2. blood pressure.
    3. impulse conduction.
    4. myocardial contractility.

16. The delivery of a synchronized shock to terminate atrial or ventricular tachyarrhythmias is called:
    1. a pacemaker.
    2. cardiac catheterization.
    3. angioplasty.
    4. cardioversion.

17. During open-heart surgery, the patient's core temperature is reduced to decrease the body's need for:
    1. oxygen.
    2. sodium.
    3. potassium.
    4. ATP.

18. The substernal pain resulting from lack of oxygen to the myocardium is called:
    1. heartburn.
    2 dyspnea.
    3. pleurisy.
    4. angina pectoris.

19. Nurses should be alert to complaints of decreased exercise tolerance and dyspnea in African-American males because they are at risk for:
    1. hypertension.
    2. cardiomyopathy.
    3. endocarditis.
    4. mitral valve stenosis.

20. Which drug is administered to dilate coronary arteries and increase blood flow to the damaged area of a patient with AMI?
    1. Nitroglycerin
    2. Furosemide
    3. Dipyridamole (Persantine)
    4. Streptokinase

21. Which veins are generally used in coronary artery bypass surgery as grafts? Select all that apply.
    1. Subclavian
    2. Femoral
    3. Internal mammary
    4. Saphenous

22. What are the reasons for placing patients with HF in a semi-Fowler's or high-Fowler's position? Select all that apply.
    1. Decrease cardiac workload
    2. Decrease aspiration
    3. Lessen fatigue
    4. Decrease pain
    5. Increase oxygenation to the myocardium

23. The most common adverse effects of diuretic therapy for patients with HF are:
    1. hypertension and tachycardia.
    2. fluid and electrolyte imbalances.
    3. headache and oliguria.
    4. confusion and weakness.

24. A common finding in patients with right-sided HF is:
    1. increased urinary output.
    2. dependent edema.
    3. weight loss.
    4. cough.

25. The most common site for organisms to accumulate in patients with infective endocarditis is the:
    1. mitral valve.
    2. tricuspid valve.
    3. aortic valve.
    4. pulmonary valve.

26. The main drugs used for endocarditis are:
    1. cardiac glycosides.
    2. diuretics.
    3. calcium channel blockers.
    4. antimicrobials.

27. The hallmark symptom of pericarditis is:
    1. chest pain.
    2. headache.
    3. hypertension.
    4. indigestion.

28. A procedure in which a peripherally inserted catheter is passed into an occluded artery and a balloon is inflated to dilate the artery is:
    1. percutaneous transluminal angioplasty (PCTA).
    2. coronary atherectomy.
    3. intracoronary stent placement.
    4. laser angioplasty.

29. Lifelong medications that must be given to patients with heart transplants include:
    1. antihistamines.
    2. analgesics.
    3. antimicrobials.
    4. immunosuppressives.

30. The two major valve problems of the heart are stenosis and:
    1. inflammation.
    2. regurgitation.
    3. emboli.
    4. hemorrhage.

31. Before each dose of digitalis, the apical pulse is counted for 1 full minute; the drug is withheld and the physician notified if the pulse is below:
    1. 60 bpm.
    2. 70 bpm.
    3. 72 bpm.
    4. 80 bpm.

32. Which are actions of antidysrhythmic drugs? Select all that apply.
    1. Increasing contractility
    2. Enhancing inotropism
    3. Depressing automaticity
    4. Stimulating the SA node
    5. Slowing impulse conduction
    6. Increasing resistance to premature contraction

33. An automatic implantable cardioverter-defibrillator is used to:
    1. improve contractility in people with cardiomyopathy.
    2. decrease the risk of sudden cardiac death in people with recurrent life-threatening dysrhythmias.
    3. convert patients in cardiac arrest to normal sinus rhythm.
    4. support cardiac function in patients awaiting heart transplants.

34. The internal cardiac defibrillator is used to treat patients with life-threatening, recurrent:
    1. hypertension.
    2. aortic stenosis.
    3. ventricular fibrillation.
    4. endocarditis.

35. A Swan-Ganz catheter is inserted into the pulmonary artery to measure:
    1. tricuspid valve function.
    2. right-sided heart pressure.
    3. mitral valve stenosis.
    4. aortic stenosis.

36. How should the nurse document a pulse that is easily obliterated by slight finger pressure, which returns as the pressure is released?
    1. Absent
    2. Nonpalpable
    3. Weak or thready
    4. Bounding

37. Which heart sound is normal in children and young adults but is pathologic if it is heard after the age of 30?
    1. S_1
    2. S_2
    3. S_3, ventricular gallop
    4. S_4, atrial gallop

38. What type of drug therapy is used after an AMI to prevent strokes?
    1. Cardiac glycosides
    2. Antidysrhythmics
    3. Antiplatelets
    4. Nitrates

39. The most widely used drugs in the treatment of HF are:
    1. cardiac glycosides.
    2. antianginals.
    3. antidysrhythmics.
    4. adrenergic beta-blockers.

40. The first medication given to patients with chest pain is:
    1. morphine.
    2. aspirin.
    3. Demerol.
    4. nitroglycerin.

41. Which herb taken to lower plasma lipids may increase the effects of anticoagulants and insulin?
    1. Kava kava
    2. Ephedra
    3. Garlic
    4. Aloe

42. If dietary control does not reduce cholesterol sufficiently, treatment may include:
    1. antihypertensives.
    2. antidysrhythmics.
    3. antianginals.
    4. lipid-lowering agents.

43. Questran, Lopid, and niacin are drugs classified as:
    1. cardiac glycosides.
    2. nitrates.
    3. lipid-lowering drugs.
    4. antiplatelets.

44. Which is an age-related change to blood vessels?
    1. Vessels become thinner.
    2. Systolic blood pressure increases.
    3. Pulse pressure decreases.
    4. Veins constrict.

45. The pain of heart problems may radiate or may be referred to other areas. Which are areas to which pain may radiate? Select all that apply.
    1. Down either arm
    2. Just below the sternum
    3. Umbilicus
    4. Jaw

46. What are reasons that PTCA may be a preferred treatment over bypass surgery? Select all that apply.
    1. Done under local anesthesia instead of general anesthesia
    2. Less invasive than bypass surgery
    3. Faster recovery time
    4. Tiny holes are drilled in the myocardium using a laser

47. Which drugs decrease cardiac contractility?
    1. Beta blockers
    2. Catecholamines
    3. Antiplatelets
    4. Thrombolytics

PART III: CHALLENGE YOURSELF!

T. Getting Ready for NCLEX.

Choose the most appropriate answer or select all that apply.

1. Which of the following drugs are used to treat angina? Select all that apply.
   1. Antidysrhythmics
   2. Nitrates
   3. Beta-adrenergic blockers
   4. Antiplatelets
   5. Calcium channel blockers
   6. Diuretics

2. Which of the following are words that patients with stable angina use to describe anginal pain? Select all that apply.
   1. Burning
   2. Squeezing
   3. Aching
   4. Dull
   5. Vise-like
   6. Smothering

3. Which findings would the nurse expect to observe in patients with mitral stenosis? Select all that apply.
   1. Bradycardia
   2. Tachypnea
   3. Increasing pulse pressure
   4. Jugular vein distention
   5. Wheezing lung sounds
   6. Rumbling, low-pitched murmur sounds

4. Which nursing diagnoses are likely to be present in a patient with AMI? Select all that apply.
   1. Ineffective thermoregulation
   2. Decreased cardiac output
   3. Anxiety
   4. Pain
   5. Risk for infection

5. When the nurse is asking cardiac patients about their diets, which areas of intake should the nurse especially record information? Select all that apply.
   1. Calcium
   2. Vitamin D
   3. Salt
   4. Protein
   5. Fat
   6. Iron

6. Which are modifiable risk factors for atherosclerosis? Select all that apply.
   1. Tobacco use
   2. High blood pressure
   3. Sedentary lifestyle
   4. Age
   5. Heredity
   6. Ethnicity
   7. Obesity

7. Heparin dosage for the patient with a cardiac disorder is adjusted according to the patient's:
   1. hemoglobin.
   2. prothrombin time.
   3. partial thromboplastin time.
   4. hematocrit.

Nursing Care Plan.

Refer to Nursing Care Plan, The Patient with Heart Failure, p. 703 in the textbook, and answer questions 8-13.

8. Which abnormal findings were found on physical examination for this patient related to heart failure?

   1. _____

   2. _____

   3. _____

   4. _____

   5. _____

   6. _____

   7. _____

   8. _____

   9. _____

   10. _____

9. What is the priority nursing diagnosis for this patient?

10. Why is this patient more susceptible to adverse drug effects?

11. If she is started on digitalis, what are early signs of digitalis toxicity that the nurse would be watching for?

12. Why is it important for her to remain on bedrest?

13. Which tasks can be assigned to unlicensed assistive personnel?

Vascular Disorders

 Go to http://evolve.elsevier.com/Linton/medsurg/ for additional activities and exercises.

NCLEX CATEGORIES:

Safe and Effective Care Environment:
Coordinated Care, Safety and Infection Control

Health Promotion and Maintenance

Psychosocial Integrity

Physiological Integrity: Basic Care and Comfort, Pharmacological Therapies, Reduction of Risk Potential, Physiological Adaptation

OBJECTIVES

1. Identify specific anatomic and physiologic factors that affect the vascular system and tissue oxygenation.
2. Indicate appropriate parameters for assessing a patient with peripheral vascular disease, aneurysm, and aortic dissection.
3. Discuss tests and procedures used to diagnose selected vascular disorders and the nursing considerations for each.
4. Describe the pathophysiology, signs and symptoms, complications, and medical or surgical treatments for selected vascular disorders.
5. Assist in developing a plan of care for patients with selected vascular disorders.

PART I: MASTERING THE BASICS

A. Key Terms.
Match the definition in the numbered column with the most appropriate term in the lettered column.

1. _____ Sudden obstruction of an artery by a floating clot or foreign material

2. _____ An abnormal sensation

3. _____ Concentration of the blood

4. _____ Development of a clot in the presence of venous inflammation

5. _____ Deficient blood flow due to obstruction or constriction of blood vessels

6. _____ Increase in blood vessel diameter

7. _____ Development of venous thrombi without venous inflammation

8. _____ Inflammation of a vein

9. _____ Coolness in an area of the body due to decreased blood flow

10. _____ Thickness of the blood

11. _____ Development or presence of a thrombus

12. _____ Dilated segment of an artery caused by weakness and stretching of the vessel wall

13. _____ Murmur detected by auscultation

A. Thrombophlebitis
B. Thrombosis
C. Phlebothrombosis
D. Embolism
E. Phlebitis
F. Paresthesia
G. Bruit
H. Ischemia
I. Aneurysm
J. Hemoconcentration
K. Poikilothermy
L. Vasodilation
M. Viscosity

B. Vascular System.

Match the definition or description in the numbered column with the most appropriate term in the lettered column. Some terms may be used more than once, and some may not be used.

1. _____ Vessels that return blood to the heart
2. _____ The two main trunks of these vessels are the thoracic duct and the right lymphatic duct
3. _____ Thick-walled, elastic structures
4. _____ Equipped with valves that aid in the transportation of blood against gravity
5. _____ Formed by a single layer of endothelial cells
6. _____ Vessels that carry blood away from the heart
7. _____ Transfer of oxygen and nutrients between the blood and the tissue cells occurs here
8. _____ Thin-walled vessels that collect and drain fluid from the peripheral tissues and transport the fluid to the venous system

A. Veins
B. Valves
C. Leaflets
D. Capillaries
E. Lymph vessels
F. Arteries
G. Lymph nodes

C. Peripheral Resistance.

Indicate for each factor in the numbered column whether it (A) increases or (B) decreases peripheral resistance.

1. _____ Sympathetic nervous system stimulation
2. _____ Epinephrine
3. _____ Angiotensin
4. _____ Vasoconstriction
5. _____ Viscous blood
6. _____ Vasodilation
7. _____ Histamine
8. _____ Prostaglandins

D. Peripheral Vascular Disease.

Match the description in the numbered column with the 6 Ps—characteristics of peripheral vascular disease in the lettered column. Answers may be used more than once.

1. _____ Decreased temperature at an ischemic site
2. _____ Paleness apparent over an area of reduced blood supply
3. _____ Associated with intermittent claudication
4. _____ Detected by palpating the affected and surrounding areas
5. _____ Determined by palpating peripheral pulses for rate, rhythm, and quality
6. _____ Abnormal sensation such as numbness, tingling, or crawling sensation
7. _____ Impairment of motor function
8. _____ Characterized by "pins and needles" sensation
9. _____ Described by patients as tenderness, heaviness, or fullness in the extremity

A. Pain
B. Pulselessness
C. Poikilothermy
D. Pallor
E. Paresthesia
F. Paralysis

E. Physical Examination.

Match the statement in the numbered column with the most appropriate term in the lettered column. Some terms may be used more than once, and some may not be used.

1. _____ A test to evaluate the pain response in the calf area that may help to determine venous thrombosis
2. _____ A test used to determine the patency of the ulnar and radial artery
3. _____ Sounds made when blood flowing through the arteries sounds like turbulent, fast-moving fluid
4. _____ Brown pigmentation sites with flaky skin over the edematous areas of the ankles

A. Bruits
B. Babinski's reflex
C. Allen's test
D. Moro's reflex
E. Homans sign
F. Stasis dermatitis

F. Diagnostic Procedures.
Match the statements in the numbered column with the most appropriate term in the lettered column. Some terms may not be used.

1. _____ A noninvasive, inexpensive diagnostic tool in which sound waves are directed toward the artery or vein being tested

2. _____ A noninvasive examination that measures the blood volume and graphs changes in the flow of blood and is often used for patients too ill to undergo arteriography

3. _____ Associated with the segmental limb pressure test and pulse volume measurement test

4. _____ An invasive procedure that requires the injection of dye into the vascular system

5. _____ A test that measures pulse volumes before and after exercise

A. Pressure measurement
B. Treadmill test
C. Angiography
D. Doppler ultrasound
E. Plethysmography

G. Surgical Procedures.

1. Match the description or definition in the numbered column with the most appropriate term in the lettered column.

   1. _____ The injection of a chemical that irritates the venous endothelium for patients with varicose veins
   2. _____ A procedure that is done to relieve arterial stenosis in people who are poor surgical risks
   3. _____ A procedure used to remove varicose veins
   4. _____ An incision into the obstructed vessel to strip away emboli and

atherosclerotic plaque followed by surgical closure of the vessel
5. _____ The excision of the sympathetic ganglia; used for patients with intermittent claudication
6. _____ The removal of a blood clot located in a large vessel

A. Sympathectomy
B. Percutaneous transluminal angioplasty (PCTA)
C. Embolectomy
D Sclerotherapy
E. Vein ligation and stripping
F. Endarterectomy

H. Drug Therapy.
Which are classifications of drugs that are used in the general management of peripheral vascular disease to improve peripheral circulation? Select all that apply.
1. Antimicrobials
2. Diuretics
3. Anticoagulants
4. Thrombolytics

I. Drug Therapy.
Which drugs are used to treat Raynaud disease? Select all that apply.
1. Thrombolytics
2. Calcium channel blockers
3. Anticoagulants
4. Bosentan (endothelin receptor antagonist)
5. Sildenafil (phosphodiesterase inhibitor)
6. Vasodilators
7. Analgesics
8. Antidysrhythmics
9. Beta adrenergic blockers

J. Anticoagulants.
List two primary anticoagulants and their antidotes.

1. Oral drug and antidote: _____

   _____

2. Parenteral drug and antidote: _____

   _____

K. Tissue Layers of Veins and Arteries.

Using Figure 36-2 (textbook p. 725) and the word bank below, label the structures of the artery, vein, and capillary using the following numbers. Structures may be used more than once.

1. Tunica adventitia
2. Endothelial cells
3. Tunica media
4. External elastic membrane

5. Tunica intima
6. Internal elastic membrane
7. Valve

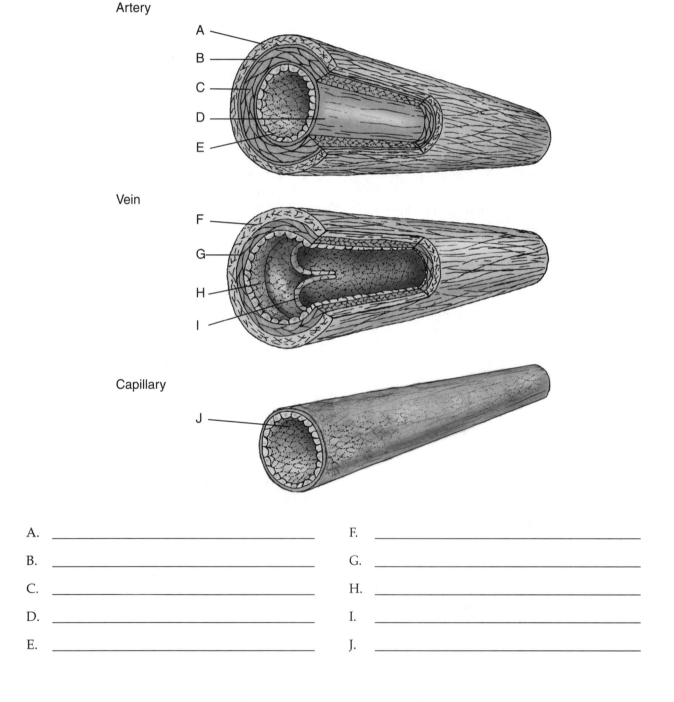

Artery

Vein

Capillary

A. _____
B. _____
C. _____
D. _____
E. _____

F. _____
G. _____
H. _____
I. _____
J. _____

L. Venous Return.

1. Using Figure 36-8 (textbook p. 746) and the word bank below, label the veins involved in varicosities using the following numbers.

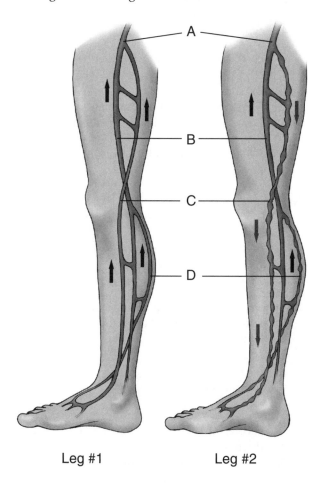

Leg #1   Leg #2

1. Small saphenous veins
2. Great saphenous veins
3. External iliac veins
4. Femoral veins

A. _____

B. _____

C. _____

D. _____

2. Which leg represents varicosities and retrograde venous flow?

3. Which are factors contributing to varicosities? Select all that apply.
   1. Hereditary weakness
   2. Aging
   3. Pregnancy
   4. Prolonged standing
   5. Orthostatic hypotension

4. What are common sites for varicosities? Select all that apply.
   1. Esophageal veins
   2. Renal veins
   3. Coronary veins
   4. Peripheral veins
   5. Hemorrhoidal veins

PART II: PUTTING IT ALL TOGETHER

M. Multiple Choice/Multiple Response.
Choose the most appropriate answer or select all that apply.

1. Any interruption of the blood flow to the distal regions of the body, as occurs in peripheral vascular disease (PVD), results in:
   1. kidney failure.
   2. cardiac shock.
   3. dyspnea.
   4. hypoxia.

2. The nervous system that acts on the smooth muscles of vessels, resulting in dilation and constriction of the artery walls, is the:
   1. autonomic.
   2. somatic.
   3. central.
   4. cranial.

3. The primary result of aging on the peripheral vessels is:
   1. vasoconstriction of arteries.
   2. vasodilation of veins.
   3. increased elasticity of vessel walls.
   4. stiffening of vessel walls.

4. Which of the following are caused by aging in the vascular system? Select all that apply.
   1. Decreased cardiac output
   2. Tachycardia
   3. Increased peripheral resistance
   4. Hypertension
   5. Slowing of the heart rate
   6. Decrease in stroke volume

5. The transportation of oxygen is compromised in the aging patient by decreased:
   1. hematocrit.
   2. WBC count.
   3. hemoglobin.
   4. cardiac enzymes.

6. PVD is a common complication of:
   1. pneumonia.
   2. myocardial infarction.
   3. diabetes.
   4. influenza.

7. A patient with PVD is experiencing a limb-threatening ischemia. Amputation of the limb may be necessary because of the development of:
   1. cyanosis.
   2. tissue necrosis.
   3. fractures.
   4. hypersensitivity.

8. Skin temperature is palpated in patients with PVD to determine the existence of:
   1. infection.
   2. bleeding.
   3. cyanosis.
   4. ischemia.

9. In the evaluation of edema, when the thumb is depressed in the area for 5 seconds and the depression of the thumb remains in the edematous area, the edema is said to be:
   1. 1+.
   2. 2+.
   3. 3+.
   4. pitting.

10. Nurses should teach patients with PVD to stop smoking because smoking causes:
    1. intermittent claudication.
    2. skin ulceration.
    3. vasoconstriction.
    4. vasodilation.

11. The primary function of intermittent pneumatic compression devices is to prevent:
    1. infection.
    2. hemorrhage.
    3. deep vein thrombosis.
    4. cyanosis.

12. Which position should be avoided by patients with PVD?
    1. Extended standing
    2. Elevation of lower extremities
    3. Lowering extremities below the level of the heart
    4. Elevation of extremities to a nondependent position

13. Which works as a vasodilator that promotes arterial flow to the peripheral tissues?
    1. TED hose
    2. Intermittent pneumatic compression
    3. Heat
    4. Cold

14. Elevation of the extremity following surgery for patients with PVD aids in the prevention of:
    1. hemorrhage.
    2. edema.
    3. hypotension.
    4. ulceration.

15. Thrombolytic therapy is employed to:
    1. shorten the clotting time.
    2. increase clot formation.
    3. prevent the formation of new clots.
    4. dissolve an existing clot.

16. The use of vasodilators results in increased blood flow by relaxing the vascular smooth muscle and causing:
    1. increased clotting time.
    2. decreased elasticity in vessels.
    3. decreased resistance in vessels.
    4. increased narrowing in vessels.

17. A serious risk with a diagnosis of deep vein thrombosis is the development of:
    1. hemorrhage.
    2. pneumonia.
    3. pulmonary embolus.
    4. infection.

18. Which are the primary diagnostic examinations used in the detection of thrombus formation? Select all that apply.
    1. Venography
    2. ECG
    3. Myelography
    4. Angioplasty
    5. Plethysmography
    6. Doppler ultrasound

19. The placement of antiembolism hose on patients with thrombosis is done to improve circulation and to prevent:
    1. infection.
    2. stasis.
    3. hemorrhage.
    4. ulceration.

20. A life-threatening event that requires immediate attention is:
    1. arterial embolism.
    2. thrombophlebitis.
    3. varicose vein disease.
    4. thrombosis.

21. The absence of a peripheral pulse below the occlusive area is a clinical manifestation of:
    1. Raynaud disease.
    2. aneurysms.
    3. peripheral arterial occlusive disease.
    4. thrombophlebitis.

22. During repair of an abdominal aneurysm, the aorta is clamped for a period of time. This poses a risk of:
    1. dyspnea.
    2. renal failure.
    3. pneumonia.
    4. incontinence.

23. Varicose veins develop as a result of faulty:
    1. elasticity.
    2. smooth muscle.
    3. thickness.
    4. valves.

24. Chronic venous insufficiency may develop from:
    1. varicose veins.
    2. plaque formations.
    3. thrombophlebitis.
    4. aortic dissection.

25. Signs of chronic venous insufficiency include edema of lower legs and:
    1. redness.
    2. infection.
    3. stasis dermatitis.
    4. cyanosis.

26. The medical management of lymphangitis necessitates the administration of:
    1. antimicrobial agents.
    2. thrombolytic agents.
    3. anticoagulants.
    4. analgesics.

27. Elastic support hose are utilized for several months following an acute attack of lymphangitis to prevent the formation of:
    1. infection.
    2. hemorrhage.
    3. lymphedema.
    4. dermatitis.

28. The primary age-related change in peripheral vessels is:
    1. thrombosis.
    2. arteriosclerosis.
    3. varicose vein disease.
    4. chronic venous insufficiency.

29. Aging in the vascular system causes:
    1. increased hemoglobin.
    2. increased stroke volume.
    3. increased heart rate.
    4. decreased cardiac output.

30. Intermittent pneumatic compression is used for patients:
    1. with paresthesia.
    2. with intermittent claudication.
    3. on bedrest following surgery.
    4. on moderate exercise programs.

31. Which medications intensify anticoagulant effects?
    1. Antacids
    2. Barbiturates
    3. Oral contraceptives
    4. NSAIDs

32. Which herbal remedy decreases the effectiveness of warfarin?
    1. Garlic
    2. Ginger root
    3. St. John's wort
    4. Ginkgo

33. Intermittent claudication is the classic sign of:
    1. hypertension.
    2. arterial embolism.
    3. deep vein thrombosis.
    4. PVD.

34. Buerger's disease (thromboangiitis obliterans) is uncommon in people living in:
    1. India.
    2. Korea.
    3. Japan.
    4. the United States.

35. Chronically cold hands and numbness are symptoms of:
    1. Buerger's disease.
    2. Raynaud disease.
    3. atherosclerosis.
    4. deep vein thrombosis.

36. An alternative therapy for vasospastic episodes of Raynaud disease is:
    1. guided imagery.
    2. meditation.
    3. biofeedback.
    4. yoga.

37. Occupations requiring prolonged standing and the aging process increase the risk for:
    1. PVD.
    2. varicosities.
    3. aneurysms.
    4. aortic dissection.

38. Which groups experience an increased incidence of Raynaud disease? Select all that apply.
    1. Men
    2. Women
    3. People who live in a hot climate
    4. People who live in a cold climate

39. What factors (called *Virchow's triad*) contribute to venous thrombus formation? Select all that apply.
    1. Stasis of the blood
    2. Damage to the vessel walls
    3. Hypertension
    4. Hypercoagulability

40. What are symptoms of a deep vein thrombosis in the lower leg? Select all that apply.
    1. Area is edematous.
    2. Area is cool.
    3. Area is dry.
    4. Area is tender to touch.

41. What percentage of patients with deep vein thrombosis have no visible signs or symptoms?
    1. 10%
    2. 20%
    3. 45%
    4. 50%

42. What is the most serious complication of deep vein thrombosis?
    1. Hemorrhage
    2. Venous stasis
    3. Pulmonary embolism
    4. Hypovolemic shock

43. Explain why care must be taken when using heat on patients with peripheral vascular disease.

44. Which are complications of aneurysms? Select all that apply.
    1. Emboli
    2. Infection
    3. Rupture
    4. Thrombus forms, obstructing blood flow
    5. Pressure on surrounding structures
    6. Liver failure

45. Which are primary diagnostic examinations used in the detection of venous thrombi? Select all that apply.
    1. Doppler ultrasonography
    2. Duplex ultrasonography
    3. Exercise treadmill test
    4. Venography

PART III: CHALLENGE YOURSELF!

N. Getting Ready for NCLEX.

Choose the most appropriate answer or select all that apply.

1. Which are characteristics of venous insufficiency in the legs? Select all that apply.
   1. Capillary refill greater than 3 seconds
   2. Lower leg edema
   3. Pale skin color when elevated
   4. Varicose veins may be visible
   5. Dark reddish color in dependent position
   6. Bronze-brown pigmentation
   7. Cool skin
   8. Intermittent claudication or rest pain
   9. Dull ache, heaviness in calf or thigh
   10. Absent peripheral pulses

2. Match the nursing diagnosis in the numbered column for a patient with venous thrombosis with the appropriate "related to" statement in the lettered column.

   1. _____ Impaired skin integrity
   2. _____ Acute pain
   3. _____ Activity intolerance
   4. _____ Ineffective tissue perfusion

   A. Impaired circulation and tissue ischemia
   B. Venous stasis
   C. Ineffective peripheral circulation
   D. Leg pain or swelling

3. What are risk factors for the development of deep vein thrombosis? Select all that apply.
   1. Prescribed bedrest
   2. Obesity
   3. Malnourishment
   4. Use of oral contraceptives
   5. Use of anticoagulants
   6. Prescribed cast for fractures
   7. Surgery under general anesthesia for patients over 40
   8. Use of alcohol

4. What is the treatment for deep vein thrombosis during the acute phase? Select all that apply.
   1. Frequent ambulation initially
   2. Elevate extremity
   3. Apply warm compresses
   4. Anticoagulant therapy
   5. Antiembolism hose

5. When are anticoagulants and thrombolytic drugs contraindicated? Select all that apply.
   1. Venous thrombosis
   2. Active bleeding
   3. Recent surgery
   4. Patients on bedrest
   5. Uncontrolled hypertension

6. If pain or severe skin color changes occur during exercises with PVD patients, the nurse should:
   1. encourage the exercises to be done gradually.
   2. stop the exercises immediately.
   3. ambulate the patient to promote venous return.
   4. administer muscle relaxants as ordered.

7. Disappearance of a peripheral pulse during the postoperative care of patients with PVD alerts the nurse to the development of a:
   1. thrombotic occlusion.
   2. massive hemorrhage.
   3. severe infection.
   4. varicose vein.

8. Patients with thrombosis should not be massaged or rubbed because of the possible development of:
   1. severe infection.
   2. hemorrhage.
   3. skin breakdown.
   4. pulmonary emboli.

9. A patient complains of severe aching pain in his left foot after lying quietly in bed. This type of pain is a symptom of:
   1. severe arterial occlusion.
   2. PVD.
   3. deep vein thrombosis.
   4. Raynaud disease.

10. A priority in caring for patients with PVD is:
    1. pain management.
    2. stress management.
    3. regular exercise.
    4. a low-sodium diet.

11. When intermittent claudication occurs, the patient should:
    1. stop smoking.
    2. avoid constrictive clothing.
    3. use antiembolism hose.
    4. stop exercise.

12. Patients taking vasodilators for PVD must be monitored for:
    1. hypotension.
    2. hemorrhage.
    3. increased vascular resistance.
    4. hypocalcemia.

13. Which food should be avoided in patients with PVD?
    1. Grapefruit
    2. Ham
    3. Milk
    4. Pasta

14. What is related to the ineffective tissue perfusion nursing diagnosis for a patient with Raynaud disease?
    1. Compromised circulation
    2. Vascular occlusion
    3. Graft thrombosis
    4. Vasoconstriction

Nursing Care Plan.

Refer to Nursing Care Plan, The Patient with a Venous Stasis Ulcer, p. 750 in the textbook, and answer questions 15-21.

15. Which eight findings on the physical examination are abnormal?

    1. _____
    2. _____
    3. _____
    4. _____
    5. _____
    6. _____
    7. _____
    8. _____

16. How does this patient describe his pain?

17. What is a risk factor of PVD for this patient?

18. What is the priority nursing diagnosis?

19. What are steps this patient can take to lessen his pain?

20. Which tasks can be assigned to unlicensed assistive personnel? Select all that apply.
    1. Check vital signs.
    2. Instruct the patient in measures to improve circulation.
    3. Assess condition of ulcer, peripheral pulses, skin color and warmth, pain, and edema.
    4. Teach hygienic techniques of handwashing and wound care.
    5. Teach signs and symptoms of infection that should be reported to physician.
    6. Teach pain relief measures.
    7. Explain the use of analgesics.
    8. Assist the patient with ambulation.
    9. Document the condition of the ulcer during each clinic visit.
    10. Weigh the patient.

Hypertension

 Go to http://evolve.elsevier.com/Linton/medsurg/ for additional activities and exercises.

NCLEX CATEGORIES:

Health Promotion and Maintenance

Physiological Integrity: Basic Care and Comfort, Pharmacological Therapies, Reduction of Risk Potential, Physiological Adaptation

OBJECTIVES

1. Define hypertension.
2. Explain the physiology of blood pressure regulation.
3. Discuss the risk factors, signs and symptoms, diagnosis, treatment, and complications of hypertension.
4. Identify the nursing considerations when administering selected antihypertensive drugs.
5. List the data to be obtained in the nursing assessment of a person with known or suspected hypertension.
6. Identify the nursing diagnoses, goals, and outcome criteria for the patient with hypertension.
7. Describe the nursing interventions for the patient with hypertension.

PART I: MASTERING THE BASICS

A. Key Terms.

Match the definition in the numbered column with the most appropriate term in the lettered column.

1. _____ Sudden drop in systolic blood pressure when changing from a lying or sitting position to a standing position
2. _____ Stationary blood clot
3. _____ Nosebleed
4. _____ Persistent elevation of arterial blood pressure of 140/90 mm Hg or greater
5. _____ Fainting

6. _____ Enlargement
7. _____ Abnormal amounts of lipids or lipoproteins in the blood

A. Hypertension
B. Syncope
C. Thrombus
D. Dyslipidemia
E. Orthostatic hypotension
F. Epistaxis
G. Hypertrophy

B. Risk Factors.

What are significant risk factors for primary (essential) hypertension? Select all that apply.

1. Varicose veins
2. Dyslipidemia
3. Tobacco use
4. Obesity
5. Thrombophlebitis

C. Drug Therapy.

Match the names of the drugs in the numbered column with the correct classification of drugs in the lettered column.

1. _____ Prazosin (Minipress), doxazosin (Cardura)
2. _____ Hydrochlorothiazide (HCTZ), furosemide (Lasix)
3. _____ Losartan potassium (Cozaar), valsartan (Diovan)
4. _____ Clonidine (Catapres), methyldopa (Aldomet)
5. _____ Propranolol (Inderal), atenolol (Tenormin)
6. _____ Hydralazine (Apresoline)

7. _____   Captopril (Capoten) and enalapril (Vasotec)

8. _____   Verapamil (Calan) and diltiazem (Cardizem)

A. Calcium channel blockers
B. Beta blockers
C. Direct vasodilators
D. Angiotensin II receptor antagonists
E. Diuretics
F. Alpha-adrenergic receptor blockers
G. Centrally acting drugs (alpha 2 agonists)
H. ACE inhibitors

D. Drug Therapy.

Match the actions of the drugs in the numbered column with the correct classification of drugs in the lettered column. Some classifications may be used more than once.

1. _____   Blocks effects of norepinephrine, causing vasodilation

2. _____   Decrease fluid retention by decreasing the production of aldosterone

3. _____   Reduce blood pressure by blocking the beta effects of catecholamines

4. _____   Acts on central nervous system (CNS) to block vasoconstriction

5. _____   Block receptors for angiotensin II and reduce aldosterone secretion

6. _____   Reduce blood volume through promotion of renal excretion of sodium and water

7. _____   Block the movement of calcium into cardiac and vascular smooth muscle cells, reducing heart rate, decreasing force of cardiac contraction, and dilating peripheral blood vessels

8. _____   Relax vascular smooth muscle, causing vasodilation

9. _____   Prevent the conversion of angiotensin I to angiotensin II, a potent vasoconstrictor, decreasing peripheral resistance

A. Centrally acting drugs (alpha 2 agonists)
B. Calcium channel blockers
C. Alpha-adrenergic receptor blockers
D. ACE inhibitors

E. Direct vasodilators
F. Beta-adrenergic receptor blockers
G. Diuretics
H. Angiotensin II receptor antagonists

E. Complications.

1. Using this figure, list four body structures (A–D) damaged by long-term blood pressure elevation.

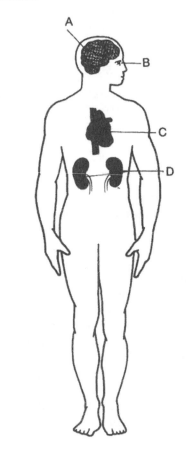

A. _____

B. _____

C. _____

D. _____

2. As blood pressure rises, what are complications that occur? Select all that apply.
   1. Heart failure
   2. Heart attack
   3. Blindness
   4. Kidney disease
   5. Hypoglycemia

3. What are long-term effects of hypertension on the eyes? Select all that apply.
   1. Retinal hemorrhages
   2. Pupil dilation
   3. Papilledema
   4. Narrowing of retinal arterioles

4. What are long-term effects of hypertension on the heart? Select all that apply.
   1. Angina
   2. Myocardial infarction
   3. Vasodilation
   4. Coronary artery disease

5. What are long-term effects of hypertension on the brain? Select all that apply.
   1. Dehydration
   2. Transient ischemic attacks
   3. Strokes

6. At what age do complications of hypertension increase?
   1. 20 years
   2. 30 years
   3. 40 years
   4. 50 years

PART II: PUTTING IT ALL TOGETHER

F. Multiple Choice/Multiple Response.

Choose the most appropriate answer or select all that apply.

1. The most common cardiovascular problem in the United States today is:
   1. arteriosclerosis.
   2. coronary artery disease.
   3. myocardial infarction.
   4. hypertension.

2. The cause of primary (essential) hypertension is:
   1. kidney disease.
   2. drugs.
   3. pregnancy.
   4. unknown.

3. Hypertension is usually detected in which age group?
   1. 20–29
   2. 30–50
   3. 51–60
   4. over 60

4. A blood pressure of 135/87 mm Hg is considered to be:
   1. hypertension, stage 1.
   2. normal.
   3. prehypertension.
   4. hypertension, stage 2.

5. In which risk group is a hypertensive patient who smokes half a pack of cigarettes a day and who has no heart disease or heart damage classified?
   1. Risk A
   2. Risk B
   3. Risk C
   4. Risk D

6. Isolated systolic blood pressure elevations of 160 mm Hg in older adults are most often due to:
   1. decreased cardiac output.
   2. atherosclerosis.
   3. increased peripheral vascular resistance.
   4. increased pulse pressure.

7. The diameter of blood vessels is regulated primarily by:
   1. the heart muscle.
   2. adrenal gland hormones.
   3. the vasomotor center.
   4. thyroid gland hormones.

8. Patients with systolic pressures between 120 and 139 mm Hg and with diastolic pressures between 80 and 89 mm Hg are said to:
   1. have normal hypertension.
   2. be in Risk Group B.
   3. have prehypertension.
   4. have Stage I hypertension.

9. Beta blockers are contraindicated in patients with:
   1. hypertension.
   2. edema.
   3. osteoporosis.
   4. asthma.

10. Which group of patients responds better to diuretics as treatment for hypertension?
    1. Caucasians
    2. African-Americans
    3. Asians
    4. Hispanics

11. Older patients taking antihypertensives are more susceptible to orthostatic hypotension, increasing their risk for:
    1. confusion.
    2. myocardial infarction.
    3. falls.
    4. congestive heart failure.

12. When body position is changed from supine to standing, the systolic pressure normally:
    1. rises about 5 mm Hg.
    2. rises about 10 mm Hg.
    3. falls about 5 mm Hg.
    4. falls about 10 mm Hg.

13. People with increased blood pressure should not take over-the-counter:
    1. analgesics.
    2. cold remedies.
    3. antacids.
    4. laxatives.

14. A common side effect of many antihypertensives is:
    1. GI distress.
    2. sexual dysfunction.
    3. respiratory depression.
    4. rebound hypertension.

15. Without appropriate treatment, the patient in hypertensive crisis may develop:
    1. cerebrovascular accident.
    2. hyperglycemia.
    3. respiratory acidosis.
    4. adrenal insufficiency.

16. What percentage of people with hypertension do not know they have it?
    1. 10%
    2. 20%
    3. 30%
    4. 40%

17. Although 59% of people with hypertension are being treated, in what percentage of people is hypertension controlled?
    1. 20%
    2. 28%
    3. 34%
    4. 42%

18. What is the medical treatment goal for patients with diabetes or renal disease?
    1. Lower than 110/70 mm Hg
    2. 120/80 mm Hg
    3. 130/80 mm Hg
    4. 140/90 mm Hg

19. Which drug is recommended for initial therapy for hypertension, according to JNC-7?
    1. Thiazide-type diuretic
    2. ACE inhibitor
    3. Calcium channel blocker
    4. Beta-adrenergic blocker

20. How does a blood pressure cuff which is too small affect the blood pressure reading?
    1. False high reading
    2. False low reading
    3. Systolic reading too high
    4. Diastolic reading too low

21. Patients taking antihypertensive medications are encouraged to rise slowly from a lying or sitting position in order to prevent:
    1. syncope.
    2. orthostatic hypotension.
    3. hypertensive crisis.
    4. confusion.

22. What is the percentage of people with hypertension who have primary or essential hypertension?
    1. 10–15%
    2. 25–30%
    3. 45–50%
    4. 90–95%

23. What is the effect of epinephrine on blood vessels? Select all that apply.
    1. Dilates blood vessels
    2. Increases blood pressure
    3. Pulse pressure widens
    4. Increases force of cardiac contraction
    5. Heart rate increases

24. Which statements are true about blood pressure? Select all that apply.
    1. When body position is altered from supine to standing, the diastolic blood pressure increases.
    2. In response to increased peripheral vascular resistance, the systolic pressure decreases.
    3. When there is narrowing of the arteries and arterioles, peripheral vascular resistance increases.
    4. When body position is altered from supine to standing, the systolic pressure normally falls.

25. Which factors contribute to hypertension? Select all that apply.
    1. Cardiac stimulation
    2. Retention of fluid
    3. Vasodilation

26. Which stimulants may contribute to hypertension? Select all that apply.
    1. Caffeine
    2. Nicotine
    3. Alcohol
    4. Amphetamines

27. Which are symptoms of hypertensive crisis? Select all that apply.
    1. Nausea
    2. Restlessness
    3. Drowsiness
    4. Blurred vision

28. Which of the following are lifestyle modifications related to exercise that are benefits for patients with high blood pressure? Select all that apply.
    1. Reduces water in the body, decreasing the circulating blood volume
    2. Decreases blood glucose and cholesterol levels, increasing sense of well-being
    3. Eliminates vasoconstriction caused by nicotine
    4. Reduces stress and lowers blood pressure
    5. Improves cardiac efficiency by increasing cardiac output and decreasing peripheral vascular resistance
    6. Reduces blood pressure by reducing the workload of the heart

29. Match the side effect or caution in the numbered column with the correct classification of drugs in the lettered column. Some classifications may be used more than once.
    1. _____ Palpitations, dizziness, headache, drowsiness
    2. _____ Hypoglycemia
    3. _____ Hyponatremia and hypokalemia
    4. _____ Flushing, dizziness, headache
    5. _____ Skin rash, cough
    6. _____ Use cautiously in patients with asthma and diabetes
    7. _____ Fluid volume deficit
    8. _____ Dry mouth, weakness

    A. Centrally acting drugs
    B. Beta blockers
    C. Calcium channel blockers
    D. Alpha-adrenergic receptor blockers
    E. Diuretics
    F. ACE inhibitors

30. What is the leading cause of death in people with hypertension?
    1. Stroke
    2. Kidney failure
    3. Cardiac disease
    4. Pneumonia

31. Refer to Table 37-1, p. 755 in the textbook.

    1. What is the category for a person with blood pressure of 150/95 mm Hg?

    2. What is the category for a person with blood pressure of 122/84 mm Hg?

    3. What is the category for a person with blood pressure of 118/78 mm Hg?

    4. What is the category for a person with blood pressure of 180/110 mm Hg?

PART III: CHALLENGE YOURSELF!

G. Getting Ready for NCLEX.

Choose the most appropriate answer or select all that apply.

1. How does aging affect blood pressure? Select all that apply.
   1. Increased elasticity of arteries
   2. Decreased cardiac output
   3. Increased peripheral vascular resistance
   4. Decreased systolic blood pressure
   5. Pulse pressure widens

2. Which food groups are emphasized in the DASH diet? Select all that apply.
   1. Vegetables
   2. Fruits
   3. Nuts and seeds
   4. Whole milk

3. Which blood studies are usually ordered for people with hypertension? Select all that apply.
   1. Hematocrit
   2. Glucose
   3. Potassium
   4. Calcium
   5. Creatine
   6. Prothrombin time
   7. Thyroid function
   8. Lipid profile

4. Which of the following are teaching points for patients with orthostatic hypotension? Select all that apply.
   1. Eat a low-sodium diet.
   2. Avoid prolonged standing.
   3. Avoid cholesterol in diet.
   4. Avoid hot baths and showers.
   5. Rise slowly.

5. What are causes of secondary hypertension? Select all that apply.
   1. Renal disease
   2. Sedentary lifestyle
   3. Tobacco use
   4. Narrowing of the aorta
   5. Increased intracranial pressure

6. An older patient taking furosemide (Lasix) for hypertension complains of muscle weakness, confusion, and irritability. Which patient teaching is correct for this patient?
   1. Decrease sodium in the diet.
   2. Increase potassium in the diet.
   3. Increase fluid intake.
   4. Decrease vitamin K intake.

7. When people with diabetes are taking beta blockers for hypertension, the only sign of hypoglycemia may be:
   1. diaphoresis.
   2. fatigue.
   3. hunger.
   4. excessive thirst.

8. Older patients taking beta blockers are at greater risk than younger people for:
   1. bradycardia.
   2. hypoglycemia.
   3. bronchoconstriction.
   4. GI upset.

9. If a patient's diastolic pressure is 120 mm Hg, the nurse should:
   1. reassess it in 10 minutes.
   2. reassess it in 30 minutes.
   3. notify the physician.
   4. encourage the patient to stay on bedrest.

10. What may occur if antihypertensive drugs are stopped abruptly?
    1. Hypotensive crisis
    2. Orthostatic hypotension
    3. Rebound hypertension
    4. Bradycardia

11. Refer to Table 37-2, p. 759 in the textbook.
    1. What is the average systolic blood pressure reduction range for a person who walks briskly 30 minutes per day, most days of the week?

    2. What is the average systolic blood pressure reduction range for a person who adopts the DASH eating plan?

    3. What is the average systolic blood pressure reduction range for a person who maintains body weight with a body mass index between 18.5–24.9 kg/m²?

Digestive Tract Disorders

chapter **38**

 Go to http://evolve.elsevier.com/Linton/medsurg/ for additional activities and exercises.

NCLEX CATEGORIES:

Safe and Effective Care Environment:
Coordinated Care, Safety and Infection Control

Health Promotion and Maintenance

Psychosocial Integrity

Physiological Integrity: Basic Care and Comfort, Pharmacological Therapies, Reduction of Risk Potential, Physiological Adaptation

OBJECTIVES

1. Identify the nursing responsibilities in the care of patients undergoing diagnostic tests and procedures for disorders of the digestive tract.
2. List the data to be included in the nursing assessment of the patient with a digestive disorder.
3. Describe the nursing care of patients with gastrointestinal intubation and decompression, tube feedings, total parenteral nutrition, digestive tract surgery, and drug therapy for digestive disorders.
4. Describe the pathophysiology, signs and symptoms, complications, and medical treatment of selected digestive disorders.
5. Assist in developing nursing care plans for patients receiving treatment for digestive disorders.

PART I: MASTERING THE BASICS

A. Key Terms. Mouth Disorders.

Match the definition in the numbered column with the most appropriate term in the lettered column.

1. _____ Difficulty swallowing
2. _____ Indigestion
3. _____ Inflammation of the oral mucosa
4. _____ Tooth decay

A. Stomatitis
B. Dysphagia
C. Caries
D. Dyspepsia

B. Key Terms. Esophageal Disorders.

Match or complete the statements in the numbered column with the most appropriate term in the lettered column. Some terms may be used more than once, and some terms may not be used.

1. _____ Inflammation of the esophagus caused by acidic gastric fluids
2. _____ Procedure used to assess bowel sounds
3. _____ Hiatal hernia is thought to be caused by weakness in the _____.
4. _____ The opening in the diaphragm through which the esophagus passes is the esophageal _____.
5. _____ Direct examination of the esophagus with an endoscope
6. _____ The procedure used to detect the presence of air, fluid, or masses in tissues is known as _____.
7. _____ The protrusion of the lower esophagus and stomach upward through the diaphragm into the chest

8. _____ A surgical procedure that strengthens the lower esophageal sphincter by suturing the fundus of the stomach around the esophagus and anchoring it below the diaphragm

A. Hiatus
B. Pyloric sphincter
C. Hiatal hernia
D. Esophagoscopy
E. Gastrectomy
F. Esophagitis
G. Heartburn
H. Palpation
I. Stomatitis
J. Auscultation
K. Fundoplication
L. Percussion
M. Lower esophageal sphincter

C. Bariatric Surgery.

1. Which are true statements about the Roux-en-Y gastric bypass (RNYGBP) procedure? Select all that apply.
    1. Procedure for decreasing size of stomach by creating a small upper pouch that receives food from the esophagus and connecting the pouch to the jejunum
    2. Complications of this bariatric procedure include dumping syndrome and iron and calcium deficiencies
    3. The newest restrictive bariatric procedure involving the laparoscopic placement of an adjustable band around the fundus of the stomach, creating a small pouch
    4. Restrictive bariatric surgery procedure that decreases the stomach capacity and bypasses much of the absorptive section of the GI tract
    5. Bariatric procedure in which the stomach is stapled to reduce its capacity, leaving a small opening for food to move from the small pouch into the lower stomach
    6. Best-tolerated bariatric surgery procedure with low rate of complications

D. Key Terms. Intestinal Disorders.

Match the statement in the numbered column with the most appropriate term in the lettered column.

1. _____ A common symptom of malabsorption is the presence of excessive fat in the stool
2. _____ A condition in which the large intestine loses the ability to contract effectively enough to propel the fecal mass toward the rectum
3. _____ The passage of loose, liquid stools with increased frequency
4. _____ Increased pressure in the chest and abdominal cavities caused by straining to have a bowel movement
5. _____ A term used to describe a condition in which one or more nutrients are not digested or absorbed
6. _____ A condition in which a person has hard, dry, infrequent stools that are passed with difficulty
7. _____ The retention of a large mass of stool in the rectum that the patient is unable to pass

A. Valsalva's maneuver
B. Diarrhea
C. Fecal impaction
D. Steatorrhea
E. Constipation
F. Malabsorption
G. Megacolon

E. Key Terms. Abdominal Hernia Disorders.

Complete the statements in the numbered column with the most appropriate term in the lettered column.

1. _____ The repair of the muscle defect in abdominal hernia by suturing
2. _____ A pad placed over the hernia to provide support for weak muscles, for patients who cannot tolerate the stress of surgical hernia repair
3. _____ The bulging portion of the large intestine pushing through the abdominal wall
4. _____ Weak location where hernias occur, in addition to the lower inguinal areas of the abdomen

A. Umbilicus
B. Hernia
C. Truss
D. Herniorrhaphy

F. Drug Therapy.
Match the drugs in the numbered column with their actions in the lettered column.

1. _____ Anticholinergics
2. _____ H$_2$-receptor antagonists
3. _____ Antiemetics
4. _____ Antacids
5. _____ Mucosal barriers (cytoprotective)
6. _____ Antidiarrheals
7. _____ Antibacterials
8. _____ Antifungals
9. _____ Proton pump inhibitors
10. _____ 5-HR receptor antagonists

A. Treat ulcerative colitis and *H. pylori*
B. Neutralize gastric acid
C. Cling to the surface of the ulcer and protect it so that healing can take place
D. Treat yeast infections in the mouth
E. Decrease hydrochloric acid production by competing at receptor sites
F. Prevent and treat nausea
G. Decrease intestinal motility so liquid portion of feces is reabsorbed
H. Reduce gastrointestinal motility and secretions; block acetylcholine
I. Prevent nausea and vomiting caused by chemotherapy
J. Inhibit gastric acid secretion and are used in peptic ulcer disease and GERD

G. Digestive Tract.

In the Figure 38-1 (p. 770) below, label the parts (A–W) of the digestive tract.

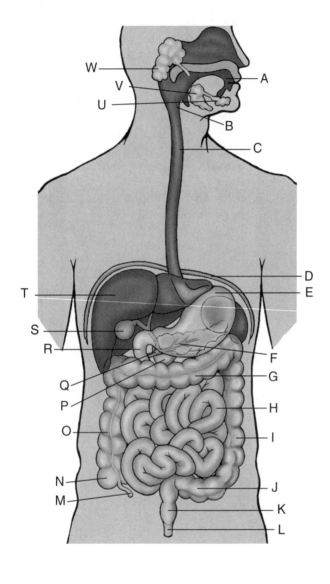

A. _____

B. _____

C. _____

D. _____

E. _____

F. _____

G. _____

H. _____

I. _____

J. _____

K. _____

L. _____

M. _____

N. _____

O. _____

P. _____

Q. _____

R. _____

S. _____

T. _____

U. _____

V. _____

W. _____

H. GI Tubes.

1. Using Figure 38-5 (p. 780) below, label the gastrointestinal tubes using the letters below.
   1. Miller-Abbott tube _____
   2. Sengstaken-Blakemore tube _____
   3. Levin tube _____
   4. Salem sump tube _____
   5. Cantor tube _____

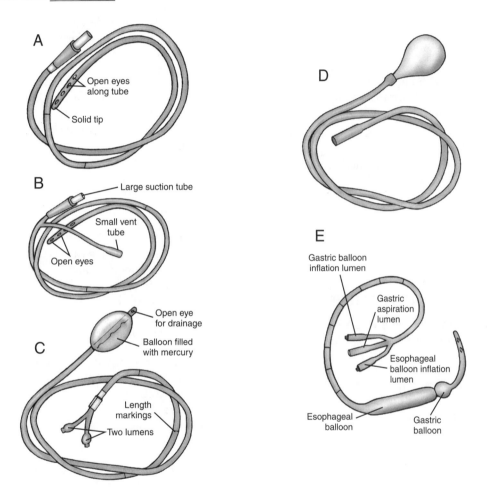

2. Which nasogastric tubes are used for gastric decompression (GI suction)?

3. Which nasoenteric tubes are weighted and used for intestinal decompressions?

4. Which esophageal-gastric balloon tube is used to control bleeding in the esophagus, usually in patients with severe complications of liver disease?

I. Intestinal Disorders.

Match the statements in the numbered column with the most appropriate term in the lettered column.

1. _____ A test which, in addition to colonoscopy, allows the physician to confirm the presence of diverticula

2. _____ A break in the wall of the stomach or the duodenum that permits digestive fluids to leak into the peritoneal cavity

3. _____ A common complication of peptic ulcers

4. _____ In addition to bloody diarrhea, the other most common symptom of inflammatory bowel disease

5. _____ A complication of diverticulitis in which an abnormal opening develops between the colon and the bladder

A. Hemorrhage
B. Barium enema
C. Perforation
D. Fistula
E. Abdominal pain

PART II: PUTTING IT ALL TOGETHER

J. Multiple Choice/Multiple Response.

Choose the most appropriate answer or select all that apply.

1. The type of acid-base imbalance that results from prolonged vomiting is:
   1. metabolic acidosis.
   2. metabolic alkalosis.
   3. respiratory acidosis.
   4. respiratory alkalosis.

2. Normal bowel sounds include:
   1. minimal clicks and gurgles.
   2. clicks and gurgles 5–30 times/minute.
   3. steady, consistent gurgling sounds.
   4. no sounds for 1 full minute.

3. Which herb is effective in calming an upset stomach, reducing flatulence, and preventing motion sickness?
   1. Ginkgo
   2. Ginseng
   3. Ginger root
   4. Garlic

4. After insertion of a gastric tube, feedings are not started until:
   1. the patient requests food.
   2. adequate oxygen levels are achieved on blood gases.
   3. placement of tube is certain.
   4. oral fluids are tolerated.

5. Severe or prolonged vomiting puts the patient at risk for:
   1. fluid volume deficit.
   2. altered tissue perfusion.
   3. hemorrhage.
   4. infection.

6. Sudden, sharp pain starting in the midepigastric region and spreading across the entire abdomen in patients with peptic ulcer may indicate:
   1. infection.
   2. perforation.
   3. dyspnea.
   4. kidney failure.

7. If the patient's abdomen becomes rigid and tender and he or she draws the knees up to the chest, this may indicate:
   1. peritonitis.
   2. perforation.
   3. kidney failure.
   4. pyloric obstruction.

8. The most prominent symptom of pyloric obstruction is persistent:
   1. eructation.
   2. heartburn.
   3. vomiting.
   4. hemorrhage.

9. A major complication of appendicitis is:
   1. diarrhea.
   2. constipation.
   3. fluid volume deficit.
   4. peritonitis.

10. The classic symptom of appendicitis is pain at:
    1. McBurney's point.
    2. the xiphoid process.
    3. right hypochondriac region.
    4. inguinal node.

11. When appendicitis is suspected, the patient is allowed:
    1. clear liquids.
    2. full liquids.
    3. nothing by mouth.
    4. soft foods.

12. In addition to deficient fluid volume, patients with peritonitis may go into shock because of:
    1. edema.
    2. convulsions.
    3. septicemia.
    4. paralysis.

13. Following abdominoperineal resection, a procedure that cleans, soothes, and increases circulation to the perineum is:
    1. use of a TENS unit.
    2. Kegel exercises.
    3. the sitz bath.
    4. débridement.

14. What is the cause of most peptic ulcers?
    1. *Helicobacter pylori*
    2. *E. coli*
    3. Stress
    4. Infection

15. *Ephedra sinica* (Ma Huang) should not be used as an over-the-counter weight loss product by a person with:
    1. a urinary tract infection.
    2. arthritis.
    3. dermatitis.
    4. hypertension.

16. Which natural substance can help control diarrhea?
    1. Garlic
    2. Rice water
    3. Kava kava
    4. *Ephedra sinica*

17. Which type of laxative may not be effective for several days?
    1. Bulk-producing laxative
    2. Intestinal stimulant
    3. Osmotic suppository
    4. Stool softener

18. The major nutritional goal of therapy for diarrhea is to replace:
    1. potassium.
    2. sodium.
    3. calcium.
    4. fluids.

19. Which is a sign of intestinal rupture in a patient with intestinal obstruction?
    1. Sudden vomiting of blood
    2. Sudden sharp pain
    3. Sudden increased temperature and chills
    4. Sudden diarrhea

20. The Roux-en-Y gastric bypass and the vertical-banded gastroplasty are restrictive procedures used to treat:
    1. peptic ulcer.
    2. extreme obesity.
    3. stomach cancer.
    4. hiatal hernia.

21. Which are results of the simple gastroplasty (stomach stapling) bariatric procedure? Select all that apply.
    1. Results in more weight loss than other procedures
    2. Does not cause dumping syndrome
    3. Does not cause malabsorption
    4. The capacity of the stomach is reduced, leaving a small opening for food to move from small pouch into lower stomach

22. What is the most serious complication of gastric endoscopy?
    1. Shock
    2. Pulmonary embolism
    3. Infection
    4. Perforation of digestive tract

23. What is the most serious complication of gastric ulcers?
    1. Infection
    2. Hemorrhage
    3. Shock
    4. Intractable pain

24. Why is the head of the bed elevated during tube feedings to patients?
    1. Prevent hemorrhage
    2. Prevent dumping syndrome
    3. Prevent aspiration
    4. Prevent hypotension

25. Which of the following are normal age-related changes of the digestive tract? Select all that apply.
    1. Gums recede
    2. Taste buds increase
    3. Walls of the esophagus and stomach thin
    4. Increased stomach secretions
    5. Atrophy of muscle layer and mucosa in large intestine
    6. Constipation
    7. Tooth loss
    8. Esophageal sphincters are more rigid
    9. Anal sphincter strength decreases
    10. Vitamin A absorption decreases

26. Which factors may cause constipation in older adults? Select all that apply.
    1. Low fluid intake
    2. Inactivity
    3. Hyperthyroidism
    4. Depression
    5. Medications

27. Which of the following statements are true about capsule endoscopy? Select all that apply.
    1. Transmits video images of the entire digestive tract
    2. May detect obscure GI bleeding
    3. Detects inflammation caused by NSAIDs and radiotherapy
    4. Measures HCl and pepsin secreted in the stomach
    5. Detects parasitic infections
    6. Detects small bowel tumors
    7. Patients fast overnight before swallowing the capsule

28. Which are terms used to describe bowel sounds? Select all that apply.
    1. Crackles
    2. Present or absent
    3. High-pitched
    4. Gurgling
    5. Increased or decreased

29. Which of the following describe the first stage of dumping syndrome? Select all that apply.
    1. Occurs 1–3 hours after eating.
    2. Patient experiences abdominal fullness and nausea within 10–20 minutes of eating.
    3. Patient feels flushed and faint.
    4. Symptoms in this stage are probably caused by distention of the small intestine by the consumed food and fluids.
    5. Patient's heart rate races and patient breaks into a sweat as a result of pooling of blood in the abdominal organs.
    6. Symptoms in this stage are a result of hypoglycemia caused by an exaggerated rise in insulin secretion in response to the rapid delivery of carbohydrates into the intestine.

30. Which of the following disorders may result in the patient's experiencing deficient fluid volume? Select all that apply.
    1. Abdominal hernia
    2. Diarrhea
    3. Inflammatory bowel disease
    4. Nausea and vomiting
    5. Gastritis
    6. Peptic ulcer
    7. Stomach cancer

31. A patient has just been admitted to the hospital with appendicitis. What is the priority nursing diagnosis for this patient?
    1. Acute pain related to abdominal cramping and rectal irritation
    2. Risk for infection (peritonitis) related to rupture
    3. Deficient fluid volume
    4. Anxiety related to threat of serious illness

32. Which patient has the greatest risk for injury related to wound dehiscence?
    1. Patient with diverticulosis
    2. Patient with hiatal hernia
    3. Patient with intestinal obstruction
    4. Patient with abdominal hernia repair

33. Which patient is most likely to experience decreased cardiac output related to hypovolemia secondary to dumping syndrome?
    1. Patient with abdominal hernia
    2. Patient with anorexia
    3. Patient who has had gastric surgery
    4. Patient with peritonitis

34. What is the diet recommended for acute diarrhea?
    1. Clear liquids
    2. Nothing by mouth
    3. Soft diet
    4. Bland diet

35. A male patient has had an abdominal hernia repair. What is a common complication of this procedure?
    1. Fever
    2. Vomiting
    3. Scrotal swelling
    4. Bradycardia

PART III: CHALLENGE YOURSELF!

K. Getting Ready for NCLEX.

Choose the most appropriate answer or select all that apply.

1. The vomiting patient who is also unconscious or who has impaired swallowing is at risk for aspiration and should be placed in which position?
   1. Lying flat in bed
   2. With head of bed elevated at least 90 degrees
   3. Side-lying
   4. With head of bed slightly elevated; for example, at 30 degrees

2. To prevent nighttime reflux, the sleeping position for patients with hiatal hernia should be:
   1. side-lying.
   2. with head of bed at 90-degree angle.
   3. flat.
   4. with head of bed elevated 6–12 inches.

3. Pain is severe for several postoperative days following abdominoperineal resection. At first, the patient will probably be most comfortable in which position?
   1. Supine
   2. Side-lying
   3. Prone
   4. Fowler's

4. Which type of diet is prescribed for moderate inflammatory bowel disease?
   1. Low-residue diet
   2. High-fiber diet
   3. Low-potassium diet
   4. Low-salt diet

5. Which side effect of opiates (such as morphine) result in opiates not being given to patients with diverticulosis?
   1. Respiratory depression
   2. Constipation
   3. Hypersensitivity
   4. Diarrhea

6. What is a complication that occurs following gastric surgery or when tube feedings of concentrated formula are given rapidly?
   1. Dumping syndrome
   2. Orthostatic hypotension
   3. Diuresis
   4. Diarrhea

7. Which factors can cause persistent vomiting in patients with vertical banded gastroplasty? Select all that apply.
   1. Rupture of the staple line
   2. Erosion of the band into the stomach tissue
   3. Infection
   4. Hemorrhage
   5. Consuming solids too rapidly
   6. Distention of walls of functional pouch

8. Which are interventions for the bariatric surgical patient related to imbalanced nutrition? Select all that apply.
   1. Imaging studies are done just after the patient is fed to assure that there are no leaks in the surgical sites.
   2. The patient is advanced from water to full liquids, and then to clear liquids.
   3. Once solid food is permitted, the typical diet is 800–1200 calories per day.
   4. Small, frequent meals are recommended.
   5. The meals are high in protein.
   6. The meals are low in fat and high in carbohydrates.

9. Which are special needs of the obese surgical patient? Select all that apply.
    1. Risk of postoperative atelectasis and pneumonia
    2. Risk of deep vein thrombosis and pulmonary emboli
    3. Increased pressure ulcers
    4. Increased risk for hemorrhage

10. A patient has had an abdominal hernia repair, and is experiencing signs and symptoms of strangulation. Which are signs and symptoms of strangulation? Select all that apply.
    1. Nausea
    2. Vomiting
    3. Coffee ground emesis
    4. Pain
    5. Black, tarry stools
    6. Fever
    7. Tachycardia

11. Which aspects of care should the nurse teach the patient who experiences dumping syndrome? Select all that apply.
    1. Follow a diet low in fat and protein.
    2. Drink fluids between meals, not with them.
    3. Lie down for about 30 minutes after meals.
    4. Follow a low-carbohydrate diet.

Nursing Care Plan.
Refer to Nursing Care Plan, The Patient with a Peptic Ulcer, p. 810 in the textbook, and answer questions 12-21.

12. What is the priority nursing diagnosis?

13. What are this patient's risk factors for duodenal ulcers?

14. What findings indicate the presence of duodenal ulcers?

15. What diet is this patient on?

16. What are signs and symptoms of bleeding the nurse would be monitoring with this patient? Select all that apply.
    1. Clay-colored stools
    2. Bradycardia
    3. Pallor
    4. Hypotension

17. If hemorrhage occurs in this patient, what will the nurse do?

18. What is the main symptom of perforation for which the nurse would monitor?

19. What is the main sign of pyloric obstruction for which the nurse would monitor in this patient?

20. What are the basic types of medications for peptic ulcer disease? Select all that apply.
    1. Proton pump inhibitors
    2. H_2 antagonists
    3. Antacids
    4. Anticoagulants
    5. Mucosal barrier agents

21. What is triple therapy (two antibiotics and a proton pump inhibitor) used to treat?

Disorders of the Liver, Gallbladder, and Pancreas

e Go to http://evolve.elsevier.com/Linton/medsurg/ for additional activities and exercises.

NCLEX CATEGORIES:

Safe and Effective Care Environment:
Coordinated Care, Safety and Infection Control

Health Promotion and Maintenance

Psychosocial Integrity

Physiological Integrity: Basic Care and Comfort, Pharmacological Therapies, Reduction of Risk Potential, Physiological Adaptation

OBJECTIVES

1. Identify nursing assessment data related to the functions of the liver, gallbladder, and pancreas.
2. Identify the nurse's role in tests and procedures performed to diagnose disorders of the liver, gallbladder, and pancreas.
3. Describe the care of the patient who has an esophageal balloon tube in place.
4. Explain the pathology, signs and symptoms, diagnosis, complications, and medical treatment of selected disorders of the liver, gallbladder, and pancreas.
5. Assist in developing a nursing care plan for the patient with liver, gallbladder, or pancreatic dysfunction.

PART I: MASTERING THE BASICS

A. Key Terms.
Match the definition in the numbered column with the most appropriate term in the lettered column.

1. _____ Chronic, progressive liver disease
2. _____ Accumulation of excess fluid in the peritoneal cavity

3. _____ Removal of ascitic fluid from the peritoneal cavity
4. _____ Enlargement of the liver
5. _____ Removal of the gallbladder
6. _____ Presence of gallstones in the gallbladder
7. _____ Obstruction in common bile duct
8. _____ Excess fat in stools
9. _____ Jaundice
10. _____ Enlargement of breast tissue in males

A. Paracentesis
B. Steatorrhea
C. Hepatomegaly
D. Icterus
E. Cirrhosis
F. Gynecomastia
G. Cholecystectomy
H. Choledocholithiasis
I. Cholelithiasis
J. Ascites

B. Anatomy and Physiology.
Match the statements in the numbered column with the most appropriate term in the lettered column. Some terms may not be used.

1. _____ Organ where bile is produced
2. _____ Specialized reticuloendothelial cells in the liver that ingest old red blood cells and bacteria
3. _____ Passage that delivers bile to the small intestine from the gallbladder
4. _____ A product of the normal breakdown of old red blood cells in the liver
5. _____ The vessel that delivers blood from the aorta to the liver

6. _____   The vessel that delivers blood from the intestines to the liver

7. _____   Passage that delivers bile produced in the liver into the gallbladder for storage

8. _____   Organ where bile is stored

A. Bilirubin
B. Portal vein
C. Kupffer cells
D. Gallbladder
E. Hepatic artery
F. Pancreatic duct
G. Common bile duct
H. Liver
I. Cystic duct
J. Jaundice

C. Diagnostic Procedures.

Match the statements in the numbered column with the most appropriate term in the lettered column.

1. _____   A procedure in which a radioactive substance is injected into a vein and visualized in a radiograph to reveal tumors and abscesses

2. _____   The use of sound waves to create an image of the liver, spleen, pancreas, gallbladder, and biliary system that is noninvasive and painless

3. _____   A procedure that involves removal of a small specimen of liver tissue for examination

4. _____   A primary complication of liver biopsy that occurs because of the liver's rich blood supply and potential for impaired coagulation

5. _____   A primary complication of liver biopsy that occurs if the lung is accidentally punctured during the biopsy

A. Liver biopsy
B. Pneumothorax
C. Ultrasonography
D. Liver scan
E. Hemorrhage

D. Hepatitis.

Match the statements in the numbered column with the most appropriate term in the lettered column. Answers may be used more than once.

1. _____   The most common type of hepatitis

2. _____   Infectious hepatitis or epidemic hepatitis, transmitted by water, food, or contaminated medical equipment

3. _____   Serum hepatitis transmitted in body fluids

A. Hepatitis A
B. Hepatitis B

E. Cirrhosis.

Match the definition or description in the numbered column with the most appropriate term in the lettered column. Some terms may be used more than once.

1. _____   Obstructive cirrhosis that develops as a result of obstruction to bile flow

2. _____   Results from venous congestion and hypoxia

3. _____   Liver enlarges, becomes "knobby," and shrinks later

A. Alcoholic cirrhosis (Laennec's disease)
B. Biliary cirrhosis
C. Cardiac cirrhosis

F. Cirrhosis Complications.

Match the effects of cirrhosis complications in the numbered column with the most appropriate complication of cirrhosis in the lettered column. Some terms may be used more than once, and some may not be used.

1. _____   Results in leaking of lymph fluid and albumin-rich fluid from the diseased liver

2. _____   Renal failure following diuretic therapy, paracentesis, or GI hemorrhage

3. _____   Caused by excessive ammonia in the blood, resulting in cognitive disturbances

4. _____   May cause fatal hemorrhage

5. _____   Development of collateral vessels

A. Hepatic encephalopathy
B. Esophageal varices
C. Portal hypertension
D. Hepatorenal syndrome
E. Ascites

G. Gallstones.

In Figure 39-9 (p. 860) below, label the anatomic parts (A–G).

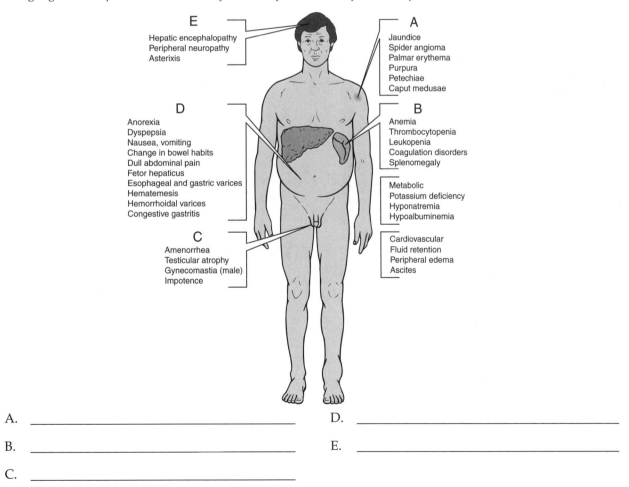

A. _____

B. _____

C. _____

D. _____

E. _____

F. _____

G. _____

H. Cirrhosis.

Using Figure 39-5 (p. 842) below, list the five areas of clinical manifestations of cirrhosis.

E
Hepatic encephalopathy
Peripheral neuropathy
Asterixis

A
Jaundice
Spider angioma
Palmar erythema
Purpura
Petechiae
Caput medusae

D
Anorexia
Dyspepsia
Nausea, vomiting
Change in bowel habits
Dull abdominal pain
Fetor hepaticus
Esophageal and gastric varices
Hematemesis
Hemorrhoidal varices
Congestive gastritis

B
Anemia
Thrombocytopenia
Leukopenia
Coagulation disorders
Splenomegaly

Metabolic
Potassium deficiency
Hyponatremia
Hypoalbuminemia

Cardiovascular
Fluid retention
Peripheral edema
Ascites

C
Amenorrhea
Testicular atrophy
Gynecomastia (male)
Impotence

A. _____   D. _____

B. _____   E. _____

C. _____

PART II: PUTTING IT ALL TOGETHER

I. Multiple Choice/Multiple Response.

Choose the most appropriate answer or select all that apply.

1. Patients with liver disease are at increased risk for drug:
   1. incompatibilities.
   2. toxicities.
   3. idiosyncrasies.
   4. synthesis.

2. Clay-colored stools are characteristic of:
   1. bile obstruction.
   2. pancreatitis.
   3. gastritis.
   4. Crohn's disease.

3. Which are included in the prescribed diet for patients with hepatitis? Select all that apply.
   1. high carbohydrates.
   2. low carbohydrates
   3. high vitamins
   4. moderate to high protein
   5. low protein
   6. low to moderate fat

4. Patients with hepatitis may have impaired skin integrity due to:
   1. jaundice.
   2. pruritus or scratching.
   3. nausea and vomiting.
   4. fluid volume deficit.

5. Which drugs may be ordered for pruritus in patients with hepatitis?
   1. Antihistamines
   2. Antiemetics
   3. Antibiotics
   4. Analgesics

6. Health care workers who work with hospitalized patients should receive:
   1. hepatitis B vaccinations.
   2. herpes zoster vaccine
   3. influenza virus vaccine.
   4. immune globulin.

7. The medical management of ascites aims to promote reabsorption and elimination of the fluid by means of salt restriction and:
   1. antihistamines.
   2. analgesics.
   3. diuretics.
   4. antibiotics.

8. Potential complications of peritoneal-venous shunts used to allow ascitic fluid to drain from the abdomen and return to the bloodstream are tubing obstruction and:
   1. jaundice.
   2. peripheral neuropathy.
   3. pruritus.
   4. peritonitis.

9. The patient with cirrhosis is at great risk for injury or hemorrhage due to impaired:
   1. coagulation.
   2. immunity.
   3. skin integrity.
   4. breathing patterns.

10. What may happen when there is upward movement of the esophageal balloon in the patient with cirrhosis?
    1. Impaired circulation
    2. Airway obstruction
    3. Cardiac shock
    4. Perforated intestine

11. When the patient's bile duct responds to obstruction from gallstones with spasms in an effort to move the stone, the intense spasmodic pain would be documented as:
    1. ascites pain.
    2. cholelithiasis.
    3. biliary colic.
    4. biliary obstruction.

12. A common symptom of cholecystitis is right upper quadrant pain that radiates to the:
    1. sternum.
    2. shoulder.
    3. umbilicus.
    4. jaw.

13. When the cholecystectomy patient first returns from surgery, the drainage from the T-tube may be bloody, but it should soon become:
    1. dark amber.
    2. clay-colored.
    3. bright red.
    4. greenish brown.

14. Patients with obstructed bile flow may have a deficiency of vitamin:
    1. A.
    2. C.
    3. D.
    4. K.

15. A patient had an endoscopic sphincterotomy and developed pancreatitis as a complication, caused by accidental entry of the endoscope into the pancreatic duct. Early signs of pancreatitis in this patient would be:
    1. jaundice and confusion.
    2. nausea and vomiting.
    3. ascites and hypertension.
    4. pain and fever.

16. A gland that has both endocrine and exocrine functions is the:
    1. pancreas.
    2. adrenal gland.
    3. thyroid gland.
    4. sebaceous gland.

17. Vitamin K is needed for the production of:
    1. bile.
    2. calcium.
    3. prothrombin.
    4. thyroxine.

18. Specific blood studies used to assess pancreatic function include serum:
    1. bilirubin.
    2. amylase.
    3. prothrombin.
    4. albumin.

19. The most prominent symptom of pancreatitis is:
    1. jaundice.
    2. abdominal pain.
    3. hypertension.
    4. diarrhea.

20. Which of the following is recommended for patients with acute pancreatitis to remove the stimulus for secretion of pancreatic fluid?
    1. Nothing by mouth
    2. Low-fat diet
    3. Clear-liquid diet
    4. Low-sodium diet

21. Which drugs do patients with chronic pancreatitis need to take in order to digest food?
    1. Analgesics
    2. Anticholinergics
    3. Antiemetics
    4. Pancreatic enzymes

22. An early sign of shock that may occur in patients with pancreatitis include:
    1. restlessness.
    2. bradycardia.
    3. hypotension.
    4. easy bruising.

23. Which herb can harm the liver?
    1. Garlic
    2. Ginkgo
    3. Comfrey
    4. Ginseng

24. The bile channels in the liver are compressed in patients with hepatitis, resulting in elevated:
    1. serum creatinine.
    2. BUN.
    3. bilirubin.
    4. hemoglobin.

25. Which cultural group has the highest rate of death from cirrhosis of the liver?
    1. Hispanics
    2. African-Americans
    3. Caucasians
    4. Asians

26. The medical treatment of hepatic encephalopathy is directed toward:
    1. raising hemoglobin.
    2. reducing ammonia formation.
    3. decreasing urea.
    4. increasing prothrombin time.

27. In patients with hepatitis and/or cirrhosis, most of the calories should come from:
    1. carbohydrates.
    2. protein.
    3. saturated fats.
    4. unsaturated fats.

28. Which is a common lab finding consistent with hepatitis?
    1. Decreased levels of serum enzymes (AST, ALT, GT)
    2. Prolonged prothrombin time
    3. High albumin
    4. Low gamma globulin

29. Which group of drugs is now being used in the treatment of patients with hepatitis (HBV and HBC)?
    1. Antimicrobials
    2. Antivirals
    3. Anticoagulants
    4. Anticholinergics

30. Which of the following are true statements about hepatitis? Select all that apply.
    1. The first phase of hepatitis, which lasts from 1–21 days, is when the patient is most infectious.
    2. The second phase of hepatitis, which lasts from 2–4 weeks, is characterized by jaundice and clay-colored stools.
    3. There is an elevation in serum amylase when bile channels are compressed due to inflammation in the liver.
    4. The third phase of hepatitis, when there is fatigue, malaise, and liver enlargement, lasts for several months.

31. Which is a symptom common in cirrhosis that is characterized by tingling or numbness in the extremities thought to be caused by vitamin B deficiencies?
    1. Peripheral neuropathy
    2. Hepatic encephalopathy
    3. Portal hypertension
    4. Ascites

PART III: CHALLENGE YOURSELF!

J. Getting Ready for NCLEX.

Choose the most appropriate answer or select all that apply.

1. Which are interventions for a patient who has just had a liver biopsy? Select all that apply.
   1. Check pressure dressing every 15 minutes for the first hour, every 30 minutes for the next hour, and then hourly.
   2. Monitor the patient for signs of blood loss, which include bradycardia and hypertension.
   3. Keep the patient on the right side at least 2 hours.
   4. The patient may be kept flat up to 14 hours.

2. What are primary complications the nurse would watch for in a patient with a liver biopsy? Select all that apply.
   1. Hemorrhage
   2. Pneumothorax
   3. Hypertensive crisis
   4. Increased intracranial pressure

3. Which of the following results of blood tests and procedures are consistent with cirrhosis? Select all that apply.
   1. Elevated serum and urine bilirubin
   2. Decreased serum enzymes
   3. Increased total serum protein
   4. Decreased cholesterol
   5. Prolonged prothrombin time

4. What neurologic symptoms are caused by a failing liver and excessive ammonia in the blood? Select all that apply.
   1. Cognitive disturbances
   2. Declining level of consciousness
   3. Changes in neuromuscular function
   4. Numbness and tingling in extremities
   5. Edema in extremities

5. The nurse should explain to patients with hepatitis that rest is necessary to allow the liver to heal by:
   1. producing more white blood cells to fight infection.
   2. producing more platelets to assist in clotting.
   3. regenerating new cells to replace damaged cells.
   4. regenerating new blood vessels to replace damaged ones.

6. The nurse should be alert for signs of fluid retention in patients with hepatitis, which include increasing abdominal girth, rising blood pressure, and:
   1. dry mucous membranes.
   2. tachycardia.
   3. edema.
   4. concentrated urine.

7. The patient with hepatitis may be self-conscious about his or her appearance because of:
   1. cyanosis.
   2. redness.
   3. ulcerations.
   4. jaundice.

8. The best position for patients with ascites to help them breathe more easily is:
   1. side-lying.
   2. prone.
   3. supine.
   4. with the head of the bed elevated.

9. What type of diet is recommended for patients with cholecystitis to decrease attacks of biliary colic?
   1. Low protein
   2. Low fat
   3. Low carbohydrate
   4. Low salt

10. When patients with pancreatitis are on TPN in order to restrict oral intake and reduce pancreatic fluid secretion, the nurse must monitor for:
    1. hyperkalemia.
    2. hypernatremia.
    3. hyperchloremia.
    4. hyperglycemia

11. Which of the following are signs of bile duct obstruction that should be taught to patients? Select all that apply.
    1. Blood in the stool
    2. Dark urine
    3. Jaundice
    4. Steatorrhea

12. A patient is admitted to the hospital with cholelithiasis. Which problems should the nurse anticipate in patients with cholelithiasis? Select all that apply.
    1. Acute pain related to biliary colic
    2. Risk for injury (bleeding) related to vitamin K deficiency
    3. Risk for impaired skin integrity related to edema
    4. Disturbed thought processes related to elevated blood ammonia
    5. Risk for infection related to tissue necrosis

13. Which are common problems for patients with cirrhosis? Select all that apply.
    1. Acute pain related to biliary obstruction
    2. Risk for injury related to impaired coagulation
    3. Deficient fluid volume related to gastrointestinal suction
    4. Ineffective breathing patterns related to ascites
    5. Risk for impaired skin integrity related to hypoproteinemia

Nursing Care Plan.
Refer to Nursing Care Plan, The Patient with Pancreatitis, p. 871 in the textbook, and answer questions 14-19.

14. What is the priority nursing diagnosis for this patient?

15. What are the patient's risk factors?

16. What data was collected about this patient, indicating the presence of pancreatitis?

17. What are causes of pancreatitis? Select all that apply.
    1. Biliary tract disorders
    2. Alcoholism
    3. Peptic ulcer disease
    4. Hyperthyroidism
    5. Smoking

18. Which are common complications of pancreatitis? Select all that apply.
    1. Pseudocyst
    2. Abscess
    3. Hypercalcemia
    4. Renal complications

19. After oral intake is resumed, what are nutritional interventions for patients with pancreatitis to avoid stimulating the pancreas and promote healing? Select all that apply.
    1. Full liquid
    2. Bland
    3. High carbohydrate
    4. High fat
    5. Small feedings

Urologic Disorders

 Go to http://evolve.elsevier.com/Linton/medsurg/ for additional activities and exercises.

NCLEX CATEGORIES:

Safe and Effective Care Environment:
Coordinated Care, Safety and Infection Control

Health Promotion and Maintenance

Psychosocial Integrity

Physiological Integrity: Basic Care and Comfort, Pharmacological Therapies, Reduction of Risk Potential, Physiological Adaptation

OBJECTIVES

1. List the data to be collected when assessing a patient who has a urologic disorder.
2. Describe the diagnostic tests and procedures for patients with urologic disorders.
3. Explain the nursing responsibilities for patients having tests and procedures to diagnose urologic disorders.
4. Describe the nursing responsibilities for common therapeutic measures used to treat urologic disorders.
5. Explain the pathophysiology, signs and symptoms, complications, and treatment of disorders of the kidney, ureters, bladder, and urethra.
6. Assist in developing a nursing care plan for patients with urologic disorders.

PART I: MASTERING THE BASICS

A. Key Terms.
Match the description in the numbered column with the most appropriate term in the lettered column.

1. _____ Incision of organ or duct to remove calculi
2. _____ Inflammation of the urinary bladder

3. _____ Inflammation of the capillary loops in the glomeruli
4. _____ Removal of bladder
5. _____ Noninvasive procedure to break up calculi
6. _____ Removal of a kidney
7. _____ Process by which thick blood is removed from the body and circulated through an artificial kidney

A. Cystectomy
B. Cystitis
C. Glomerulonephritis
D. Hemodialysis
E. Lithotomy
F. Lithotripsy
G. Nephrectomy

B. Physiology.
Match the description or definition in the numbered column with the most appropriate term in the lettered column. Some terms may be used more than once.

1. _____ Causes reabsorption of water in the renal tubules, decreasing urine volume
2. _____ Released in response to inadequate renal blood flow or low arterial pressure
3. _____ The hormone secreted in the kidneys that stimulates the bone marrow to produce red blood cells
4. _____ The hormone that is released from the pituitary gland when stimulated by hypertonic plasma

A. Erythropoietin
B. Renin
C. Antidiuretic hormone

C. Diagnostic Procedures.

Match the statements in the numbered column with the most appropriate term in the lettered column.

1. _____ A general indicator of the kidneys' ability to excrete urea; values are raised by high-protein diets, gastrointestinal bleeding, dehydration, and some drugs

2. _____ The best laboratory test of overall kidney function

3. _____ Measures the rate of urine flow during voiding

4. _____ Outlines the contour of the bladder and shows reflux of urine

5. _____ Dye is injected IV, radiographs of kidney, ureters, and bladder are taken; used to assess kidney function

A. Blood urea nitrogen (BUN)
B. Creatinine clearance
C. Cystogram
D. Intravenous pyelogram
E. Urodynamic study

D. Urologic Disorders.

Match the statement in the numbered column with the most appropriate term in the lettered column.

1. _____ Condition in which calculi are formed in the kidneys.

2 _____ Inflammation of the renal pelvis.

3. _____ Hereditary disorder in which grape-like cysts replace normal kidney tissue

4. _____ Removal of a calculus from the renal pelvis

5. _____ Formation of calculi in the urinary tract

6. _____ Formation of calculi in the kidneys

A. Inflammation of the capillary loops in the glomeruli
B. Pyelolithotomy
C. Glomerulonephritis
D. Urolithiasis
E. Nephrolithiasis
F. Pyelonephritis

E. Diagnostic Procedures.

Match the description or definition in the numbered column with the appropriate diagnostic test in the lettered column.

1. _____ Examination of voided urine (or from catheter) specimen for pH, blood, glucose, and protein

2. _____ Clean-catch or midstream urine specimen is collected to determine which antibiotics will be effective against the specific organisms found in the culture

3. _____ Collection of urine for 12 or 24 hours, which is an estimate of the glomerular filtration rate

4. _____ A blood test that is a general indicator of the kidneys' ability to excrete urea

5. _____ A blood test that is indicative of the kidney's ability to excrete wastes

6. _____ A blood test that may show elevated sodium and potassium levels and decreased calcium levels, which indicate renal failure

A. Creatinine clearance
B. Serum creatinine
C. Urinalysis
D. Serum electrolytes
E. Blood urea nitrogen (BUN)
F. Urine sensitivity

F. Drug Therapy.

For the following drugs, indicate whether it is used to treat (A) oliguria or (B) hyperkalemia.

1. _____ Hypertonic glucose and insulin

2. _____ Furosemide (Lasix)

3. _____ Sodium bicarbonate

4. _____ Calcium gluconate

5. _____ Sodium polystyrene sulfonate (Kayexalate)

G. Age-Related Changes.

1. Which are true statements about age-related changes in the kidneys? Select all that apply.
    1. The function of kidneys remains normal.
    2. The renal blood flow increases.
    3. The glomerular filtration rate declines.
    4. The antidiuretic hormone's effect on tubules is that the tubules are more responsive.
    5. The kidney's ability to concentrate and dilute urine decreases.
    6. The incidence of nocturia decreases.

2. Which are true statements about age-related changes of the bladder? Select all that apply.
    1. Bladder muscles are weaker.
    2. Connective tissue in the bladder decreases.
    3. Capacity of bladder decreases
    4. Emptying function of bladder is incomplete.

H. Urine Characteristics.

Match the description in the numbered column with the appropriate term in the lettered column. Answers may be used more than once.

1. _____ Hematuria in acidic urine
2. _____ Small amounts of blood or bacterial infection
3. _____ Excessive fluid intake
4. _____ Chronic renal failure
5. _____ Normal
6. _____ Hematuria in alkaline urine
7. _____ Diabetes mellitus

A. Straw-colored
B. Bright red
C. Tea-colored
D. Cloudy or hazy appearance
E. Colorless

I. Urinary System.

In Figure 40-1 (p. 880) below, label the parts (A–H) of the urinary system.

A. _____

B. _____

C. _____

D. _____

E. _____

F. _____

G. _____

H. _____

PART II: PUTTING IT ALL TOGETHER

J. Multiple Choice/Multiple Response.

Choose the most appropriate answer or select all that apply.

1. Glomerular filtrate and blood plasma are essentially the same, except that the filtrate does not have:
   1. water.
   2. sodium.
   3. potassium.
   4. proteins.

2. As the blood passes through the glomerulus, which element is too large to pass through the semipermeable membrane?
   1. Serum sodium
   2. Serum potassium
   3. Plasma protein
   4. Glucose

3. The normal pH of urine is:
   1. 1.0–3.0.
   2. 4.5–8.0.
   3. 8.5–10.0.
   4. 10.5–3.0.

4. The body normally excretes how many liters of urine per day?
   1. 0.5 liter
   2. 1–2 liters
   3. 5 liters
   4. 7–10 liters

5. Two substances that are present in blood but not normally present in urine are:
   1. sodium and chloride.
   2. glucose and protein.
   3. calcium and magnesium.
   4. potassium and bicarbonate.

6. Glomerular damage may be indicated by the presence of which of the following in the urine?
   1. Sodium
   2. Chloride
   3. Protein
   4. Potassium

7. The presence of how much urine usually causes the urge to urinate?
   1. 100–150 ml
   2. 200–400 ml
   3. 500–600 ml
   4. 800–1000 ml

8. Blood pressure is regulated through fluid volume maintenance and release of the hormone:
   1. aldosterone.
   2. renin.
   3. antidiuretic hormone.
   4. parathormone.

9. A change in blood volume will result in a change in:
   1. body temperature.
   2. heart rate.
   3. blood pressure.
   4. respiratory rate.

10. Decreased oxygen in renal blood triggers the secretion of:
    1. aldosterone.
    2. antidiuretic hormone.
    3. epinephrine.
    4. erythropoietin.

11. Patients in renal failure have a deficiency of erythropoietin, which causes them to have:
    1. pneumonia.
    2. anemia.
    3. seizures.
    4. hypertension.

12. A common age-related problem in males related to the urinary system is:
    1. urethral obstruction.
    2. incontinence.
    3. relaxed pelvic musculature.
    4. lack of testosterone.

13. If crystals on the skin are observed during the examination of patients with urinary disorders, this is recorded as:
    1. ashen skin.
    2. edema.
    3. uremic frost.
    4. scaly skin.

14. Tissue turgor is evaluated in patients with urinary disorders to detect:
    1. uremic frost.
    2. Kussmaul's respirations.
    3. infection.
    4. dehydration.

15. If patients with urinary disorders have an odor of urine on their breath, this may indicate:
    1. urinary tract infection.
    2. kidney failure.
    3. cardiac failure.
    4. diabetes mellitus.

16. Patients with urinary disorders who have potassium imbalances may have:
    1. uremic frost.
    2. heart irregularities.
    3. hypertension.
    4. rapid respirations.

17. The edema found in renal failure is described as:
    1. dependent.
    2. peripheral.
    3. pitting.
    4. generalized.

18. In patients with renal failure, the skin over edematous areas is likely to be described as:
    1. warm and moist.
    2. dry and flushed.
    3. pink and intact.
    4. pale and thick.

19. Normally, urine is sterile and slightly:
    1. alkaline.
    2. acidic.
    3. pyuric.
    4. hematuric.

20. A diagnostic test for the identification of microorganisms present in urine is:
    1. blood urea nitrogen.
    2. urinalysis.
    3. urine culture.
    4. creatinine clearance.

21. Which blood test needs to be within normal limits before a renal biopsy is performed?
    1. Electrolytes
    2. Blood urea nitrogen
    3. Serum creatinine
    4. Clotting studies

22. After a renal biopsy, what is the most important side effect to watch for?
    1. Infection
    2. Dyspnea
    3. Bleeding
    4. Fatigue

23. Following cystoscopy, at first the urine will be:
    1. colorless.
    2. pink-tinged.
    3. tea-colored.
    4. orange.

24. Following cystoscopy, urine should lighten to its usual color within:
    1. 4–6 hours.
    2. 8–10 hours.
    3. 24–48 hours.
    4. 60–72 hours.

25. Following cystoscopy, belladonna and opium suppositories may be ordered to reduce:
    1. bladder spasm.
    2. hematuria.
    3. infection.
    4. back pain.

26. Bladder perforation is rare following cystoscopy, but it may be indicated by severe:
    1. hematuria.
    2. abdominal pain.
    3. tachycardia.
    4. hypotension.

27. The most common health care–associated infections are:
    1. skin infections.
    2. wound infections.
    3. urinary tract infections.
    4. blood infections.

28. A patient has urethritis. Which are common symptoms the nurse would expect to find? Select all that apply.
    1. Dysuria
    2. Frequency
    3. Dull flank pain
    4. Hematuria
    5. Bladder spasms
    6. Urgency

29. The pain of urethritis may be reduced by:
    1. antiemetics.
    2. back massage.
    3. sitz baths.
    4. meditation.

30. The passage of renal calculi is facilitated by:
    1. bedrest.
    2. opiates.
    3. restricted fluids.
    4. ambulation.

31. Which is a common symptom of pyelonephritis?
    1. Polyuria
    2. Hypotension
    3. Bradycardia
    4. Flank pain

32. The most common type of glomerulonephritis follows a respiratory tract infection caused by:
    1. staphylococcus.
    2. a virus.
    3. a fungus.
    4. streptococcus.

33. A patient has acute glomerulonephritis. Which medications are used in the treatment of this patient? Select all that apply.
    1. Diuretics
    2. Antihistamines
    3. Anticholinergics
    4. Antihypertensives
    5. Antibiotics

34. A patient is in the acute phase of glomerulonephritis. Bedrest is ordered to prevent or treat heart failure and severe hypertension that result from:
    1. fluid volume deficit.
    2. fluid overload.
    3. altered renal tissue perfusion.
    4. respiratory distress.

35. A common nursing diagnosis for patients with acute glomerulonephritis is:
    1. Fluid volume deficit.
    2. Fluid volume excess.
    3. Altered renal tissue perfusion.
    4. High risk for injury.

36. In which of the following groups is the incidence of uric acid stones high?
    1. Jewish males
    2. Caucasian females
    3. African-American females
    4. Hispanic males

37. When a person is dehydrated, the kidneys conserve water, causing urine to be:
    1. dilute.
    2. cloudy.
    3. alkaline.
    4. concentrated.

38. A major nursing concern for patients with renal calculi is:
    1. frequent ambulation.
    2. emotional support.
    3. range-of-motion exercises.
    4. pain relief.

39. The treatment of choice for renal cancer is:
    1. lithotripsy.
    2. radical nephrectomy.
    3. cystectomy.
    4. nephrostomy.

40. The location of the flank incision following nephrectomy causes pain with expansion of the:
    1. abdomen.
    2. pelvis.
    3. cerebrum.
    4. thorax.

41. Which is the most common malignancy of the urinary tract?
    1. Cancer of the kidney
    2. Cervical cancer
    3. Bladder cancer
    4. Liver cancer

42. The most frequent symptom of bladder cancer is intermittent:
    1. glycosuria.
    2. proteinuria.
    3. pyuria.
    4. hematuria.

43. When the bladder is removed completely, urinary diversion is sometimes provided, which allows urine to be excreted through the:
    1. urethra.
    2. ileal conduit.
    3. ureter.
    4. cystoscopy.

44. Which is the most effective means of assessing changes in fluid status of patients in acute renal failure?
    1. Monitoring edema
    2. Recording intake and output
    3. Weighing daily
    4. Taking vital signs

45. When 90–95% of kidney function is lost, the patient is considered to be in:
    1. acute renal failure.
    2. chronic renal failure.
    3. renal shock.
    4. renal oliguria.

46. The most life-threatening effect of renal failure is:
    1. hypernatremia.
    2. hyponatremia.
    3. hyperkalemia.
    4. hypokalemia.

47. When a kidney is obtained from a living related donor, the 1-year survival rate for transplantation is about:
    1. 30–33%
    2. 65–70%.
    3. 75–80%.
    4. 95–97%.

48. Which mediation is the transplant recipient given to control the body's response to foreign tissue?
    1. Analgesics
    2. Immunosuppressants
    3. Anticholinergics
    4. Antihistamines

49. Which specific nursing diagnosis is related to the possibility of organ rejection after renal transplantation?
    1. Risk for injury
    2. Altered role performance
    3. Anxiety
    4. Diarrhea

50. Complications of lithotripsy include:
    1. bruising.
    2. congestive heart failure.
    3. dyspnea.
    4. thrombus.

51. Risk factors for bladder cancer include:
    1. obesity.
    2. cigarette smoking.
    3. a high-purine diet.
    4. a sedentary lifestyle.

52. Which procedure is contraindicated in patients with known renal insufficiency or diabetes mellitus?
    1. Intravenous pyelogram (IVP)
    2. Flat plate
    3. Renal scan
    4. Ultrasonography

53. Which statements are true regarding diagnostic procedures for kidney disorders? Select all that apply.
    1. With normally functioning kidneys, the serum creatinine level is very high.
    2. A general indicator of the kidneys' ability to excrete urea is the BUN test.
    3. A better measurement of kidney functioning than the BUN because it is elevated only in kidney disorders is the serum creatinine.
    4. With normally functioning kidneys, the urine creatinine level is high.
    5. Two tests that are compared to each other and that should be opposite each other if kidneys are functioning normally are the creatinine clearance and the serum creatinine.

54. Which of the following statements about kidney disorders are true? Select all that apply.
    1. Itching can be caused by the accumulation of calcium phosphate crystals and urea in the skin.
    2. When a calculus obstructs urine flow, the urine may back up into the kidney, causing hydronephrosis.
    3. In patients with hydronephrosis, urine is usually strained and examined for bacteria.
    4. Most patients with chronic kidney failure retain water and sodium.

55. Which are symptoms of an allergic reaction to iodine dye used for intravenous pyelogram procedures? Select all that apply.
    1. Edema
    2. Hives
    3. Urticaria
    4. Swollen parotid glands

PART III: CHALLENGE YOURSELF!

K. Getting Ready for NCLEX.

Choose the most appropriate answer or select all that apply.

1. Which are signs of blood loss for which the nurse observes when a patient with kidney disease returns from undergoing angiography? Select all that apply.
   1. Bradycardia
   2. Restlessness
   3. Dyspnea
   4. Bleeding at injection site

2. The eyes of a patient with a urinary disorders are examined and periorbital edema is present. What is the reason for periorbital edema in this patient?
   1. Dehydration
   2. Fluid retention
   3. Uremic frost
   4. Kussmaul's respirations

3. If patients with urinary disorders have dyspnea, this may be a sign of:
   1. dehydration.
   2. uremic frost.
   3. potassium imbalance.
   4. fluid overload.

4. Inspection of the genitalia during the examination of patients with urinary disorders must always be done utilizing:
   1. auscultation.
   2. palpation.
   3. Standard Precautions.
   4. aseptic technique

5. To measure residual volume, the patient must be catheterized immediately after voiding. Which of the following is an abnormal finding?
   1. 5 ml
   2. 10 ml
   3. 25 ml
   4. 75 ml

6. Following urologic surgery, which of the following outputs should be reported to the physician?
   1. Less than 30 ml/hour
   2. Less than 50 ml/hour
   3. Less than 70 ml/hour
   4. Less than 100 ml/hour

7. An older patient with pyelonephritis experiences a suddenly increased fluid volume. Which complication may develop for which the nurse must monitor?
   1. Hypotension
   2. Congestive heart failure
   3. Seizures
   4. Thrombophlebitis

8. When the patient with renal calculi is discharged, what will the nurse teach about prevention of renal calculi? Select all that apply.
   1. Continue a high fluid intake (4L of fluids daily unless contraindicated)
   2. Drink most of the fluids during the day to prevent nocturia.
   3. Advise the patient to drink two glasses of water before bed and two glasses when awakening at night.
   4. Watch for signs of heart failure.

9. A patient has had a nephrectomy and is protecting his chest by not breathing deeply. For which related complication must the nurse monitor?
   1. Hemorrhage
   2. Infection
   3. Atelectasis
   4. Shock

10. Preoperative care for a patient undergoing an ileal or sigmoid conduit includes thorough preparation of the intestinal tract. Which antibiotic is administered that is not absorbed from the intestinal tract?
    1. Keflex
    2. Penicillin
    3. Neomycin
    4. Tetracycline

11. Which signs of dehydration would the nurse monitor in the patient who has had a renal transplant? Select all that apply.
    1. Thready pulse
    2. Bounding pulse
    3. Poor tissue turgor
    4. Hypertension
    5. Hypotension
    6. High fever

12. Which diet is recommended for patients with chronic kidney disease that will reduce the accumulation of urea? Select all that apply.
    1. High calcium
    2. High carbohydrates
    3. Low fat
    4. Low protein
    5. Low sodium

Nursing Care Plan.

Refer to Nursing Care Plan, The Patient with Renal Calculi, p. 905 in the textbook, and answer questions 13-18.

13. What are four abnormal findings on the physical examination for this patient?

14. How does this patient describe his pain after lithotripsy?

15. Which is a factor in this patient's history that fosters the development of calculi?

16. What is the priority nursing diagnosis?

17. What are the nursing interventions to alleviate pain in this patient? Select all that apply.
    1. Administer analgesics as ordered.
    2. Strain all urine to collect calculi fragments.
    3. Position changes to enhance analgesia.
    4. Administer antispasmodics as ordered.
    5. Administer antiemetics as ordered.
    6. Assess the abdomen and groin area for bruising.

18. Which tasks can be assigned to unlicensed assistive personnel for this patient? Select all that apply.
    1. Measure intake and output.
    2. Report low output to the nurse.
    3. Assess respiratory effort: rate, effort, breath sounds.
    4. Monitor vital signs.
    5. Teach patient about importance of consuming fluids over a 24-hour period.

Connective Tissue Disorders

 Go to http://evolve.elsevier.com/Linton/medsurg/ for additional activities and exercises.

NCLEX CATEGORIES:

Safe and Effective Care Environment:
Coordinated Care, Safety and Infection Control

Health Promotion and Maintenance

Psychosocial Integrity

Physiological Integrity: Basic Care and Comfort, Pharmacological Therapies, Reduction of Risk Potential, Physiological Adaptation

OBJECTIVES

1. Define connective tissue.
2. Describe the function of connective tissue.
3. Describe the characteristics and prevalence of connective tissue diseases.
4. Describe the diagnostic tests and procedures used for assessing connective tissue diseases.
5. Discuss the drugs used to treat connective tissue diseases.
6. Describe the pathophysiology and treatment of osteoarthritis (degenerative joint disease), rheumatoid arthritis, osteoporosis, gout, progressive systemic sclerosis, polymyositis, bursitis, carpal tunnel syndrome, ankylosing spondylitis, polymyalgia rheumatica, Reiter syndrome, Behçet syndrome, and Sjögren syndrome.
7. Identify the data to be collected in the nursing assessment of a patient with a connective tissue disorder.
8. Assist in developing a nursing care plan for a patient whose life has been affected by a connective tissue disease.

PART I: MASTERING THE BASICS

A. Key Terms.

Match the definition in the numbered column with the most appropriate term in the lettered column.

1. _____ Instrument used to measure joint range of motion
2. _____ Within the joint
3. _____ Elevated level of uric acid in the blood
4. _____ Deposit of sodium urate crystals under the skin
5. _____ Protrusions of the distal interphalangeal finger joints; associated with osteoarthritis
6. _____ Enlarged proximal interphalangeal joints of the fingers
7. _____ Granulation of tissue surrounding cores of fibrous debris
8. _____ Plastic repair of a joint
9. _____ Inflammation of blood vessels
10. _____ Crackling sound or sensation
11. _____ Joint immobility

A. Hyperuricemia
B. Ankylosis
C. Tophus
D. Vasculitis
E. Intra-articular
F. Heberden nodes
G. Crepitus
H. Goniometer
I. Rheumatoid nodule
J. Bouchard nodes
K. Arthroplasty

B. Diagnostic Tests.

Match the purpose or description in the numbered column with the appropriate diagnostic test in the lettered column. Some tests may not be used.

1. _____ Determines presence of inflammation; increased with rheumatoid arthritis (RA) and decreased with osteoarthritis

2. _____ Detection of blood dyscrasias; decreased values in RA and systemic lupus erythematosus (SLE)

3. _____ Increased values with infection, tissue necrosis, and inflammation; sometimes decreased values in SLE

4. _____ Determines the presence of antibodies; present in patients with RA

5. _____ Assesses renal function; elevated values in SLE, scleroderma, and polyarteritis

6. _____ Detects active inflammation, as in RA and SLE

7. _____ Measures presence of antibodies that react with a variety of nuclear antibodies; positive in SLE, RA, scleroderma, Raynaud disease, Sjögren syndrome

A. C-reactive protein
B. Rheumatoid factor (RF)
C. Erythrocyte sedimentation rate (ESR)
D. White blood cell count (WBC)
E. Antinuclear antibodies (ANA)
F. Red blood cell count (RBC)
G. Platelet count
H. Creatinine

C. Radiologic Tests.

Match the purpose or description in the numbered column with the appropriate radiologic test in the lettered column. Some tests may not be used.

1. _____ Intravenous radioactive material that is taken up by bone is injected for visualization of entire skeletal system; procedure detects malignancies, osteoporosis, osteomyelitis, and some fractures

2. _____ Determines density, texture, and alignment of bones; assesses soft tissue involvement

3. _____ Scans the soft tissues and bones by use of both radiographs and computers; determines presence of tumors or some spinal fractures

4. _____ Examines soft tissue joint structures; performed most commonly on shoulder or knee when a traumatic injury is suspected and determines presence of bone chips, torn ligaments, or other loose bodies

5. _____ Contrast medium injected directly into vertebral disk being examined

6. _____ Soft tissue visualization produced by sound waves

7. _____ A noninvasive procedure that makes use of magnetic energy sources to view soft tissue

A. Ultrasound
B. Magnetic resonance imaging (MRI)
C. Radiography
D. Discography
E. Nuclear scintigraphy (bone scan)
F. PET
G. Computed tomography (CT) scan
H. Arthrography

D. Drug Therapy.

Match the description in the numbered column with the drug classification(s) in the lettered column. Some answers may have more than one drug classification.

1. _____ Examples are Indocin and Clinoril.

2. _____ Examples are methotrexate (Folex) and sulfasalazine (Azulfidine).

3. _____ Examples are allopurinol and probenecid.

4. _____ Examples are etanercept (Enbrel) and infliximab (Remicade).

5. _____ Examples are Fosamax, calcitonin (Miacalcin), and raloxifene (Evista).

6. _____ Examples are hydrocortisone and prednisone.

7. _____ Example is celecoxib (Celebrex).

8. _____ Examples are aspirin, naproxen, and ibuprofen.

9. _____ Main side effect is GI bleeding.

10. _____ Indicated for severe ankylosing spondylitis and painful shoulders.

11. _____ A monoclonal antibody that neutralizes activity of tumor necrosis factor, decreasing inflammation. Used to treat RA.

12. _____ Drugs that inhibit synthesis of uric acid or increase urinary excretion of uric acid.

13. _____ Antiinflammatory drugs that suppress normal immune response.

A. First-generation nonsteroidal antiinflammatory drugs (NSAIDs)
B. Second-generation nonsteroidal antiinflammatory drugs: COX-2 inhibitors
C. Indole analogues
D. Glucocorticoids
E. Disease-modifying antirheumatic drugs (DMARDs)
F. Biologic response modifiers, antiarthritic
G. Antigout agents
H. Bone resorption inhibitors

E. Osteoarthritis.
Match the statement in the numbered column with the most appropriate term in the lettered column. Some terms may be used more than once, and some terms may not be used.

1. _____ A device that is used after joint replacement surgery to move the joints through a set range of motions at a set rate of movements per minute

2. _____ The most common form of arthritis, which is also called *degenerative joint disease*

3. _____ The surgical treatment of choice for OA

4. _____ Disorder in which joint activities are compromised because the basic structure of the cartilage is altered

5. _____ The primary indication for total joint replacement in patients with OA

6. _____ A condition that generally affects joints under pressure (such as the spine and knees)

A. Total joint replacement
B. Physical therapy
C. Continuous passive movement machine
D. Osteoarthritis (OA)
E. Ankylosing spondylitis
F. Intractable pain

F. Rheumatoid Arthritis.
Match the statement in the numbered column with the most appropriate term in the lettered column. Some terms may be used more than once, and some terms may not be used.

1. _____ Disorder in which the synovium thickens and fluid accumulates in the joint spaces of patients

2. _____ A loss of joint mobility occurring in RA

3. _____ Disorder in which morning stiffness lasting more than 1 hour is a common symptom

4. _____ Inflammation of blood vessels affected by RA

5. _____ Subcutaneous nodules over bony prominences, which are often present in RA

6. _____ Inflammation of sacs at joints treated by lidocaine injections for temporary relief

7. _____ Compression of the median nerve in the wrist, causing pain and tenderness

8. _____ A chronic, progressive inflammatory disease

A. Rheumatoid arthritis (RA)
B. Osteoarthritis
C. Rheumatoid nodules
D. Bursitis
E. Vasculitis
F. Polymyositis
G. Ankylosis
H. Carpal tunnel syndrome

G. Connective Tissue Disorders.
Complete the statements in the numbered column with the most appropriate term in the lettered column. Some terms may be used more than once, and some terms may not be used.

1. _____ A disease characterized by dry mouth, dry eyes, and dry vagina

2. _____ A condition in which there is loss of bone mass, making the patient susceptible to fractures

3. _____ A common site of fractures due to osteoporosis, in addition to the wrist and vertebrae

4. _____   A technique for measuring bone mass

5. _____   A systemic disease characterized by the deposition of urate crystals in the joints and other body tissues

6. _____   An excessive rate of uric acid production or decreased uric acid excretion by the kidneys

7. _____   The joint commonly affected by gout

8. _____   Substance not recommended in diet for patients with gout

A. Absorptiometry
B. Hyperuricemia
C. Purine
D. Hip
E. Systemic lupus erythematosus
F. Sjögren syndrome
G. Osteoporosis
H. Gout
I. Great toe

H. Connective Tissue Disorders.

Complete the statement in or match the numbered column with the most appropriate term in the lettered column. Some terms may be used more than once.

1. _____   Decreased elasticity, stenosis, and occlusion of vessels

2. _____   An inflammatory disease that primarily affects the vertebral column, causing spinal deformities

3. _____   The management of Raynaud phenomenon is aimed at elimination of anything that causes _____.

4. _____   Scleroderma may be brought into remission with high doses of immunosuppressants or _____.

5. _____   A condition characterized by inflammation and damage to blood vessels that is present in nearly all connective tissue diseases

6. _____   A condition characterized by degeneration of articular cartilage

7. _____   The primary symptom of polymyositis

8. _____   A chronic multisystem disease that draws its name from the characteristic hardening of the skin

A. Muscle weakness
B. Osteoarthritis
C. Vasculitis
D. Steroids
E. Progressive systemic sclerosis (scleroderma)
F. Ankylosing spondylitis
G. Vasospasm
H. Dermatomyositis
I. Polymyositis

I. Synovial Joint.

In Figure 41-1 (p. 939) below, label the major structures (A–H) of the normal diarthroidal joint.

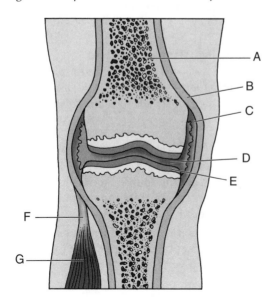

A. _____

B. _____

C. _____

D _____

E. _____

F. _____

G. _____

PART II: PUTTING IT ALL TOGETHER

J. Multiple Choice/Multiple Response.

Choose the most appropriate answer or select all that apply.

1. Important changes in the connective tissue of the body that occur with aging include loss of bone strength and bone:
   1. nutrients.
   2. mass.
   3. vitamins.
   4. minerals.

2. Age-related joint changes are related primarily to changes in:
   1. blood volume.
   2. bone strength.
   3. bone mass.
   4. cartilage.

3. When assessing patients for joint pain and range of motion, the nurse watches for signs of pain and listens for the crackling sound called:
   1. bursitis.
   2. grinding.
   3. crepitus.
   4. scraping.

4. Which blood test results would the nurse expect to see increase in patients with RA and decrease in patients with OA?
   1. C-reactive protein
   2. Creatinine
   3. White blood cell count
   4. Erythrocyte sedimentation rate (ESR)

5. Which categories of drugs are used in the treatment of arthritis? Select all that apply.
   1. Nonsteroidal antiinflammatory drugs (NSAIDs)
   2. Glucocorticoids
   3. Disease-modifying antirheumatic drugs (DMARDS)
   4. Diuretics

6. Following joint replacement surgery, a continuous passive motion (CPM) machine may be used to prevent formation of scar tissue and promote:
   1. phagocytosis.
   2. clotting.
   3. flexibility.
   4. circulation.

7. Often the pain in OA can be controlled with:
   1. beta blockers.
   2. salicylates.
   3. anticholinergics.
   4. narcotics.

8. Which is a nursing diagnosis that patients with OA often may have related to pain and limited range of motion?
   1. Ineffective coping
   2. Altered self-esteem
   3. Impaired tissue perfusion
   4. Impaired physical mobility

9. A patient has had knee replacement surgery. Which are interventions that reduce the risk of deep vein thrombosis? Select all that apply.
   1. Antiembolic stockings
   2. Pneumatic compression devices
   3. Anticoagulants
   4. Placement of pillows under legs
   5. Exercises to flex and extend the toes, feet, and ankles hourly

10. A patient who has had hip surgery is showing signs of cerebral blood vessel occlusion, headache, confusion, and loss of consciousness. The nurse will monitor this patient for:
    1. deep vein thrombosis.
    2. hemorrhage.
    3. fat embolus.
    4. neuropathy.

11. How should the nurse document the manifestation of pressure caused by edema or constrictive dressings following joint replacement surgery that is causing nerve damage?
    1. Paresthesia
    2. Infection
    3. Positive Homans sign
    4. Hemorrhage

12. Which drugs are administered to patients with joint replacements who are at risk for infection?
    1. Antihistamines
    2. Antimicrobials
    3. Antiemetics
    4. Anticoagulants

13. Which factor slows bone loss and improves strength, balance, and reaction time (reducing the risk of falls and fractures)?
    1. Vitamin D
    2. Increased fluid intake
    3. Regular exercise
    4. Protein

14. Patients with gout may have altered urinary elimination related to:
    1. dehydration.
    2. restricted fluid intake.
    3. kidney stones.
    4. edema.

15. To prevent the complication of kidney stones in patients with gout, patients are advised to:
    1. protect affected joints from trauma.
    2. keep walking pathways lighted and free from obstacles.
    3. obtain assistance with activities of daily living.
    4. drink at least eight glasses of fluid daily.

16. When a patient has pain from RA, which group is most likely to face pain stoically?
    1. Dominican Republican
    2. German
    3. Caucasian American
    4. Italian

17. When a patient is taking NSAIDs for RA, the nurse monitors the patient for:
    1. fatigue.
    2. edema.
    3. bruising.
    4. infection.

18. Which antiinflammatory drugs slow the progression of RA?
    1. COX-2 inhibitors
    2. Disease-modifying antirheumatic drugs (DMARDs)
    3. Biologic response modifiers (BRMs)
    4. Glucocorticoids

19. Which are symptoms of RA? Select all that apply.
    1. Fatigue
    2. Morning stiffness lasting more than 1 hour
    3. Muscle aches
    4. Increased temperature
    5. Hypotension
    6. Tingling in extremities

PART III: CHALLENGE YOURSELF!

K. Getting Ready for NCLEX.

Choose the most appropriate answer or select all that apply.

1. When mobility is severely impaired following hip replacement surgery, which of the following are complications for which the patient is at risk? Select all that apply.
   1. Contractures
   2. Pulmonary and circulatory complications
   3. Urinary retention
   4. Constipation
   5. Hemorrhage
   6. Skin breakdown

2. Which nursing diagnoses are common in patients with gout? Select all that apply.
   1. Acute pain related to joint inflammation
   2. Chronic pain related to swelling and tenderness
   3. Risk for trauma related to loss of bone strength
   4. Risk for injury related to improper alignment
   5. Chronic pain with motion related to loss of smooth joint surfaces
   6. Impaired urinary elimination related to urate kidney stones

3. A patient with RA is taking ibuprofen. Which are the expected outcomes of this drug for this patient? Select all that apply.
   1. Reduce pain
   2. Decrease inflammation
   3. Prevent joint damage
   4. Slow progress of the disease

4. Symptoms of salicylate toxicity in older adults may be atypical; instead of the common symptoms of gastrointestinal complaints or ototoxicity, the older person may exhibit:
   1. drowsiness.
   2. confusion.
   3. malaise.
   4. hypotension.

5. Which of the following may promote independence and safety for the patient who has poor hip mobility? Select all that apply.
   1. Bathroom grab bars
   2. Seat in the shower
   3. Antiembolic stockings
   4. Raised toilet seat
   5. Use of sterile technique

6. A nursing diagnosis following total joint replacement that is related to improper alignment, dislocated prosthesis, and/or weakness is:
   1. Altered peripheral tissue perfusion.
   2. Risk for injury.
   3. Risk for infection.
   4. Knowledge deficit.

7. A patient with uncontrolled pain is reluctant to participate in rehabilitation measures following total joint replacement surgery. Which intervention may improve patient participation?
   1. Assess nerve and circulatory status before exercises.
   2. Check vital signs at least every 4 hours.
   3. Assist patient in and out of bed.
   4. Administer analgesics 30 minutes to 1 hour before exercises.

8. Prosthetic joints can become dislocated if they are not maintained in proper alignment. After hip replacement surgery, the affected leg must be kept in a position of:
   1. abduction.
   2. adduction.
   3. slight elevation.
   4. supination.

9. Body areas distal to the operative joint are monitored for circulatory adequacy by assessing warmth, color, and:
   1. peripheral pulses.
   2. ulceration.
   3. skin necrosis.
   4. wound drainage.

10. Pillows and pads should not be placed under the legs of patients with joint replacements in order to reduce the risk of:
    1. ulceration.
    2. gangrene.
    3. deep vein thrombosis.
    4. infection.

11. After joint replacement, the patient often has ineffective tissue perfusion and is at risk for:
    1. headache.
    2. hemorrhage.
    3. seizure.
    4. pneumonia.

12. If the nurse suspects that a dressing is too tight and is causing nerve damage, the nurse monitors sensations:
    1. at the wound site.
    2. proximal to the joint.
    3. distal to the joint.
    4. within the joint.

13. A nursing intervention related to the patient's high risk for infection is that the nurse will:
    1. place the call light in easy reach.
    2. instruct patient to keep legs slightly abducted.
    3. use strict sterile technique for dressing changes.
    4. assess nerve and circulatory status.

14. A measure to control morning pain and stiffness in patients with RA is to:
    1. take a warm shower.
    2. increase intake of fluids.
    3. eat foods low in purines.
    4. apply ice.

15. An important teaching point for patients taking antigout medications is to:
    1. increase potassium intake.
    2. avoid foods high in vitamin K.
    3. rise slowly from a sitting position.
    4. increase fluids.

16. Which food should be avoided in patients with acute gout?
    1. Sardines
    2. Aged cheese
    3. Bananas
    4. Orange juice

Nursing Care Plan.
Refer to Nursing Care Plan, The Patient with a Total Hip Replacement, p. 941 in the textbook, and answer questions 17-20.

17. What are the four priority problems for which this patient is at risk?

    1. _____

    2. _____

    3. _____

    4. _____

18. What are this patient's risk factors related to osteoarthritis (OA) that resulted in the need for total hip replacement surgery?

    1. _____

    2. _____

19. What are three interventions related to prevention of injury concerning dislocation for this patient?

    1. _____

    2. _____

    3. _____

20. What tasks for this patient could be assigned to unlicensed assistive personnel?

    1. _____

    2. _____

    3. _____

    4. _____

    5. _____

Fractures

 Go to http://evolve.elsevier.com/Linton/medsurg/ for additional activities and exercises.

NCLEX CATEGORIES:

Safe and Effective Care Environment:
Coordinated Care, Safety and Infection Control

Health Promotion and Maintenance

Psychosocial Integrity

Physiological Integrity: Basic Care and Comfort, Pharmacological Therapies, Reduction of Risk Potential, Physiological Adaptation

OBJECTIVES

1. Identify the types of fractures.
2. Describe the five stages of the healing process.
3. Discuss the major complications of fractures, their signs and symptoms, and their management.
4. Compare the types of medical treatment for fractures, particularly reduction and fixation.
5. Describe common therapeutic measures for fractures, including casts, traction, crutches, walkers, and canes.
6. Discuss the nursing care of a patient with a fracture.
7. Describe specific types of fractures, including hip fractures, Colles fractures, and pelvic fractures.

PART I: MASTERING THE BASICS

A. Key Terms. Fractures.
Match the definition in the numbered column with the most appropriate term in the lettered column.

1. _____ Fracture in which the fragments of the broken bone break through the skin

2. _____ Fracture in which the break extends across the entire bone, dividing it into two separate pieces

3. _____ Fracture in which the bone breaks only partially across, leaving some portion of the bone intact

4. _____ Fracture caused by either sudden force or prolonged stress

5. _____ Break or disruption in the continuity of a bone

6. _____ Fracture in which the bone is broken or crushed into small pieces

7. _____ Fracture in which the bone is broken on one side but only bent on the other; most common in children

8. _____ Fracture in which the broken bone does not break through the skin

A. Closed or simple fracture
B. Incomplete fracture
C. Fracture
D. Complete fracture
E. Stress fracture
F. Open or compound fracture
G. Comminuted fracture
H. Greenstick fracture

B. Complications.
Match the definition in the numbered column with the most appropriate term in the lettered column.

1. _____ Condition in which fat globules are released from the marrow of the broken bone into the bloodstream, migrate to the lungs, and cause pulmonary edema

2. _____ Serious complication of a fracture caused by internal or external pressure to the affected area, resulting in decreased blood flow, pain, and tissue damage

3. _____ Failure of a fracture to heal

4. _____ Procedure done during the open reduction surgical procedure to attach the fragments of the broken bone together when reduction alone is not feasible

5. _____ Process of bringing the ends of the broken bone into proper alignment

6. _____ Nonsurgical realignment of the bones to their previous anatomic position using traction, angulation, rotation, or a combination of these

7. _____ Surgical procedure in which an incision is made at the fracture site, usually on patients with open (compound) or comminuted fractures, to cleanse the area of fragments and debris

8. _____ Process in which immature bone cells are gradually replaced by mature bone cells

9. _____ Healing of fracture does not occur in the normally expected time

10. _____ Improper alignment of a fracture resulting in deformity

A. Compartment syndrome
B. Open reduction
C. Fixation
D. Delayed union
E. Nonunion
F. Bone remodeling
G. Closed reduction or manipulation
H. Fat embolism
I. Reduction
J. Malunion

C. Casts.

Complete the statements in the numbered column with the most appropriate term in the lettered column. Some terms may be used more than once.

1. _____ A cast used for breaks in the forearm, elbow, or humerus

2. _____ A cast used for fracture of the distal femur, knee, or lower leg

3. _____ A cast that encircles the trunk; used for stable spine injuries of thoracic or lumbar spine

4. _____ A cast that encases the trunk plus two extremities; used for fractures of the femur, acetabulum, or pelvis

5. _____ Used for fractures of the foot, ankle, or distal tibia or fibula

6. _____ Used for injury to the knee or knee dislocation

7. _____ Used for soft tissue injury to knee, allowing knee to bend

8. _____ Used for fracture of the hand or wrist

A. Body jacket cast
B. Short arm cast
C. Short leg cast
D. Bilateral long leg hip spica cast
E. Long leg cast
F. Long arm cast
G. Cast brace

D. Traction.

Match the statements in the numbered column with the most appropriate term in the lettered column. Some terms may be used more than once.

1. _____ A pulling force on a fractured extremity to provide alignment of the broken bone fragments

2. _____ Traction applied directly to a bone

3. _____ Traction applied directly to the skin

4. _____ A type of traction used for immobilization of fractures of the cervical vertebrae

5. _____ A type of traction used for hip and knee contractures, muscle spasms, and alignment of hip fractures

6. _____ A type of traction in which tongs are inserted into either side of the skull

A. Skin traction
B. Buck's traction
C. Crutchfield's traction
D. Skeletal traction
E. Traction

E. Fracture Healing.

Place the stages of fracture healing in the correct order. Refer to Figure 42-2, p. 962 in the textbook.

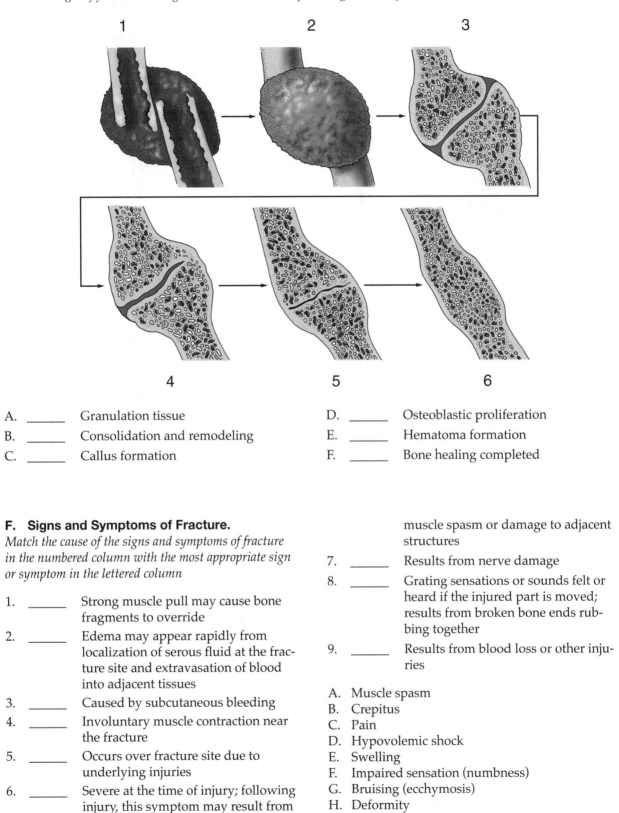

1	2	3
4	5	6

A. _____ Granulation tissue

B. _____ Consolidation and remodeling

C. _____ Callus formation

D. _____ Osteoblastic proliferation

E. _____ Hematoma formation

F. _____ Bone healing completed

F. Signs and Symptoms of Fracture.

Match the cause of the signs and symptoms of fracture in the numbered column with the most appropriate sign or symptom in the lettered column

1. _____ Strong muscle pull may cause bone fragments to override

2. _____ Edema may appear rapidly from localization of serous fluid at the fracture site and extravasation of blood into adjacent tissues

3. _____ Caused by subcutaneous bleeding

4. _____ Involuntary muscle contraction near the fracture

5. _____ Occurs over fracture site due to underlying injuries

6. _____ Severe at the time of injury; following injury, this symptom may result from muscle spasm or damage to adjacent structures

7. _____ Results from nerve damage

8. _____ Grating sensations or sounds felt or heard if the injured part is moved; results from broken bone ends rubbing together

9. _____ Results from blood loss or other injuries

A. Muscle spasm
B. Crepitus
C. Pain
D. Hypovolemic shock
E. Swelling
F. Impaired sensation (numbness)
G. Bruising (ecchymosis)
H. Deformity
I. Tenderness

G. Types of Fractures.

1. In Figure 42-1 (p. 961) below, label each type of fracture (A–L) with numbers from the following list.

1. Greenstick
2. Oblique
3. Transverse
4. Displaced
5. Longitudinal
6. Stress

7. Comminuted (fragmented)
8. Interarticular
9. Spiral
10. Avulsion
11. Impacted
12. Pathologic

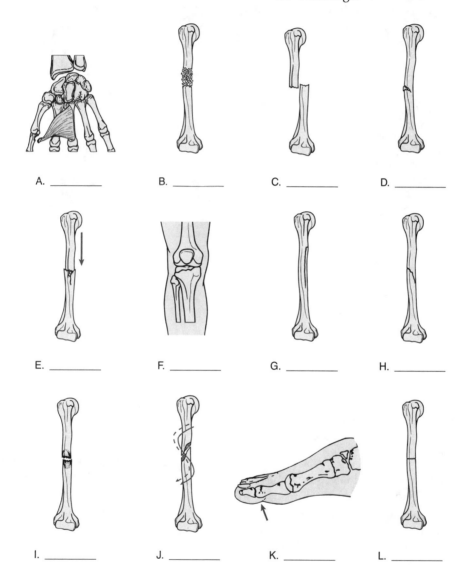

A. _____   B. _____   C. _____   D. _____

E. _____   F. _____   G. _____   H. _____

I. _____   J. _____   K. _____   L. _____

2. Which type of fracture is caused by a tumor in the bone?

3. Which type of fracture occurs most frequently in children?

4. Which type of fracture is often related to a sports injury, such as track?

H. Hip Fractures.

1. Using Figure 42-10 (p. 975) below, label the anatomic regions in the diagram below and the type of fractures in B–E.

A. Anatomic Regions

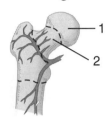

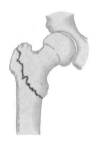

B

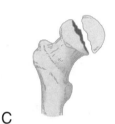

C

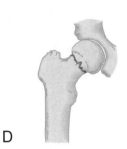

D

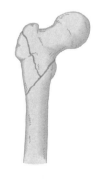

E

A. 1. _____

   2. _____

B. _____

C. _____

D. _____

E. _____

2. Where do most hip fractures occur? Select all that apply.
   1. Femoral head
   2. Femoral neck
   3. Intertrochanteric region
   4. Subtrochanteric region

3. What percentage of women by the age of 90 have sustained a hip fracture?
   1. 10%
   2. 20%
   3. 30%
   4. 40%

4. What are signs and symptoms of a hip fracture? Select all that apply.
   1. History of a fall
   2. Severe pain and tenderness in the region of the fracture site
   3. Bleeding at the fracture site
   4. Internal rotation of the hip on the affected side

5. What is the standard treatment for hip fractures? Select all that apply.
   1. Traction
   2. External fixation
   3. Femoral head replacement
   4. Total hip replacement

I.   Skin Traction.

1.   In Figure 42-7 (p. 969) below, label each type of traction (A–E) using the following list.

  1.   _____   Head halter traction
  2.   _____   Pelvic traction
  3.   _____   Russell's traction
  4.   _____   Buck's traction
  5.   _____   Balanced suspension traction

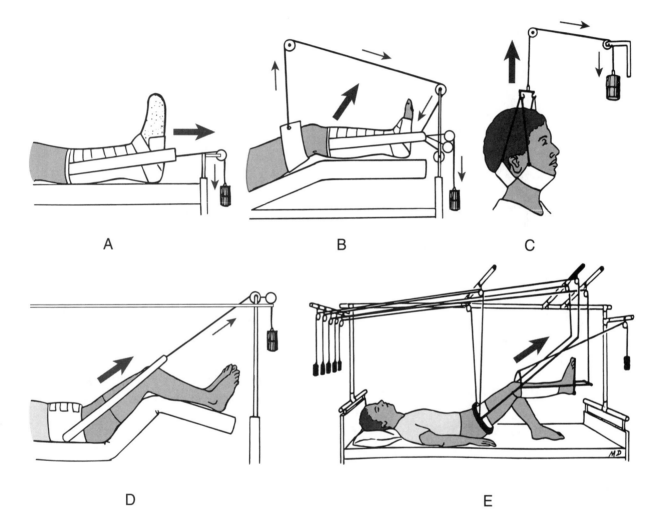

A   B   C

D   E

2.   What are the purposes of traction? Select all that apply.
   1.   Prevent or correct deformity
   2.   Decrease muscle spasm
   3.   Promote rest
   4.   Clean the area of fragments and debris
   5.   Use of rods, pins and metal plates to align bone fragments and keep them in place for healing
   6.   Maintain the position of the diseased or injured part

PART II: PUTTING IT ALL TOGETHER

J. Multiple Choice/Multiple Response.

Choose the most appropriate answer or select all that apply.

1. In adults, the bones most commonly fractured are:
    1. femurs.
    2. ribs.
    3. pelvic bones.
    4. wrists.

2. In young and middle-aged adults, the most common fractures are those of the:
    1. femur.
    2. rib.
    3. wrist.
    4. pelvis.

3. The most common fractures in older adults are fractures of the wrist and:
    1. femur.
    2. rib.
    3. hip.
    4. shoulder.

4. Which is a characteristic of fat embolism following a fracture?
    1. Bradycardia
    2. Decreased respirations
    3. Oliguria
    4. Petechiae

5. The most common diagnostic test used to reveal bone disruption, deformity, or malignancy following a fracture is:
    1. myelography.
    2. standard radiography.
    3. ultrasonography.
    4. bone scan.

6. The use of rods, pins, nails, screws, or metal plates to align bone fragments is called:
    1. external fixation.
    2. closed reduction.
    3. internal fixation.
    4. mechanical reduction.

7. Which are used for external fixation of extensive fractures and fractures of the extremities?
    1. External frames
    2. Rods
    3. Pins
    4. External metal plates

8. A condition in which a patient in a body cast may have feelings of claustrophobia is called:
    1. compartmental syndrome.
    2. cardiac shock.
    3. cast syndrome.
    4. fat embolus.

9. Following total hip replacement, which patient teaching is contraindicated?
    1. Do not extend the affected hip more than 90 degrees.
    2. Use an elevated toilet seat.
    3. Sit in supportive chairs.
    4. Avoid crossing the legs.

10. Crutch use may not be appropriate for older or frail patients, because it requires good:
    1. lower extremity function.
    2. cardiac function.
    3. lung expansion.
    4. upper body strength.

11. When walking with crutches, patients should put their weight on the:
    1. top of the crutches.
    2. hand grips.
    3. lower extremities.
    4. shoulders.

12. The type of gait pattern used with bilateral lower extremity prostheses is called:
    1. four-point.
    2. swing-to.
    3. swing-through.
    4. two-point.

13. When a patient is climbing stairs using crutches, which body part goes up the step first while the body is supported by the crutches?
    1. Unaffected leg
    2. Affected leg
    3. Upper extremities
    4. Spine

14. Which gait is used with a walker?
    1. Two-point
    2. Four-point
    3. Modified swing-to
    4. Modified swing-through

15. Canes should be held close to the body on the:
    1. left side.
    2. right side.
    3. affected side.
    4. unaffected side.

16. When the nurse is assessing the patient with a fracture, the affected extremity is compared with the:
    1. proximal body parts.
    2. distal body parts.
    3. unaffected extremity.
    4. normal skeleton.

17. In order to assess circulation and sensation in the affected and unaffected extremity, the nurse should perform neurovascular checks in the areas:
    1. distal to the wound.
    2. proximal to the wound.
    3. surrounding the wound.
    4. inside the wound.

18. A good indication of circulation to the extremity in patients with a fracture is:
    1. size of the wound.
    2. edema.
    3. skin color.
    4. infection.

19. If pallor is observed in the extremity of patients with fractures, this may be an indication of:
    1. infection.
    2. poor circulation.
    3. hemorrhage.
    4. skin breakdown.

20. The primary method of pain relief for patients with fractures is:
    1. application of cold to the affected part.
    2. application of heat to the affected part.
    3. wrapping the affected part with a blanket.
    4. immobilization of the affected part.

21. An appropriate intervention for patients with fractures who have impaired physical mobility is:
    1. strict aseptic technique.
    2. monitor for fever.
    3. isolation precautions.
    4. gait training.

22. Patients with fractures are at risk for impaired skin integrity; treatment measures such as casts or traction to immobilize parts may result in:
    1. pressure sores.
    2. petechiae.
    3. palmar erythema.
    4. paralysis.

23. For older patients with hip fractures, the treatment of choice is:
    1. immobilization.
    2. antibiotic therapy.
    3. surgical repair.
    4. traction.

24. Colles fracture is a break in the distal:
    1. humerus.
    2. tibia.
    3. radius.
    4. fibula.

25. Colles fractures frequently occur in older adults when they use their hands to:
    1. sew or knit.
    2. break a fall.
    3. write letters.
    4. reach for objects above their heads.

26. Interventions for Colles fractures are aimed at relieving pain and preventing edema; for the first few days, the extremity should be:
    1. below the heart.
    2. exercised.
    3. elevated.
    4. flat.

27. Patients with Colles fractures are encouraged to move their fingers and thumb to promote circulation and reduce:
    1. temperature.
    2. swelling.
    3. infection.
    4. dyspnea.

28. Patients with Colles fractures are encouraged to move their shoulders to prevent:
    1. infection.
    2. circulation.
    3. cyanosis.
    4. stiffness.

29. The most common cause of pelvic fractures in young adults is:
    1. head injury.
    2. motor vehicle accidents.
    3. falls.
    4. myocardial infarction.

30. The main cause of pelvic fractures in older adults is:
    1. motor vehicle accidents.
    2. head injury.
    3. falls.
    4. heart attacks.

31. The nurse needs to observe the patient with a pelvic fracture closely for signs of:
    1. internal trauma.
    2. bone infection.
    3. kidney failure.
    4. dyspnea.

32. Which is restricted in patients with pelvic fractures until healing is complete?
    1. Use of a trapeze while in bed
    2. Range-of-motion exercises
    3. Coughing and deep-breathing exercises
    4. Weight-bearing

33. Which are short-term complications of a fracture that the nurse should monitor during the first 3 days post-surgery? Select all that apply.
    1. Deep vein thrombosis
    2. Fat embolism
    3. Delayed union
    4. Complex regional pain syndrome
    5. Joint stiffness and contractures
    6. Compartment syndrome
    7. Shock

34. Which are common causes of osteomyelitis associated with fractures? Select all that apply.
    1. Indwelling hardware used to repair the bone
    2. Wound contamination
    3. Fat embolism
    4. Compartment syndrome

PART III: CHALLENGE YOURSELF!

K. Getting Ready for NCLEX.
Choose the most appropriate answer.

1. The nurse is taking care of a patient with a lumbar spine fracture. Which is the proper positioning for this patient?
    1. Before medical treatment, keep patient supine and immobilize patient's neck; after treatment, turn with head well-supported
    2. Avoid high sitting positions; log roll
    3. When fracture is stable or after fixation, turn to side opposite fracture
    4. Elevate head of bed to comfort; turn to side opposite fracture

2. An appropriate intervention for patients with fractures who have ineffective tissue perfusion is:
    1. strict aseptic technique.
    2. gait training.
    3. elevation of the affected part above the heart.
    4. rest periods to preserve strength.

Nursing Care Plan.
Refer to Nursing Care Plan, The Patient with a Fracture, p. 972 in the textbook, and answer questions 3-5.

3. What is the priority nursing diagnosis for this patient?

4. What are risk factors for this patient to have a fracture?

5. What tasks can be assigned to unlicensed assistive personnel?

Amputations

 Go to http://evolve.elsevier.com/Linton/medsurg/ for additional activities and exercises.

NCLEX CATEGORIES:

Safe and Effective Care Environment:
Coordinated Care, Safety and Infection Control

Health Promotion and Maintenance

Psychosocial Integrity

Physiological Integrity: Basic Care and Comfort, Pharmacological Therapies, Reduction of Risk Potential, Physiological Adaptation

OBJECTIVES

1. Identify the clinical indications for amputations.
2. Describe the different types of amputations.
3. Discuss the medical and surgical management of the amputation patient.
4. Identify appropriate nursing interventions during the preoperative and postoperative phases of care.
5. Assist in developing a nursing care plan for the amputation patient.

PART I: MASTERING THE BASICS

A. Key Terms.

Match the definition in the numbered column with the most appropriate term in the lettered column.

1. _____ Type of amputation in which a limb or portion of a limb is severed from the body and the wound is left open; a type of open amputation

2. _____ Amputation that is done over the course of several surgeries; usually done to control the spread of infection or necrosis

3. _____ Amputation in which a limb or part of a limb is removed and the wound is surgically closed

4. _____ Individual who has undergone an amputation

5. _____ Necrosis, or death of tissue, usually due to a deficient or absent blood supply; may result from inflammatory processes, injury, arteriosclerosis, frostbite, or diabetes mellitus

6. _____ Deformity or absence of a limb or limbs occurring during fetal development in the uterus

7. _____ The sensation that a limb still exists following amputation of the limb

8. _____ Amputation in which the wound is left open; usually done in cases of infection or necrosis

9. _____ Partial limb remaining after amputation

10. _____ Removal of a limb, part of a limb, or an organ; may be done by surgical means or may be the result of an accident

11. _____ Surgical reattachment of an organ to its original site; reimplantation

A. Phantom limb
B. Amputee
C. Guillotine amputation
D. Staged amputation
E. Gangrene
F. Open amputation
G. Replantation
H. Closed amputation
I. Congenital amputation
J. Amputation
K. Residual limb (stump)

B. Indications for Amputation.

Which of the following are diseases leading to impaired circulation that may result in the need for an amputation? Select all that apply.
1. Osteoporosis
2. Peripheral vascular disease
3. Diabetes mellitus
4. Arteriosclerosis

C. Open Amputation.

Which of the following are reasons for doing an open amputation instead of a closed amputation? Select all that apply.
1. Create a weight-bearing residual limb
2. Done when an actual or potential infection exists
3. Done in the case of gangrene or trauma
4. Done for non-weight–bearing residual limb amputations

D. Types of Amputations.

Match or complete the statement in the numbered column with the most appropriate term in the lettered column.

1. _____ The removal of the lower leg at the middle of the shin
2. _____ Removal of part or all of a limb during a serious accident
3. _____ Conditions that lead to the need for an amputation include trauma, disease, and _____.
4. _____ An amputation through the joint

A. Tumors
B. Traumatic amputation
C. Disarticulation
D. Below-knee amputation

E. Diagnostic Tests.

Match the indication in the numbered column with the name of the appropriate diagnostic test relating to amputation in the lettered column. Some terms may be used more than once.

1. _____ Record heat present to measure amount of blood flow to certain part of body
2. _____ Done after imaging reveals suspicious lesions
3. _____ Detects infection

4. _____ Determine nature of tumor
5. _____ Indicates volume of blood flow to extremity
6. _____ Determine presence of pulses in extremities
7. _____ Compromised circulation

A. Bone biopsy
B. Pulse volume recording (plethysmography)
C. Doppler ultrasound
D. WBC
E. Vascular studies (angiography)
F. Thermography

F. Complementary Therapies.

Which are complementary therapies that are used with analgesics to control pain in patients after surgical amputation? Select all that apply.
1. Imagery
2. Relaxation
3. Aerobic exercises
4. Meditation
5. Acupuncture

PART II: PUTTING IT ALL TOGETHER

G. Multiple Choice/Multiple Response.

Choose the most appropriate answer or select all that apply.

1. Replantation surgery is most likely to be performed on the:
   1. shoulder.
   2. hand.
   3. forearm.
   4. upper arm.

2. The purpose of giving heparin to a postoperative replantation patient is to reduce the risk of:
   1. thrombosis.
   2. edema.
   3. infection.
   4. hypersensitivity.

3. A complication of amputation due to inadequate hemostasis is:
   1. necrosis.
   2. hemorrhage.
   3. gangrene.
   4. contracture.

4. A complication of amputation manifested by redness, warmth, swelling, and exudate formation at the residual limb site due to invasion of tissues by pathogens is called:
   1. contracture.
   2. infection.
   3. edema.
   4. necrosis.

5. Which may be prevented by frequent position changes and range-of-motion exercises?
   1. Infection
   2. Hemorrhage
   3. Necrosis
   4. Contractures

6. Which is an opening of the suture line (caused by early removal of sutures or falling) that requires reclosure?
   1. Gangrene
   2. Necrosis
   3. Wound dehiscence
   4. Contracture

7. Which person will request that an amputated body part be present for burial?
   1. Roman Catholic
   2. Mormon
   3. Orthodox Jew
   4. Muslim

8. Which diagnosis is a priority in the postoperative period for a patient after surgical amputation?
   1. Disturbed body image
   2. Impaired skin integrity
   3. Pain
   4. Disturbed sensory perception

9. Which treatment for venous congestion of a replanted limb utilizes the saliva of parasites that extracts excess blood?
   1. Anticoagulants
   2. Vasodilators
   3. Leeches
   4. Local anesthetics

10. What complication can occur if pillows are placed continuously under a below-knee amputation?
    1. Infection
    2. Necrosis
    3. Phantom limb sensation
    4. Hip contractures

11. Which complications are associated with amputations? Select all that apply.
    1. Urinary retention
    2. Hemorrhage and hematoma
    3. Wound dehiscence
    4. Gangrene
    5. Hyperglycemia
    6. Contracture
    7. Infection
    8. Constipation
    9. Pulmonary complications
    10. Necrosis
    11. Phantom limb sensation
    12. Phantom limb pain

12. What are signs that indicate the medical emergency of inadequate arterial circulation following replantation? Select all that apply.
    1. No peripheral pulse
    2. Warm skin
    3. Pallor
    4. Slow capillary refill

13. Which medications may be helpful for phantom limb pain? Select all that apply.
    1. Beta blockers
    2. Anticonvulsants
    3. Antidepressants
    4. Benzodiazepines
    5. Opioids
    6. NSAIDs

PART III: CHALLENGE YOURSELF!

H. Getting Ready for NCLEX.

Choose the most appropriate answer.

1. Which statements are true regarding patient instruction for residual limb and prosthesis care? Select all that apply.
    1. Wash residual limb with soap and water every night. Rinse and dry skin thoroughly.
    2. Do not expose the residual limb to air.
    3. Keep prosthetic socket and residual limb sock clean. Use a clean sock every day.
    4. Lotions, ointments, and powders may be applied once a day.
    5. If redness or irritation develops on the residual limb, discontinue use of prosthesis and have area checked.
    6. The residual limb may shrink in size for up to 2 years after surgery. Annual visits to the prosthetist are recommended.

2. What is the indication that a postoperative amputation patient would experience readiness for enhanced self-care?
    1. Surgical incision, scar formation on a severed nerve
    2. Surgical disruption of skin integrity
    3. Expressed need to function independently after loss of limb
    4. Perceived threat of disability

3. A patient had an above-the-knee amputation 1 week ago. Which nursing interventions related to impaired physical mobility are indicated for this patient to prevent contractures? Select all that apply.
    1. Active and passive range-of-motion exercises
    2. Check temperature; watch for foul or unpleasant odor from stump
    3. Use of overbed trapeze
    4. Whirlpool, massage, or TENS stimulation if ordered
    5. Observe for excessive bleeding
    6. Use of imagery, acupuncture, analgesics
    7. Wrap bandage smoothly; elevate residual limb
    8. Avoid prolonged flexion of the hip

4. Which are appropriate outcome criteria for a postoperative patient following amputation? Select all that apply.
    1. Patient accepts limb loss; demonstrates proper care of residual limb
    2. Bright red bleeding is expected at first in Hemovac, followed by reddish-brown drainage
    3. Patient carries out daily activities without excessive fatigue
    4. Treatment for phantom limb pain includes diversional activities and transcutaneous electrical nerve stimulation (TENS).

5. Which are nursing interventions for the older adult who has had an amputation? Select all that apply.
    1. Emphasize high-calorie and high-protein diet
    2. Skip unnecessary details when teaching
    3. Provide a prosthesis with extra padding and support to patients with diabetes
    4. Recognize that poor vision and decreased sensation may keep older people from recognizing complications
    5. Explain that phantom pain is a serious complication that should be reported to the physician

6. Which are nursing measures for a patient with a replanted limb that promote circulation to the replanted limb? Select all that apply.
    1. Elevate limb above the level of the heart.
    2. Avoid caffeine for 7–10 days postoperatively.
    3. Enforce no smoking.
    4. Maintain room temperature at 80° F to prevent vasoconstriction.
    5. Wear loose clothing.

Nursing Care Plan.
Refer to Nursing Care Plan, The Patient with an Upper Extremity Amputation, p. 985 in the textbook, and answer questions 7-9.

7. What is the priority nursing diagnosis for this patient?

8. What were risk factors that led to this patient's need for an upper extremity amputation?

9. What tasks can be assigned to unlicensed assistive personnel?

Pituitary and Adrenal Disorders

 Go to http://evolve.elsevier.com/Linton/medsurg/ for additional activities and exercises.

NCLEX CATEGORIES:

Safe and Effective Care Environment:
Coordinated Care, Safety and Infection Control

Health Promotion and Maintenance

Psychosocial Integrity

Physiological Integrity: Basic Care and Comfort, Pharmacological Therapies, Reduction of Risk Potential, Physiological Adaptation

OBJECTIVES

1. Identify data to be collected for the nursing assessment of the adrenal and pituitary glands.
2. Describe the tests and procedures used to diagnose disorders of the adrenal and pituitary glands.
3. Describe the pathophysiology and medical treatment of adrenocortical insufficiency, excess adrenocortical hormones, hypopituitarism, diabetes insipidus, and pituitary tumors.
4. Assist in developing nursing care plans for patients with selected disorders of the adrenal and pituitary glands.

PART I: MASTERING THE BASICS

A. Key Terms.

Match the definition in the numbered column with the most appropriate term in the lettered column.

1. _____ Ductless gland that produces an internal secretion discharged into the lymph or bloodstream and circulated to all parts of the body; hormones, the active substances of these glands, cause an effect on certain organs or tissues

2. _____ Disease resulting from a deficiency of adrenocorticotropic hormone (ACTH)

caused by destruction or dysfunction of the adrenal glands; characterized by increased pigmentation of the skin and mucous membranes, weakness, fatigue, hypotension, nausea, weight loss, and hypoglycemia

3. _____ Disease caused by inadequate secretion of antidiuretic hormone (ADH) by the posterior pituitary gland; symptoms include excessive urination, thirst, and dehydration

4. _____ Disease of middle-aged adults resulting from overproduction of growth hormone (GH) by the anterior pituitary gland; characterized by enlargement of the facial bones, nose, lips, and jaw; also associated with decreased libido, moodiness, fatigue, muscle pains, sweating, and headache

5. _____ Type of hormone secreted by the adrenal cortex and involved in the regulation of fluid and electrolyte levels in the body

6. _____ Disorder caused by excess antidiuretic hormone production; symptoms include decreased urination, edema, and fluid overload

7. _____ Disorder resulting from excessive glucocorticoids in the body as a result of tumor or hypersecretion of the pituitary; may also be caused by prolonged administration of large doses of exogenous steroids; symptoms include fat deposits in the neck and abdomen, fatigue, weakness, edema, excess hair growth, glucose intolerances, skin discoloration, and mood swings

8. _____ Class of adrenocortical hormones that affects protein and carbohydrate metabolism and helps protect the body against stress

9. _____ Chemical (dopamine, epinephrine, norepinephrine) released at sympathetic nerve endings in response to stress

10. _____ Hormones produced by the ovaries, adrenal glands, and fetoplacental unit in females that are responsible for the development and maturation of females

11. _____ Disease caused by excessive growth hormone in children and young adolescents, resulting in excessive proportional growth

12. _____ Disease caused by the hypersecretion of glucocorticoids as a result of excessive release of adrenocorticotropic hormone by the pituitary gland

13. _____ Hormones produced by the adrenal cortex and testes that stimulate the development of male characteristics

14. _____ Surgical removal of all or part of the pituitary gland

15. _____ Epinephrine; a powerful vasoactive substance produced by the medulla or adrenal glands in times of stress or danger, allowing the body to react by fighting or fleeing

A. Acromegaly
B. Addison's disease
C. Adrenaline
D. Androgens
E. Catecholamines
F. Cushing's disease
G. Cushing's syndrome
H. Diabetes insipidus (DI)
I. Endocrine gland
J. Estrogens
K. Gigantism
L. Glucocorticoids
M. Hypophysectomy
N. Mineralocorticoids
O. Syndrome of inappropriate antidiuretic hormone (SIADH)

B. Pituitary Gland Disorders.

Match or complete the statements in the numbered column with the most appropriate term in the lettered column.

1. _____ Often the first symptom of a problem in hyperpituitarism

2. _____ Radiographic films of the skull of people with hyperpituitarism may show a large sella turcica and increased _____.

3. _____ The treatment of choice for patients with a diagnosis of pituitary tumors

4. _____ A disease that occurs in early childhood or puberty in which the diaphyses of the long bones grows to great lengths stimulated by excess GH

5. _____ A disease that appears when adults are in their 30s and 40s in which bones increase in thickness and width after epiphyseal closure

A. Gigantism
B. Hypophysectomy
C. Bone density
D. Acromegaly
E. Visual deficit

C. SIADH.

Complete the statements in the numbered column with the most appropriate term in the lettered column. Some terms may be used more than once.

1. A syndrome characterized by a water imbalance related to an increase in ADH secretion is called _____.

2. Kidneys retain fluid due to the elevation of _____.

3. Plasma volume expands when ADH is elevated in SIADH, causing an increased _____.

4. When the ADH level is elevated, the patient experiences water intoxication and the body's sodium is diluted, resulting in _____.

5. Weight gain without edema is one of the main symptoms of _____.

6. The treatment of SIADH promotes the elimination of _____.

7. In patients with SIADH, fluids are restricted and patients are given _____.

8. Patients with SIADH have fluid volume excess related to excess secretion of _____.

A. Blood pressure
B. Excess water
C. SIADH
D. Hyponatremia
E. ADH
F. Sodium chloride

D. Addison's Disease.

Complete the statements in the numbered column with the most appropriate term in the lettered column. Some terms may be used more than once.

1. Addison's disease results in the loss of aldosterone and _____.

2. A test that is necessary for a definitive diagnosis of hypoadrenalism, such as Addison's disease, is _____.

3. The mainstay of treatment of patients with Addison's disease is replacement therapy with mineralocorticoids and _____.

4. Potassium excretion is decreased when cortisol is not secreted, resulting in _____.

5. Secondary adrenal insufficiency is a result of dysfunction of the hypothalamus or the _____.

6. Decreased levels of aldosterone alter the clearance of potassium, water, and _____.

7. When sodium and water excretion rates accelerate, resulting problems are hyponatremia and _____ .

8. Acute adrenal crisis is also called _____.

9. Impaired secretion of cortisol results in decreased liver and muscle glycogen and decreased _____.

10. Secondary adrenal insufficiency leads to decreased production of cortisol and _____.

11. Primary adrenal insufficiency is also called _____.

12. Decreased supply of available glucose which occurs as a result of impaired secretion of cortisol is called _____.

13. Patients with either primary or secondary adrenal insufficiency are at risk for episodes of _____.

14. A condition that occurs because hyperkalemia promotes hydrogen ion retention is _____.

A. Hypovolemia
B. Pituitary gland
C. Addison's disease
D. Gluconeogenesis
E. Glucocorticoids
F. ACTH stimulation test
G. Hypoglycemia
H. Hyperkalemia
I. Metabolic acidosis
J. Sodium
K. Androgen
L. Cortisol
M. Addisonian crisis

E. Pituitary and Adrenal Hormones.

Match the definition or description in the numbered column with the most appropriate term in the lettered column. Some terms may be used more than once, and some may not be used.

1. _____ Stimulates the growth and development of bone, muscles, or organs

2. _____ Controls ovulation or egg release in the female and testosterone production in the male

3. _____ Controls the release of glucocorticoids and adrenal androgens

4. _____ Stimulates the development of eggs in the ovary of the female and the production of sperm in the testes of the male

5. _____ Another name for the somatotrophic hormone

6. _____ Stimulates breast milk production in the female

7. _____ Promotes pigmentation

8. _____ Another name for the lactogenic hormone

9. _____ Causes the reabsorption of water from the renal tubules of the kidney)

10. _____ Causes contractions of the uterus in labor and the release of breast milk

11. _____ Another name for vasopressin

12. _____ Controls the secretory activities of the thyroid gland

A. Luteinizing hormone
B. Thyroid-stimulating hormone
C. Oxytocin
D. Melanocyte-stimulating hormone
E. Growth hormone
F. Antidiuretic hormone
G Adrenocorticotropic hormone
H. Prolactin
I. Follicle-stimulating hormone

F. Diabetes Insipidus.
Complete the statements in the numbered column with the most appropriate term in the lettered column.

1. Increased plasma osmolarity stimulates the osmoreceptors, which in turn relay information to the cerebral cortex, causing the person to experience _____ .

2. Massive dehydration leads to severe _____ imbalances.

3. With ADH deficiency, massive dehydration occurs, which leads to decreased intravascular volume, circulatory collapse, and _____ .

4. Electrolyte imbalances contribute to circulatory collapse by causing arrhythmias and impaired contractility of the _____ .

5. Massive diuresis results in increased plasma _____ .

A. Thirst
B. Hypotension
C. Heart
D. Electrolyte
E. Osmolarity

G. Drug Therapy.
Match the descriptions of drugs used for adrenal disorders in the numbered column with the drug classification in the lettered column. Answers may be used more than once.

1. _____ Used to suppress adrenocortical function

2. _____ Stimulate reabsorption of sodium and excretion of potassium and hydrogen ions

3. _____ Stimulate the formation of glucose and promote the storage of glucose as glycogen

4. _____ Used to treat adrenal insufficiency

5. _____ Example of this category is Florinef

6. _____ Example of this category is hydrocortisone (Cortef)

A. Glucocorticoids
B. Mineralocorticoids
C. Adrenocortical cytotoxic agents

H. Diagnostic Tests.
Match the description in the numbered column with the name of the procedure in the lettered column.

1. _____ Used to detect diabetes mellitus and hyperpituitarism

2. _____ Serum levels are measured to detect elevations or deficiencies of pituitary hormones

3. _____ Given to stimulate release of ADH to detect DI

4. _____ Measures cortisol, which increases with adrenal hyperplasia and Cushing's syndrome

5. _____ Detects changes in specific gravity and osmolality after vasopressin is given; used to detect DI

6. _____ Radiographs taken to study cerebral blood flow and blood vessels

7. _____ Uses radiographs to create images of internal structures and detect tumors

A. Cerebral computed tomography scan
B. Cerebral angiogram
C. Glucose tolerance test
D. Dexamethasone suppression tests
E. Pituitary hormone serum levels
F. Hypertonic saline test
G. Fluid deprivation test

I.   Endocrine System.

Using Figure 44-1 (p. 995) below, label the organs of the endocrine system (A–G).

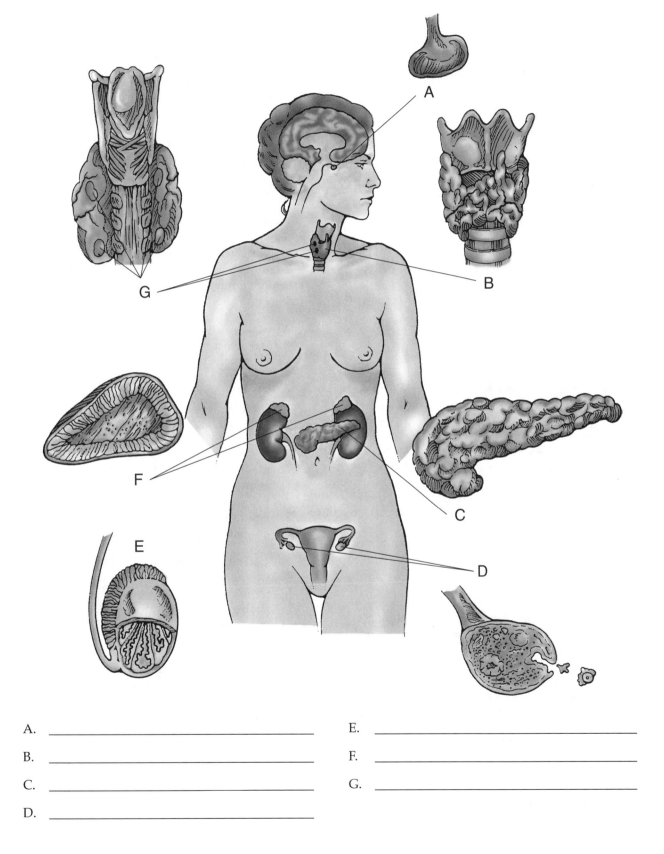

A. _____   E. _____

B. _____   F. _____

C. _____   G. _____

D. _____

PART II: PUTTING IT ALL TOGETHER

J.   Multiple Choice/Multiple Response.

Choose the most appropriate answer or select all that apply.

1. In the healthy older person, there may be increased secretion of ADH, which may lead to:
    1.   fluid imbalance.
    2.   dyspnea.
    3.   hypertension.
    4.   hypopituitarism.

2. The production of excess GH may lead to the development of:
    1.   atherosclerosis and hyperglycemia.
    2.   edema and congestive heart failure.
    3.   dyspnea and pneumonia.
    4.   oliguria and kidney failure.

3. GH antagonizes insulin and interferes with its effects, thus leading to:
    1.   hyperkalemia.
    2.   hypokalemia.
    3.   hyperglycemia.
    4.   hypoglycemia.

4. Because growth hormone mobilizes stored fat for energy, levels of free fatty acids are elevated in the bloodstream, leading to the development of:
    1.   pneumonia.
    2.   kidney failure.
    3.   hypotension.
    4.   atherosclerosis.

5. Visual problems occur in hyperpituitarism due to pressure on the:
    1.   occipital lobe.
    2.   optic nerves.
    3.   frontal lobe.
    4.   oculomotor nerves.

6. Patients with gigantism and acromegaly initially present with increased strength, progressing rapidly to complaints of:
    1.   hypotension and syncope.
    2.   weakness and fatigue.
    3.   edema and dry skin.
    4.   dehydration and bradycardia.

7. One drug commonly prescribed for patients with acromegaly is:
    1.   octreotide (Sandostatin).
    2.   furosemide (Lasix).
    3.   levothyroxine (Synthroid).
    4.   digoxin.

8. A common nursing diagnosis for patients with hyperpituitarism is:
    1.   Altered tissue perfusion.
    2.   Altered skin integrity.
    3.   High risk for infection.
    4.   Disturbed body image.

9. Bromocriptine (Parlodel) inhibits the release of prolactin and GH from:
    1.   antidiuretic hormone.
    2.   the thyroid gland.
    3.   the adrenal gland.
    4.   the pituitary gland.

10. Strict documentation of intake and output and measurement of specific gravity are important because postoperative hypophysectomy patients are at risk for:
    1.   congestive heart failure.
    2.   kidney failure.
    3.   pneumonia.
    4.   DI.

11. A bedside test can be done with a chemical strip to detect whether drainage in a postoperative hypophysectomy patient is cerebrospinal fluid (CSF), because CSF has a high content of:
    1.   glucose.
    2.   protein.
    3.   white blood cells.
    4.   red blood cells.

12. Decreased pigmentation of the skin results in:
    1.   edema.
    2.   pallor.
    3.   pruritus.
    4.   erythema.

13. The patient who has a complete hypophysectomy requires hormone replacement:
    1.   preoperatively.
    2.   during the postoperative recovery period.
    3.   for 6 months to 1 year.
    4.   for a lifetime.

14. In patients with hypopituitarism, insufficient thyroid hormone is available for normal metabolism and:
    1.   visual acuity.
    2.   muscle tone.
    3.   heat production.
    4.   bone growth.

15. If there is a lack of melanocyte-stimulating hormone, the skin exhibits decreased:
    1. sensory perception.
    2. immunity.
    3. pigmentation.
    4. thermoregulation.

16. To produce or maintain libido, secondary sexual characteristics, and well-being, males with hypopituitarism should receive:
    1. testosterone.
    2. estrogen.
    3. levothyroxine (Synthroid).
    4. bromocriptine (Parlodel).

17. Drug-related DI is often caused by:
    1. bromocriptine (Parlodel).
    2. lithium carbonate (Eskalith).
    3. levothyroxine (Synthroid).
    4. digitalis.

18. A 24-hour urine output of greater than 4 liters of fluid suggests a diagnosis of:
    1. hypertension.
    2. kidney infection.
    3. congestive heart failure.
    4. DI.

19. In order to maintain adequate blood volume in patients with DI, two measures that are required include intravenous fluid volume replacement and:
    1. diuretics.
    2. vasopressors.
    3. anticholinergics.
    4. antihistamines.

20. The level of consciousness deteriorates and the patient may have seizures or lapse into a coma when water intoxication affects the:
    1. respiratory system.
    2. urinary system.
    3. cardiovascular system.
    4. central nervous system.

21. In postmenopausal women, the primary source of endogenous estrogen is the:
    1. hypothalamus.
    2. thyroid gland.
    3. adrenal cortex.
    4. ovarian follicle.

22. A common skin finding in patients with adrenal dysfunction is:
    1. protruding bones.
    2. erythema.
    3. bronze pigmentation.
    4. pruritus.

23. An age-related change that affects the adrenal glands is that adrenal function:
    1. decreases in epinephrine.
    2. remains adequate.
    3. becomes hyperactive.
    4. increases in metabolism.

24. What is a common sign of DI?
    1. Massive diuresis
    2. Edema
    3. Hyperglycemia
    5. Oliguria

25. Which is the most common cause of Cushing's syndrome?
    1. Prolonged administration of high doses of corticosteroids
    2. Corticotropin-secreting pituitary tumor
    3. Truncal obesity
    4. Protein wasting

26. In the immediate postoperative period of adrenalectomy patients, which medication is needed to maintain blood pressure?
    1. Glucocorticoids
    2. Vasopressors
    3. Beta blockers
    4. Oxytocin

27. Indicate whether the following laboratory study results would be expected to (A) increase or (B) decrease in patients with Addison's disease.
    1. _____ Serum cortisol level
    2. _____ Fasting glucose
    3. _____ Sodium
    4. _____ Potassium
    5. _____ Blood urea nitrogen

28. Match the nursing diagnoses for patients with Cushing's syndrome in the numbered column with the most appropriate "related to" statements in the lettered column.

    1. _____ Risk for infection
    2. _____ Disturbed thought processes
    3. _____ Risk for impaired skin integrity
    4. _____ Risk for injury (fracture)
    5. _____ Disturbed body image

    A. Changes in skin and connective tissue and edema
    B. Changes in physical appearance and function
    C. Fluid and electrolyte imbalance
    D. Osteoporosis
    E. High serum cortisol levels

29. Which are appropriate nursing diagnoses for patients with Cushing's syndrome? Select all that apply.
    1. Risk for injury (fracture)
    2. Risk for impaired skin integrity
    3. Disturbed body image
    4. Fluid volume deficit
    5. Ineffective self health management
    6. Disturbed thought processes
    7. Risk for infection

30. Which of the following are age-related changes in the healthy older person regarding pituitary function? Select all that apply.
    1. Pituitary function is not adequate.
    2. ADH secretion may be increased.
    3. Ability to concentrate urine may be decreased.
    4. Risk for dehydration decreases.

31. The nurse is monitoring the postoperative hypophysectomy patient for signs and symptoms of infection. Which are signs and symptoms that may be indications of meningitis? Select all that apply.
    1. Decreased white blood cell (WBC) count
    2. Sudden rise in temperature
    3. Headache
    4. Neck rigidity

32. Which medications are given as hormone replacement therapy following a complete hypophysectomy? Select all that apply.
    1. Pituitary hormone suppressants
    2. Dopamine receptor antagonists
    3. Glucocorticoids
    4. Thyroid medications

33. The postoperative hypophysectomy patient is instructed to avoid any activities that can cause Valsalva's maneuver. Which activities may create enough intracranial pressure to disrupt the surgical site and cause CSF leakage? Select all that apply.
    1. Passive range-of-motion exercises
    2. Coughing
    3. Straining
    4. Vomiting

34. Which are manifestations of acute adrenal crisis (addisonian crisis)? Select all that apply.
    1. Bradycardia
    2. Dehydration
    3. Confusion
    4. Hyponatremia
    5. Hypoglycemia
    6. Hyperkalemia
    7. Hypertension

35. Which types of stressors can initiate acute adrenal crisis (addisonian crisis)? Select all that apply.
    1. Infection
    2. Illness
    3. Steroid therapy use
    4. Trauma

36. Which are diagnostic test results used to determine the presence of Addison's disease? Select all that apply.
    1. Decreased fasting glucose
    2. Decreased BUN
    3. Hyponatremia
    4. ECG changes of increased peaked T waves

PART III: CHALLENGE YOURSELF!

K. Getting Ready for NCLEX.

Choose the most appropriate answer or select all that apply.

1. A patient has been admitted to the hospital with Addison's disease. Which problem would the nurse expect to see in this patient?
    1. Excess fluid volume related to excess ADH secretion
    2. Risk for infection related to high serum cortisol levels
    3. Ineffective tissue perfusion related to electrolyte imbalances
    4. Fluid volume deficit related to excessive urine output

2. Changes in assessment findings following hypophysectomy that may reflect edema due to the manipulation of tissues or bleeding intracranially include:
    1. unequal pupil size.
    2. decreasing alertness.
    3. decreasing blood pressure.
    4. rising body temperature.

3. Following hypophysectomy, the nurse asks the patient to place the chin to the chest to assess for nuchal rigidity, which is associated with:
    1. bone density.
    2. meningeal irritation.
    3. cerebral edema.
    4. impaired circulation.

4. Because CSF leaks sometimes occur in postoperative hypophysectomy patients, the nurse should check:
    1. intake and output.
    2. pupil reactivity.
    3. nasal packing.
    4. vital signs.

5. Deficiency of thyroid-stimulating hormones necessitates thyroid replacement with a drug such as:
    1. octreotide acetate (Sandostatin).
    2. bromocriptine (Parlodel).
    3. levothyroxine (Synthroid).
    4. vasopressin (Pitressin Synthetic).

6. A nursing diagnosis for patients with SIADH is Risk for injury related to confusion associated with:
    1. acute adrenal insufficiency.
    2. impaired physiologic response to stress.
    3. water intoxication.
    4. decreased ADH secretion.

7. To prevent progressive cerebral edema in patients with SIADH, patients are placed in which position in bed?
    1. Semi-Fowler's
    2. Flat
    3. Fowler's
    4. Side-lying

8. The response to sodium restriction and position changes is less efficient in older adults because of declines in the secretion of plasma renin and:
    1. thyroxine.
    2. aldosterone.
    3. estrogen.
    4. androgens.

9. Signs and symptoms of hyperkalemia that should be reported to the physician by patients with Addison's disease include:
    1. dyspnea and coughing.
    2. oliguria and flank pain.
    3. constipation and fatty stools.
    4. weakness and paresthesia.

10. Which substance may be used liberally in the diet of patients with Addison's disease?
    1. Carbohydrates
    2. Salt
    3. Saturated fats
    4. Caffeine

11. What is a priority nursing diagnosis specific to the patient who has had an adrenalectomy?
    1. Ineffective tissue perfusion related to fluid volume deficit
    2. Risk for injury related to acute adrenal insufficiency
    3. Fatigue related to fluid and electrolyte imbalance
    4. Risk for injury related to infection

12. Which are appropriate nursing interventions for patients with Cushing's syndrome? Select all that apply.
    1. Avoid exposure to infections
    2. Report minor signs, such as low-grade fever, sore throat, or aches to the physician
    3. Seek a psychiatric referral if mood swings continue to be a problem
    4. Assist patient to change positions at least every 2 hours
    5. Protect patient from falls or trauma
    6. Discuss bruises, abnormal fat distribution, and hirsutism with the patient if they cause embarrassment
    7. Teach patient about the importance of continuing drug therapy under medical supervision

Nursing Care Plan.
Refer to Nursing Care Plan, The Patient with Addison's Disease, p. 1018 in the textbook, and answer questions 13-17.

13. What is the priority nursing diagnosis for this patient?

14. What is the most common cause of primary Addison's disease?

15. What are the manifestations of adrenal insufficiency exhibited by this patient? Select all that apply.
    1. Hypoglycemia
    2. Nausea, vomiting, and diarrhea
    3. Weight loss
    4. Weakness
    5. Darkening of the skin on his face and arms
    6. Irritability
    7. Dehydration
    8. Hypokalemia
    9. Hypotension

16. What type of diet is this patient on?

17. Which tasks can be assigned to unlicensed assistive personnel for this patient?

Thyroid and Parathyroid Disorders

 Go to http://evolve.elsevier.com/Linton/medsurg/ for additional activities and exercises.

NCLEX CATEGORIES:

Safe and Effective Care Environment:
Coordinated Care, Safety and Infection Control

Health Promotion and Maintenance

Psychosocial Integrity

Physiological Integrity: Basic Care and Comfort, Pharmacological Therapies, Reduction of Risk Potential, Physiological Adaptation

OBJECTIVES

1. Identify nursing assessment data related to the functions of the thyroid and parathyroid glands.
2. Describe tests and procedures used to diagnose disorders of the thyroid and parathyroid glands and nursing responsibilities relevant for each.
3. Describe the pathophysiology, signs and symptoms, complications, and treatment of hyperthyroidism, hypothyroidism, hyperparathyroidism, and hypoparathyroidism.
4. Assist in the development of nursing care plans for patients with disorders of the thyroid or parathyroid glands.

PART I: MASTERING THE BASICS

A. Key Terms.

Match the definition in the numbered column with the most appropriate term in the lettered column.

1. _____ Facial edema that develops with severe, long-term hypothyroidism; sometimes used as a synonym for hypothyroidism

2. _____ Enlargement of the thyroid gland, causing the neck to appear swollen

3. _____ Steady muscle contraction caused by hypocalcemia

4. _____ Small mass of tissue that can be palpated

5. _____ Spasmodic closure of the larynx

6. _____ Permanent mental and physical retardation caused by congenital deficiency of thyroid hormones

7. _____ Excessive metabolic stimulation caused by elevated thyroid hormone level

8. _____ Inflammation of the parotid (salivary) gland

9. _____ Inflammation of the thyroid gland

10. _____ Substance that suppresses thyroid function

11. _____ Protrusion of the eyeballs associated with hyperthyroidism

A. Goiter
B. Goitrogen
C. Exophthalmos
D. Myxedema
E. Nodule
F. Cretinism
G. Parotiditis
H. Tetany
I. Laryngospasm
J. Thyroiditis
K. Thyrotoxicosis

B. Hyperthyroidism/Hypothyroidism.

For each of the following signs or symptoms, indicate whether it is characteristic of (A) hyperthyroidism or (B) hypothyroidism.

1. _____ Heat intolerance

2. _____ Apathy

3. _____ Increased appetite

4. _____ Tachycardia

5. _____ Cold intolerance

6. _____ Weight loss

7. _____ Anorexia

8. _____ Bradycardia

9. _____ Nervousness and restlessness

10. _____ Weight gain

11. _____ Coarse, dry skin and hair

12. _____ Systolic hypertension

C. Thyroid and Parathyroid Hormones.

Complete the statements below with either (A) increases or (B) decreases.

1. _____ The effect on the pulse rate when thyroid hormones are elevated

2. _____ The effect on the body's metabolic rate when there is excess thyroxine

3. _____ The effect on retention of calcium caused by high levels of parathyroid hormone (parathormone, PTH)

4. _____ The effect on blood pressure when thyroid hormones are elevated

5. _____ The effect on the loss of phosphates by the kidneys when there are high levels of PTH

D. Complications.

Select all that apply.

1. Which are signs and symptoms of poor oxygenation due to airway obstruction that may occur after thyroidectomy? Select all that apply.
   1. Restlessness
   2. Increased pulse
   3. Increased temperature
   4. Petechiae
   5. Dyspnea
   6. Cold intolerance

2. Which are signs of laryngeal nerve damage that may occur after thyroidectomy? Select all that apply.
   1. Tachycardia
   2. Exophthalmos
   3. Inability to speak
   4. Hoarseness

3. Which are signs of severe hyperthyroidism that may occur after thyroidectomy? Select all that apply.
   1. Tetany
   2. Fever
   3. Confusion
   4. Tachycardia

4. Which are true statements about complications following thyroidectomy? Select all that apply.
   1. A complication involving injury to parathyroid glands results in tetany.
   2. Symptoms of infection that should be reported after thyroidectomy include fever, wound swelling, and foul discharge.
   3. The most serious side effect of hypocalcemia is dyspnea.
   4. Laryngospasm can be prevented by preoperative treatment with parathyroid drugs.

E. Diagnostic Tests.

Match the description in the numbered column with the diagnostic procedure in the lettered column. Answers may be used more than once.

1. _____ After radioactive iodine is given and the amount of iodine taken up is measured, a high uptake indicates hyperthyroidism.

2. _____ Provides high-quality images of thyroid and any nodules.

3. _____ An elevated T_3 serum level indicates Graves' disease.

4. _____ After iodine isotope is given, a scanner detects the pattern of uptake by the thyroid gland.

5. _____ Elevated T_4 serum levels indicate hyperthyroidism.

6. _____ Assesses response of the pituitary to thyroid-releasing hormone (TRH); differentiates types of hypothyroidism.

7. _____ Test that can differentiate benign and malignant nodules and detect other abnormalities.

8. _____ Material from thyroid nodules is aspirated and is guided by ultrasonography.

A. Serum T$_3$ and T$_4$ measurements
B. Radioactive iodine uptake test
C. Thyroid scan
D. Thyroid ultrasonography
E. Fine needle aspiration biopsy
F. TRH stimulation test

F. Drug Therapy.
Match the description in the numbered column with the drug classification in the lettered column. Answers may be used more than once.

1. _____ Used to treat hyperthyroidism by interfering with synthesis of thyroid hormones

2. _____ Concentrates in thyroid tissue for diagnostic scans

3. _____ Used to treat hypothyroidism and thyroiditis

4. _____ Reduces the size and vascularity of thyroid gland in hyperthyroidism

5. _____ Promotes calcium absorption from digestive tract

6. _____ Corrects calcium deficiency due to hypoparathyroidism

7. _____ Inhibits bone resorption and reduces serum calcium

8. _____ Increases the metabolic rate

A. Thyroid hormone replacement drugs
B. Antithyroid drugs
C. Iodides
D. Radioactive iodine
E. Calcium salts
F. Vitamin D
G. Biphosphonates

G. Neck, Thyroid, and Parathyroid glands.
Referring to Figure 45-7 (p. 1040) below, fill in the spaces with the correct letters.

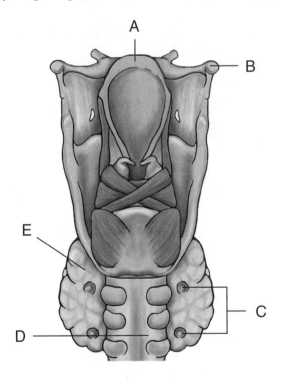

1. _____ Parathyroid glands
2. _____ Epiglottis
3. _____ Thyroid gland (posterior surface)
4. _____ Hyoid bone
5. _____ Trachea

PART II: PUTTING IT ALL TOGETHER

H. Multiple Choice/Multiple Response.

Choose the most appropriate answer or select all that apply.

1. Which is secreted when serum calcium levels are high to limit the shift of calcium from the bones into the blood?
   1. Calcitonin
   2. Thyroxine
   3. Thymine
   4. Phosphorus

2. Hyperthyroid patients often experience sleep disturbances and:
   1. sedation.
   2. bradycardia.
   3. restlessness.
   4. hypotension.

3. Poor tolerance of heat and excessive perspiration are symptoms of:
   1. hyperparathyroidism.
   2. hypoparathyroidism.
   3. hyperthyroidism.
   4. hypothyroidism.

4. If untreated, hyperthyroidism may lead to:
   1. thyrotoxicosis (thyroid storm).
   2. hypotension.
   3. bradycardia.
   4. decreased metabolism.

5. Signs of iodine toxicity include:
   1. bradycardia and hypotension.
   2. urinary retention and oliguria.
   3. esophageal ulcers and pyloric sphincter spasms.
   4. swelling and irritation of mucous membranes and increased salivation.

6. Elevated thyroid hormones result in:
   1. decreased pulse and blood pressure.
   2. increased pulse and blood pressure.
   3. decreased temperature and susceptibility to infection.
   4. increased temperature and susceptibility to infection.

7. An important nursing diagnosis for the patient with exophthalmos is:
   1. Risk for infection.
   2. Knowledge deficit (of disease process).
   3. Decreased cardiac output.
   4. Disturbed body image.

8. A complication of thyroidectomies includes injury to the parathyroid glands, which results in:
   1. bradycardia.
   2. cyanosis.
   3. tetany.
   4. headache.

9. Results of two tests that are indicative of hypocalcemia are:
   1. positive Chvostek's and Trousseau's signs.
   2. increased blood urea nitrogen and potassium levels.
   3. increased WBC and decreased RBC levels.
   4. increased phosphorus and decreased iodine levels.

10. An early symptom of tetany is:
    1. flank pain with hematuria.
    2. difficulty breathing.
    3. a tingling sensation around the mouth, fingers, and toes.
    4. muscle cramps in leg and arm muscles.

11. Graves' disease (toxic diffuse goiter) is characterized by:
    1. increased secretion of thyroid hormones.
    2. a decreased metabolic rate.
    3. intolerance to cold.
    4. constipation.

12. Which drug stains the teeth and should be sipped through a straw?
    1. Iron
    2. Saturated solution of potassium iodide (SSKI)
    3. Levothyroxine (Synthroid)
    4. Propylthiouracil

13. In patients with toxic diffuse goiter, there is a risk for injury related to:
    1. increased metabolic energy production.
    2. exophthalmos.
    3. increased thyroid hormone stimulation.
    4. intolerance to heat.

14. Lack of iodine is associated with:
    1. goiter.
    2. hypoparathyroidism.
    3. tetany.
    4. thyrotoxicosis.

15. Thyroxine (T_4), triiodothyronine (T_3), and calcitonin are hormones produced by the:
    1. adrenal gland.
    2. thymus gland.
    3. thyroid gland.
    4. parathyroid gland.

16. Which drug is used to treat hypothyroidism?
    1. SSKI
    2. Synthroid
    3. Methimazole (Tapazole)
    4. Lugol's solution

17. If thyroid enlargement is mild and thyroid hormone production is normal, what treatment is required?
    1. No treatment
    2. Radioactive iodine
    3. Antithyroid medication
    4. Thyroid replacement therapy

18. Which statements are true about hyperparathyroidism? Select all that apply.
    1. PTH plays a critical role in regulating sodium.
    2. The most notable effect of hyperparathyroidism is hypercalcemia.
    3. People who undergo kidney transplantation after being on dialysis for a long time may experience hyperparathyroidism.
    4. When the serum calcium level falls, PTH is secreted.
    5. A spasm of the facial muscle when the face is tapped over the facial nerve is Chvostek's sign.
    6. A carpopedal spasm that occurs when a blood pressure cuff is inflated beyond a patient's systolic blood pressure and is left in place for several minutes is Trousseau's sign.
    7. Potassium is an element that is an important component of strong bones and plays a vital role in the functions of nerve and tissue cells.

19. Which are manifestations of hyperparathyroidism? Select all that apply.
    1. Cramps
    2. Poor muscle tone
    3. Bone pain
    4. Demineralization
    5. Twitching
    6. Fractures

PART III: CHALLENGE YOURSELF!

I.   Getting Ready for NCLEX.

Choose the most appropriate answer or select all that apply

1. Which two things should be placed at the bedside before the patient who is having a thyroidectomy returns from surgery? Select two that apply.
   1. Thromboembolic stockings
   2. Suction equipment
   3. Emergency tracheotomy tray

2. What are two reasons that respiratory distress can result following thyroidectomy? Select two that apply.
   1. Compression of the trachea
   2. Aspiration leading to atelectasis
   3. Spasms of the larynx due to nerve damage or hypocalcemia

3. Following thyroidectomy surgery, where should the nurse check for bleeding? Select all that apply.
   1. Inspect the dressing on the front of the neck.
   2. Check behind the neck.
   3. Check in the midclavicular area.

4. A patient has had thyroidectomy surgery and asks why the surgery will be followed with radioactive iodine treatment. The nurse should respond that the purpose of this treatment is to:
   1. stimulate the thyroid gland to produce thyroxine.
   2. inhibit the thyroid-stimulating hormone produced by the pituitary gland.
   3. decrease the activity of the thyroid gland and decrease the thyroid hormones.
   4. destroy any remaining tissue that might contain malignant cells.

5. Which statements are true about hyperthyroidism? Select all that apply.
   1. Symptoms of thyrotoxicosis include tachycardia, heart failure, and hyperthermia.
   2. The two classes of drugs commonly used as antithyroid drugs are iodides and thyroid hormones.
   3. When a patient is taking drugs that interfere with thyroxine secretion, the nurse should monitor for edema, weight gain, and cold intolerance.
   4. Examples of antithyroid thioamides are methimazole (Tapazole) and propylthiouracil (PTU).
   5. One main disadvantage of the thioamides is that they can cause agranulocytosis.

6. Which patient problems are seen in patients with hyperthyroidism? Select all that apply.
   1. Hyperthermia related to increased metabolic energy production
   2. Ineffective airway clearance related to laryngeal spasm
   3. Risk for impaired skin integrity related to dryness and edema
   4. Risk for injury related to hypocalcemia
   5. Risk for injury related to weakness and decreased bone mass
   6. Risk for injury related to exophthalmos
   7. Decreased cardiac output related to excessive thyroid hormone stimulation

7. Which patient problems are seen in patients who have had a thyroidectomy? Select all that apply.
   1. Hypothermia related to cold intolerance
   2. Impaired urinary elimination related to urinary calculi
   3. Decreased cardiac output related to dysrhythmias and heart failure secondary to hypocalcemia
   4. Decreased cardiac output related to blood loss
   5. Ineffective airway clearance related to laryngeal spasm

Nursing Care Plan.
Refer to Nursing Care Plan, The Patient with Hypothyroidism, p. 1027 in the textbook, and answer questions 8-10.

8. What is the priority nursing diagnosis for this patient?

9. What data collected for this patient indicate the presence of hypothyroidism?

10. What tasks can be assigned to unlicensed assistive personnel?

Diabetes Mellitus and Hypoglycemia

chapter

46

 Go to http://evolve.elsevier.com/Linton/medsurg/ for additional activities and exercises.

NCLEX CATEGORIES:

Safe and Effective Care Environment:
Coordinated Care, Safety and Infection Control

Health Promotion and Maintenance

Psychosocial Integrity

Physiological Integrity: Basic Care and Comfort, Pharmacological Therapies, Reduction of Risk Potential, Physiological Adaptation

OBJECTIVES

1. Describe the role of insulin in the body.
2. Explain the pathophysiology of diabetes mellitus and hypoglycemia.
3. Describe the signs and symptoms of diabetes mellitus and hypoglycemia.
4. Explain tests and procedures used to diagnose diabetes mellitus and hypoglycemia.
5. Discuss treatment of diabetes mellitus and hypoglycemia.
6. Explain the difference between type 1 and type 2 diabetes mellitus.
7. Differentiate between acute hypoglycemia and diabetic ketoacidosis.
8. Describe the treatment of a patient experiencing acute hypoglycemia or diabetic ketoacidosis.
9. Describe the complications of diabetes mellitus.
10. Identify nursing interventions for a patient diagnosed with diabetes mellitus or hypoglycemia.
11. Identify nursing interventions for a patient diagnosed with ketoacidosis.

PART I: MASTERING THE BASICS

A. Key Terms.
Match or complete the statement in the numbered column with the most appropriate term in the lettered column. Some terms may not be used.

1. _____ Condition where there is an inadequate amount of insulin to meet daily requirements

2. _____ Insulin is released in the body in response to the ingestion of _____.

3. _____ Condition in which there is an absence of endogenous insulin in the body

4. _____ When insulin is absent, the blood becomes thick with glucose, causing the patient to experience _____.

5. _____ Tissue breakdown and burning of lean body mass send hunger signals to the hypothalamus; consequently, the patient experiences _____.

6. _____ The hormone that stimulates the active transport of glucose into the cells of muscle and adipose tissue

7. _____ Condition that is thought to be a precursor to diabetes mellitus

A. Insulin
B. Type 1 diabetes mellitus
C. Type 2 diabetes mellitus
D. Glycogen
E. Polydipsia
F. Carbohydrates
G. Polyphagia
H. Metabolic syndrome (insulin resistance syndrome)

B. Complications.
Match the description in the numbered column with the complication in the lettered column. Answers may be used more than once.

1. _____ Life-threatening emergency caused by a relative or absolute deficiency of insulin

2. _____ Complication in which signs and symptoms are classified as adrenergic and neuroglucopenic

3. _____ Complication caused by rough shoe linings, burns, or chemical irritation

4. _____ Symptoms range from tingling, numbness, and burning to complete loss of sensation caused by sensory and autonomic nerve impairment

5. _____ Glycosuria, along with hypertension, gradually destroy the capillaries that supply the renal glomeruli

6. _____ Characterized by macular edema

7. _____ Dangerous drop in blood glucose caused by taking too much insulin, not eating enough food, or not eating at the right time

8. _____ Results from inadequate blood supply and is experienced as sharp, stabbing pain in muscles

9. _____ Patient goes into a coma from extremely high glucose levels with no evidence of elevated ketones

10. _____ Nerve tissue involvement affects the sympathetic and parasympathetic nervous systems

A. Retinopathy
B. Nephropathy
C. Mononeuropathy
D. Polyneuropathy
E. Autonomic neuropathy
F. Neuropathic foot ulcers
G. Acute hypoglycemia
H. Diabetic ketoacidosis (DKA)
I. Hyperglycemic hyperosmolar nonketotic syndrome (HHNKS)

C. Complications of Diabetes.
Complete the statement in the numbered column with the most appropriate term in the lettered column.

1. Diabetes is the leading cause of _____.

2. With diabetic retinopathy, the vitreous humor becomes cloudy and vision is lost as a result of _____.

3. A symptom of eye problems for patients with diabetes is the presence of spots, which are called _____.

4. People with diabetes account for a large percentage of patients with renal disease, which is called _____.

5. Elevated insulin levels circulating in the blood of patients with diabetes contribute to the premature development of _____.

A. "Floaters"
B. Hemorrhage
C. Atherosclerosis
D. Nephropathy
E. End-stage renal disease (ESRD)

D. Ketoacidosis.
Complete the statement in the numbered column with the most appropriate term in the lettered column.

1. Treatment of ketoacidosis is aimed at correction of three main problems which are acidosis, dehydration, and _____.

2. The patient with ketoacidosis may have lost a large volume of fluid as the result of vomiting, hyperventilation, and _____.

3. Replacement of potassium is vital in patients with ketoacidosis because hypokalemia can lead to severe _____.

4. A life-threatening emergency caused by lack of insulin or inadequate amounts of insulin is called diabetic _____.

5. Air hunger, seen in patients with ketoacidosis, is observed as _____.

6. The movement of potassium from the extracellular compartment into the cells is enhanced by _____.

7. Ketoacidosis results in disorders in the metabolism of carbohydrates, fats, and _____.

8. The electrolyte of primary concern in ketoacidosis is _____.

A. Ketoacidosis
B. Insulin
C. Electrolyte imbalance
D. Potassium

E. Cardiac dysrhythmias
F. Kussmaul's respirations
G. Protein
H. Polyuria

E. Insulin.
Indicate whether insulin (A) increases or (B) decreases each of the following actions or conditions.

1. _____ Rate of metabolism of carbohydrates
2. _____ Conversion of glucose to glycogen
3. _____ Conversion of glycogen to glucose
4. _____ Fatty acid synthesis and conversion of fatty acids into fat
5. _____ Breakdown of adipose tissue
6. _____ Rate of glucose utilization
7. _____ Mobilization of fat
8. _____ Conversion of fats to glucose
9. _____ Protein synthesis in tissue
10. _____ Conversion of protein into glucose

F. Insulin.
Which organs of the body do not depend on insulin for the transport of glucose into them? Select all that apply.

1. Kidneys
2. Brain and nerve cells
3. Lens of the eye
4. Lungs
5. Heart
6. Exercising muscles

G. Foot Complications.
A patient with diabetes has signs of foot complications. Indicate which changes occur (A) when the nerve supply is impaired and (B) when the blood supply is impaired.

1. _____ The foot is warm and pink.
2. _____ There are no pedal pulses.
3. _____ Sensation is impaired.
4. _____ The foot is cold; foot is pale when raised and red when lowered.
5. _____ The pedal pulses are good and can be felt.
6. _____ The sensation is normal.

H. Serum Glucose Levels.
Indicate whether (A) too much or (B) not enough of the following factors causes serum glucose levels to drop.

1. _____ Insulin
2. _____ Food
3. _____ Exercise

I. Hypoglycemia.
Which are initial signs and symptoms of hypoglycemia? Select all that apply.

1. Blurred vision
2. Slurred speech
3. Shakiness
4. Nervousness
5. Bradycardia
6. Anxiety
7. Lightheadedness
8. Hunger
9. Drowsiness
10. Tingling or numbness of the lips or tongue
11. Diaphoresis
12. Disorientation

J. Diagnostic Tests.
Match the description in the numbered column with the diagnostic test in the lettered column.

1. _____ A reading greater than 200 mg/dl indicates a diagnosis of diabetes mellitus.

2. _____ Reflects glucose levels over the past few months.

3. _____ Blood is drawn at 30 minutes and 1 hour after the ingestion of glucose and then hourly for 3–5 hours when patient is suspected of having diabetes mellitus.

A. Serum glucose levels
B. Oral glucose tolerance test (OGTT)
C. Glycosylated hemoglobin (HbA_{1C}) levels

K. Insulin.

Match the description in the numbered column with the drug in the lettered column. Answers may be used more than once. Refer to Drug Therapy Table 46-1, p. 1059 in the textbook.

1. _____ Category that includes NPH and Lente insulin

2. _____ Category that includes Ultralente and insulin glargine (Lantus)

3. _____ Category that includes Humalog and NovoLog

4. _____ Category that includes Regular insulin

5. _____ Onset occurs in less than 15 minutes

6. _____ The peak occurs in 6–10 hours

7. _____ Duration is 20–36 hours

8. _____ The onset is 30 minutes–1 hour

A. Rapid-acting
B. Short-acting
C. Intermediate-acting
D. Long-acting

L. Drug Therapy.

Match the descriptions in the numbered column with the drug in the lettered column. Answers may be used more than once. Refer to Drug Therapy Table 46-2, Oral Hypoglycemics for Type 2 Diabetes, p. 1062 in the textbook.

1. _____ Drugs in this category include Actos and Avandia

2. _____ Drugs in this category include glipizide (Glucotrol) and glyburide (Diabeta)

3. _____ The main drug in this category is metformin (Glucophage)

4. _____ Drugs in this category include acarbose and miglitol

5. _____ Drugs in this category include Prandin and Starlix

6. _____ The main drug in this category is sitagliptin (Januvia)

7. _____ Three categories that stimulate pancreatic secretion of insulin

8. _____ Action is to delay absorption of carbohydrates in the intestine

9. _____ Action is to inhibit hepatic glucose production and increase insulin sensitivity

10. _____ The newest oral medicine that stimulates the pancreatic release of insulin and inhibits hepatic glucose production

11. _____ Action is to increase sensitivity in the tissues

A. Sulfonylureas (three generations)
B. Biguanides
C. Meglitinides/D-phenylalanines
D. Thiazolinediones
E. Alpha-glucosidase inhibitors
F. Dipeptidyl peptidase-4 inhibitors (DPP-4s)

PART II: PUTTING IT ALL TOGETHER

M. Multiple Choice/Multiple Response.

Choose the most appropriate answer or select all that apply.

1. Which of the following inhibits the conversion of glycogen to glucose?
   1. Fatty acids
   2. Insulin
   3. Triglycerides
   4. Ketones

2. Which herbal supplement can lower blood glucose?
   1. Ginseng
   2. Ginkgo
   3. Kava kava
   4. Ephedra

3. The diagnosis of diabetes is based on:
   1. amylase levels.
   2. red blood cell count.
   3. hemoglobin.
   4. serum glucose levels.

4. Which of the following represents normal fasting serum glucose level?
   1. 30–50 mg/dl
   2. 70–100 mg/dl
   3. 150–200 mg/dl
   4. 205–300 mg/dl

5. The American Diabetes Association recommends that 60–70% of the total daily calories should come from:
   1. protein.
   2. saturated fats.
   3. carbohydrates and monounsaturated fats.
   4. polyunsaturated fats.

6. The most commonly used insulin concentration is:
   1. U-40.
   2. U-80.
   3. U-100.
   4. U-500.

7. Regular insulin should be given:
   1. at bedtime.
   2. before meals.
   3. during meals.
   4. after meals.

8. Which injection site has the fastest rate of absorption for insulin?
   1. Upper arm
   2. Upper buttocks
   3. Abdomen
   4. Thighs

9. The two oral sulfonylurea hypoglycemic agents that are recommended for older patients are glipizide (Glucotrol) and:
   1. chlorpropamide (Diabinese).
   2. glyburide (Diabeta, Micronase).
   3. tolbutamide (Orinase).
   4. acetohexamide (Dymelor).

10. When mixing Regular and longer-acting insulins, which should be drawn into the syringe first?
    1. Regular insulin
    2. Protamine zinc insulin
    3. Ultralente U insulin
    4. Lente L insulin

11. What is the most frequent cause of hypoglycemia?
    1. Liver deficiency
    2. Alcohol
    3. Oral hypoglycemic agents
    4. Insulin

12. Which is a side effect of sulfonylureas used in the treatment of diabetes mellitus?
    1. Hyperglycemia
    2. Hypoglycemia
    3. Hyperkalemia
    4. Hypokalemia

13. Patients who require insulin injections need to self-monitor levels of:
    1. serum cholesterol.
    2. red blood cells.
    3. amylase.
    4. blood glucose.

14. Late signs of hypoglycemia include:
    1. palpitations and dyspnea.
    2. oliguria and hypotension.
    3. peripheral edema and tachypnea.
    4. confusion and unconsciousness.

15. To detect possible changes in the eyes associated with diabetes mellitus, the nurse inquires whether the patient has had floaters, blurred vision, or:
    1. hemorrhage.
    2. infection.
    3. diplopia.
    4. conjunctivitis.

16. Disturbed thought processes in diabetic patients, including confusion, anger, and decreased level of consciousness, may be due to:
    1. neuropathy.
    2. nephropathy.
    3. ketoacidosis.
    4. hyperglycemia.

17. *Hypoglycemia* is defined as a syndrome that develops when the blood glucose level falls to less than:
    1. 10–15 mg/dl.
    2. 45–50 mg/dl.
    3. 80–120 mg/dl.
    4. 200–300 mg/dl.

18. When blood glucose levels fall rapidly, the four substances that are secreted by the body in an attempt to increase glucose levels are cortisol, glucagon, growth hormone, and:
    1. antidiuretic hormone.
    2. epinephrine.
    3. aldosterone.
    4. thyroxine.

19. Early signs of hypoglycemia include:
    1. bradycardia and edema.
    2. oliguria and constipation.
    3. infection and red skin.
    4. weakness and hunger.

20. Which group of oral antidiabetic agents does not cause hypoglycemia as a side effect?
    1. Biguanides (metformin)
    2. Alpha-glucosidase inhibitors (Precose)
    3. Sulfonylureas
    4. Thiazolidinediones (Avandia)

21. Patients with hypoglycemia are at risk for injury related to:
    1. oliguria and nephropathy.
    2. polydipsia and polyphagia.
    3. dizziness and weakness.
    4. retinopathy and hypotension.

22. Hyperosmolar nonketotic coma is loss of consciousness caused by extremely high serum:
    1. ketones.
    2. glucose.
    3. calcium.
    4. potassium.

23. When a patient's serum glucose is 260 mg/dl and ketoacidosis is present, the patient should:
    1. administer glucagon.
    2. drink 8 ounces of skim milk.
    3. drink 4 ounces of concentrated orange juice.
    4. avoid exercise.

24. The patient has taken NPH insulin at 8:00 AM. At what time of day should he be provided a snack in order to prevent hypoglycemia?
    1. 9:00 AM
    2. 10:00 AM
    3. 12:00 PM
    4. 4:00 PM

25. The goal of the diabetic diet is to:
    1. limit carbohydrate intake.
    2. increase protein intake.
    3. limit total calorie intake.
    4. normalize plasma glucose levels.

26. What are areas of injection sites for insulin? Select all that apply.
    1. Buttocks
    2. Upper arm
    3. Abdomen
    4. Thighs

27. Which statements are true regarding the administration of insulin? Select all that apply.
    1. It is best to rotate sites from one area of the body to another.
    2. The site with the fastest absorption rate is the abdomen.
    3. Exercise decreases the absorption rate of insulin.
    4. Heat and massage increase the absorption rate of insulin.

28. Which insulins are clear in appearance? Select all that apply.
    1. Rapid-acting (Humalog, aspart)
    2. Short-acting (Regular)
    3. Intermediate-acting (NPH)
    4. Long-acting (Lantus)

29. Which are exogenous causes of hypoglycemia? Select all that apply.
    1. Tumors
    2. Insulin
    3. Alcohol
    4. Exercise
    5. Severe liver deficiency
    6. Oral hypoglycemic drugs

PART III: CHALLENGE YOURSELF!

N. Getting Ready for NCLEX.

Choose the most appropriate answer or select all that apply.

1. Which are risk factors for type 2 diabetes mellitus? Select all that apply.
    1. Obesity
    2. Family history of diabetes
    3. People under the age of 40
    4. Hispanic/Latino ethnicity
    5. Sedentary lifestyle
    6. Asian ethnicity
    7. Presence of acanthosis nigricans or insulin resistance condition

2. Which are causes of foot problems in the person with diabetes? Select all that apply.
    1. Impaired hormone supply
    2. Impaired blood supply
    3. Impaired nerve supply

3. A patient with diabetes asks the nurse: "How could it be that I have a large ulcer on my foot and yet I did not even know it was there? I don't feel anything, but my foot looks normal." The nurse's most appropriate response would be:
   1. "It is common for people with diabetes to have ulcers on their feet. Just elevate your feet at the end of the day."
   2. "When the nerve supply to the foot is impaired, the foot remains warm and pink, but the sensation is impaired."
   3. "This is an emergency situation. I will contact your physician."
   4. "The ulcer will heal within a week. It is important to keep it clean."

4. Which situations put the patient with diabetes at risk for ketoacidosis? Select all that apply.
   1. The patient eats too much food and does not take enough insulin
   2. The patient does not get enough exercise
   3. The patient experiences stress such as infection or surgery
   4. When diabetes mellitus has not been diagnosed

5. Which statements explain why patients receiving total parenteral nutrition or dialysis are likely to have hyperosmolar nonketotic coma? Select all that apply.
   1. IV solutions containing large amounts of glucose are administered to the patient.
   2. The digestive system is bypassed.
   3. There is no stimulus to trigger the pancreas to release insulin.
   4. Patients can go into a coma from extremely low glucose levels.

6. The nurse reads a physician's written order for a patient with diabetes that states: "Give Regular insulin, 20 units, PO, bid." What is the nurse's most appropriate response?
   1. Explain to the patient that insulin cannot be given PO and that you will call the physician to get an order to give it IM.
   2. Give the insulin PO as ordered, making sure that you give it before meals.
   3. Call the physician to clarify the order, since you know that Regular insulin is made ineffective in the gastrointestinal tract and cannot be given PO.
   4. Explain to the patient that the peak effect of Regular insulin will be in 2–3 hours.

7. A reason for avoiding long-acting oral sulfonylurea hypoglycemic agents in older patients is that decreased renal function in older adults makes them more prone to:
   1. hyponatremia.
   2. hypernatremia.
   3. hypoglycemia.
   4. hyperglycemia.

8. During the physical assessment of the diabetic patient, the nurse inspects the feet carefully for lesions, discoloration, and:
   1. edema.
   2. ability to dorsiflex.
   3. ability to evert.
   4. dehydration.

9. A nursing diagnosis for patients with diabetes is Chronic pain related to:
   1. abnormal blood glucose levels.
   2. adverse effects of drugs.
   3. neuropathy.
   4. alterations in urine output.

10. Patients with diabetes may have disturbed sensory perception related to:
    1. dietary restrictions.
    2. anxiety and fear.
    3. imbalance between food intake and activity expenditure.
    4. neurologic and circulatory changes.

11. Alterations in tactile sensations in diabetic patients may result in:
    1. burns or frostbite.
    2. floaters or diplopia.
    3. altered urine output or oliguria.
    4. abnormal blood glucose levels.

Nursing Care Plan.
Refer to Nursing Care Plan, The Patient with Type 1 Diabetes Mellitus, p. 1068 in the textbook, and answer questions 12-13.

12. What is the priority nursing diagnosis for this patient?

13. What data collected in the health history and physical examination indicate the presence of type I diabetes mellitus?

Nursing Care Plan.
Refer to Nursing Care Plan, The Patient with Type 2 Diabetes Mellitus, p. 1069 in the textbook, and answer questions 14-15.

14. What is the priority diagnosis for this patient?

15. What data collected in the health history and physical examination are related to the presence of type 2 diabetes mellitus?

Female Reproductive Disorders

chapter

47

 Go to http://evolve.elsevier.com/Linton/medsurg/ for additional activities and exercises.

NCLEX CATEGORIES:

Safe and Effective Care Environment:
Coordinated Care, Safety and Infection Control

Health Promotion and Maintenance

Psychosocial Integrity

Physiological Integrity: Basic Care and Comfort, Pharmacological Therapies, Reduction of Risk Potential, Physiological Adaptation

OBJECTIVES

1. List data to be collected when assessing the female reproductive system.
2. Describe the nursing interventions for women who are undergoing diagnostic tests and procedures for reproductive system disorders.
3. Identify the nursing interventions associated with douche, cauterization, heat therapy, and topical medications used to treat disorders of the female reproductive system.
4. Explain the pathophysiology, signs and symptoms, complications, diagnostic procedures, and medical or surgical treatment for selected disorders of the female reproductive system.
5. Assist in developing a nursing care plan for the patient with common disorders of the female reproductive system.
6. Describe the nursing interventions for the patient who is menopausal.

PART I: MASTERING THE BASICS

A. Key Terms.
Match the definition in the numbered column with the most appropriate term in the lettered column.

1. _____ Surgical excision of a fallopian tube and ovary

2. _____ Difficult or painful sexual intercourse in women
3. _____ A condition in which endometrial tissue is abnormally located outside the uterus
4. _____ Inflammation of breast tissue
5. _____ Menstrual periods characterized by profuse or prolonged bleeding
6. _____ Herniation of the urinary bladder into the vagina
7. _____ Bleeding or spotting between menstrual periods
8. _____ Surgical removal of the uterus
9. _____ Abnormal cells
10. _____ Cessation of menstruation
11. _____ Herniation of part of the rectum into the vagina
12. _____ Age at which the first menstrual period occurs
13. _____ Painful menstruation

A. Cystocele
B. Menopause
C. Dysmenorrhea
D. Endometriosis
E. Menorrhagia
F. Metrorrhagia
G. Rectocele
H. Dyspareunia
I. Hysterectomy
J. Dysplasia
K. Mastitis
L. Menarche
M. Salpingo-oophorectomy

B. Diagnostic Procedures.

Match the definition or description in the numbered column with the most appropriate term in the lettered column. Some terms may be used more than once, and some terms may not be used.

1. _____ A type of invasive surgery procedure in which a large amount of cervical tissue is removed to treat cancer

2. _____ An invasive surgical procedure that provides direct visualization of the female pelvic cavity

3. _____ A test for which specimens are collected routinely to detect cervical cancer and dysplasia

4. _____ A procedure that is commonly done before cervical biopsies

5. _____ A type of biopsy done in a physician's office or an outpatient clinic to diagnose cervical cancer

6. _____ Specimens collected to identify infections

7. _____ The procedure that is done to identify ectopic pregnancy or pelvic masses

8. _____ A test performed to diagnose uterine cancer

9. _____ A procedure in which an instrument is used to inspect the cervix under magnification and to identify abnormal and potentially cancerous tissue

10. _____ Deliberate tissue destruction by means of heat, electricity, or chemicals

11. _____ Visualization of abdominal organs in order to perform tubal ligation

A. Multiple-punch biopsy
B. Papanicolaou (Pap) smear
C. Dilation and curettage
D. Culture and smear
E. Cone biopsy
F. Aspiration biopsy
G. Endometrial biopsy
H. Culdoscopy
I. Breast biopsy
J. Colposcopy
K. Laparoscopy
L. Cauterization

C. Uterine Displacement.

Match the definition or description in the numbered column with the most appropriate term in the lettered column.

1. _____ The body of the uterus bends backward on itself

2. _____ A forward tilt of the uterus at a sharp angle to the vagina

3. _____ The uterus bends forward on itself

4. _____ A backward tilt of the uterus with the cervix pointed downward toward the anterior vaginal wall

A. Anteflexion
B. Retroversion
C. Retroflexion
D. Anteversion

D. Menstruation.

Match the term in the numbered column with the most appropriate numerical range in the lettered column. (These terms refer to the variations within normal menstrual periods.) Some ranges may be used more than once, and some may not be used.

1. _____ Length of cycle (days)
2. _____ Duration of menstruation (days)
3. _____ Amount of blood loss (ml)

A. 2–8
B. 10–14
C. 21–40
D. 40–100
E. 150–200

E. Female Reproductive System Disorders.

Which descriptions below are related to Candida albicans? *Select all that apply.*

1. Often seen with diabetes
2. A sexually transmitted infection that is the primary cause of ectopic pregnancy and infertility
3. Includes profuse, frothy, and yellow-gray discharge
4. Includes cottage cheese-like discharge
5. Protozoal infection
6. Fungal infection
7. Infection often caused by disruption of the normal vaginal flora

F. Drug Therapy.

1. Which descriptions of drug actions and uses described below are related to ovulatory stimulants? Select all that apply.
   1. Enhances bone formation
   2. Promotes secretory function in endometrium
   3. Initially increases and then decreases testosterone levels
   4. Stimulates ovarian follicular growth
   5. Treats uterine bleeding and endometriosis
   6. Used as fertility drugs
   7. Clomid and Pergonal are examples

2. Which descriptions of drug actions and uses below are related to selective estrogen receptor modulators (SERMS)? Select all that apply.
   1. Used to replace natural hormones after menopause and to treat advanced breast cancer
   2. Influences contractile activity of the uterus
   3. Inhibits production of pituitary gonadotropins
   4. Initially increases and then decreases testosterone levels; used to treat endometriosis
   5. Used to treat breast cancer
   6. Tamoxifen and Evista are examples

G. PID.

Which groups of women are especially prone to developing pelvic inflammatory disease not associated with sexually transmitted infections? Select all that apply.
   1. Women in low socioeconomic groups
   2. Women who are poorly nourished
   3. Women with compromised resistance to infection

H. Menopause.

How do the following structures change after menopause without estrogen present? Select all that apply.
   1. The uterus becomes enlarged.
   2. The vagina shortens.
   3. Vaginal tissues become drier.
   4. Breast tissue becomes more elastic.
   5. Pubic and axillary hair become sparse.
   6. Bone mass increases and becomes less flexible.
   7. Osteoporosis increases.

I. Mastectomy.

Complete the statement in the numbered column with the most appropriate term in the lettered column.

1. Mastectomy patients are at risk for injury related to _____.

2. The removal of the tumor with a margin of surrounding healthy tissue but preserving most of the breast is called _____.

3. A low-incidence cancer of the nipple and areola is _____.

4. The implantation of a tissue expander injected with saline is a type of _____

5. The removal of all breast tissue, overlying skin, axillary lymph nodes, and underlying pectoral muscles is called _____.

6. If breast cancer cells removed during surgery need estrogen for cell replication, they are said to be _____.

7. Removal of the entire breast is called _____.

A. Paget's disease
B. Radical mastectomy
C. Simple mastectomy
D. ER-positive
E. Breast reconstruction
F. Lumpectomy
G. Lymphedema

J. External Female Genitalia.

Using Figure 47-1 (p. 1078) below, label the external female genitalia (A–L) from the terms (1–12) below.

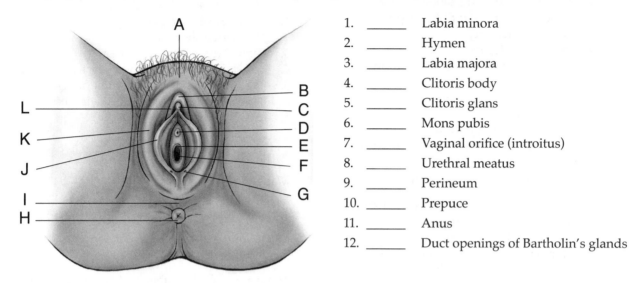

1. _____ Labia minora
2. _____ Hymen
3. _____ Labia majora
4. _____ Clitoris body
5. _____ Clitoris glans
6. _____ Mons pubis
7. _____ Vaginal orifice (introitus)
8. _____ Urethral meatus
9. _____ Perineum
10. _____ Prepuce
11. _____ Anus
12. _____ Duct openings of Bartholin's glands

K. Internal Female Genitalia.

Using Figure 47-9 (p. 1100) below, label the sites of endometriosis (A–L) from the terms provided (1–12) below.

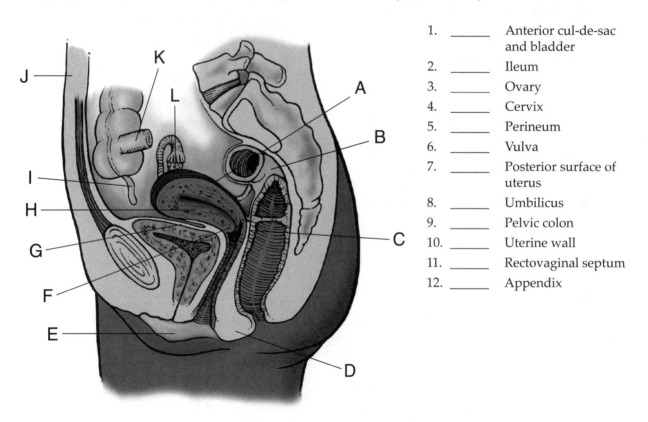

1. _____ Anterior cul-de-sac and bladder
2. _____ Ileum
3. _____ Ovary
4. _____ Cervix
5. _____ Perineum
6. _____ Vulva
7. _____ Posterior surface of uterus
8. _____ Umbilicus
9. _____ Pelvic colon
10. _____ Uterine wall
11. _____ Rectovaginal septum
12. _____ Appendix

PART II: PUTTING IT ALL TOGETHER

L. Multiple Choice/Multiple Response.

Choose the most appropriate answer or select all that apply.

1. The two main hormones produced by the ovaries are:
   1. estrogen and progesterone.
   2. testosterone and prolactin.
   3. thyroxine and oxytocin.
   4. follicle-stimulating hormone and luteinizing hormone.

2. In which position is the patient placed for a pelvic exam?
   1. Lithotomy
   2. Right side-lying
   3. Knee-chest
   4. Supine

3. Advise the patient that air entering the pelvic cavity during the culdoscopy procedure may cause pain in the:
   1. abdomen.
   2. heart.
   3. thigh.
   4. shoulder.

4. A method of deliberate tissue destruction through use of heat, electricity, or chemicals is called:
   1. culdoscopy.
   2. colposcopy.
   3. cauterization.
   4. dilation and curettage.

5. A particularly helpful type of heat application for small areas such as the vulva or perineum is:
   1. sitz baths.
   2. an electric heating pad.
   3. Aquathermia (K-pad).
   4. hot compresses.

6. For which signs must the nurse observe in patients taking sitz baths? Select all that apply.
   1. Dyspnea
   2. Faintness
   3. Dermatitis
   4. Headache
   5. Severe pain
   6. Shock

7. Dilation of large pelvic vessels during sitz baths may cause:
   1. hypertension.
   2. hypotension.
   3. pneumonia.
   4. seizures.

8. Following the administration of vaginal suppositories, the patient is asked to remain in which position for at least 15 minutes to allow the medication to be absorbed?
   1. Prone
   2. Supine
   3. Sitting
   4. Right side-lying

9. Deviations from normal menstrual cycles are viewed as:
   1. uterine bleeding disorders.
   2. vaginal hemorrhage problems.
   3. endometrial cancers.
   4. pelvic inflammatory diseases.

10. The most common characteristics of vulvitis are inflammation and:
    1. bleeding.
    2. pruritus.
    3. cheese-like discharge.
    4. pain.

11. Which are signs and symptoms of vaginitis? Select all that apply.
    1. Local swelling
    2. Itching
    3. Redness
    4. Pus
    5. Hemorrhage
    6. Ulcers
    7. Significant discharge

12. A potential complication of vulvitis and vaginitis is:
    1. hypotension.
    2. ascending infection.
    3. seizures.
    4. thrombophlebitis.

13. When Bartholin's glands are infected, the resultant edema and pus formation occlude the duct and form:
    1. tumors.
    2. cysts.
    3. warts.
    4. abscesses.

14. The most noticeable symptom of bartholinitis which causes patients to seek medical attention is:
    1. edema.
    2. pain.
    3. discharge.
    4. itching.

15. The portal of entry for organisms that cause mastitis is the:
    1. areola.
    2. mammary gland.
    3. nipple.
    4. lactating duct.

16. The most serious complication of pelvic inflammatory disease is:
    1. peritonitis.
    2. pneumonia.
    3. hemorrhage.
    4. hypertension.

17. Which are methods of treatment of pelvic inflammatory disease? Select all that apply.
    1. Application of heat
    2. Antibiotics
    3. Diuretics
    4. Antispasmodics
    5. Rest

18. Which are major symptoms of endometriosis? Select all that apply.
    1. Pain
    2. Sudden weakness
    3. Difficulty breathing
    4. Pelvic heaviness
    5. Dysmenorrhea

19. Women who are given androgenic steroids for treatment of endometriosis often experience the common side effect of:
    1. masculinizing characteristics.
    2. palpitations.
    3. insomnia.
    4. diuresis.

20. Severe and sudden abdominal pain may occur as a complication of follicular ovarian cysts due to:
    1. infection.
    2. rupture.
    3. muscle spasms.
    4. vaginitis.

21. A serious complication of a very large fibroid tumor is that it may compress the urethra, obstructing urine flow and causing secondary:
    1. vaginitis.
    2. pelvic inflammatory disease.
    3. hydronephrosis.
    4. diuresis.

22. For women with fibroid tumors who desire to become pregnant, a procedure that can be done by laser surgery to remove only the tumor is:
    1. hysterectomy.
    2. myomectomy.
    3. dilation and curettage.
    4. culdoscopy.

23. Women at risk for developing rectoceles and cystoceles are those who have experienced a weakened pubococcygeal muscle due to:
    1. extended antibiotic treatment.
    2. repeated pregnancies.
    3. effects of herpes infection.
    4. poor nutrition.

24. A treatment of small cystoceles that is aimed at improving the tone of the pubococcygeal muscle is:
    1. pelvic floor (Kegel) exercises.
    2. surgical intervention (A and P repair).
    3. vaginal hysterectomy.
    4. increased fluid intake.

25. Which of the following is an established risk factor for breast cancer?
    1. Age of first baby 24 years or older
    2. Age 12 years or older at menarche
    3. Radiation exposure
    4. Age over 50

26. It is recommended that yearly mammograms be done every year beginning at age:
    1. 35.
    2. 40.
    3. 50.
    4. 65.

27. A common problem for mastectomy patients is:
    1. disturbed sleep pattern.
    2. decreased cardiac output.
    3. functional incontinence.
    4. disturbed body image.

28. An important aspect of postoperative care after mastectomy is directed toward the prevention and minimization of:
    1. lymphedema.
    2. hemorrhage.
    3. hypertension.
    4. nausea.

29. The high mortality from ovarian cancer is due to the fact that:
    1. symptoms are multiple and serious.
    2. it is asymptomatic in early stages.
    3. abnormal cell growth occurs in one ovary.
    4. it is diagnosed around the time of menopause concurrent with ascites.

30. Diminished ovarian function associated with aging causes cessation of ovulation as well as decreased production of:
    1. thyroxine.
    2. estrogen.
    3. epinephrine.
    4. prolactin.

31. A women is said to be postmenopausal when she has not had a menstrual period for:
    1. 3 months.
    2. 1 year.
    3. 2 years.
    4. 5 years.

32. Some women experience surgical menopause, which occurs as a result of surgical removal of the:
    1. ovaries.
    2. uterus.
    3. vagina.
    4. cervix.

33. The type of drug therapy prescribed promptly for surgical menopause to decrease menopausal symptoms is:
    1. diuretics.
    2. steroids.
    3. estrogen.
    4. analgesics.

34. The symptom of hot flashes that may accompany menopause is due to:
    1. increased menstrual bleeding.
    2. vasodilation.
    3. abdominal cramps.
    4. increased body temperature.

35. The treatment of choice for large and symptomatic cystoceles and rectoceles is:
    1. hysterectomy.
    2. myomectomy.
    3. Kegel exercises.
    4. A and P repair.

36. The incidence of fibroid tumors is increased among women who are:
    1. African-American.
    2. Caucasian.
    3. Asian.
    4. Hispanic.

37. Recent findings from the Women's Health Initiative (2002) indicate that combination estrogen–progestin therapy increases the risk of breast cancer and:
    1. osteoporosis.
    2. endometriosis.
    3. coronary heart disease.
    4. amenorrhea.

38. Mastectomy patients are at risk for injury related to:
    1. infectious drainage.
    2. tissue trauma.
    3. possible abscess formation.
    4. lymphedema.

39. Which are signs and symptoms of menopause? Select all that apply.
    1. Vaginal dryness
    2. Drowsiness
    3. Headache
    4. Hot flashes
    5. Depression

40. Which are signs and symptoms of pelvic inflammatory disease? Select all that apply.
    1. Nausea and vomiting
    2. Abdominal pain
    3. Fever and chills
    4. Hypotension
    5. Dysuria
    6. Irregular bleeding
    7. Foul-smelling vaginal discharge
    8. Dyspareunia

41. Which are common side effects of danazol, which may be given to patients with endometriosis? Select all that apply.
    1. Irregular bleeding
    2. Fever and chills
    3. Voice deepening
    4. Hirsutism
    5. Clitoral enlargement
    6. Vaginal atrophy and dryness
    7. Thromboembolism

42. Which drug is given to patients with endometriosis because it inhibits endometrial proliferation?
    1. Oral contraceptives
    2. Ovulatory stimulants
    3. Androgens
    4. SERMs

43. In addition to lower back and pelvic discomfort and recurrent bladder infections, what are symptoms that women with cystoceles are likely to experience? Select all that apply.
    1. Dyspareunia
    2. Stress incontinence
    3. Irregular bleeding
    4. Incomplete bladder emptying

44. What are ways ovarian cancer metastasizes? Select all that apply.
    1. Direct invasion
    2. Pleural fluid
    3. Lymphatic and venous systems
    4. Peritoneal fluid

PART III: CHALLENGE YOURSELF!

M. Getting Ready for NCLEX.

Choose the most appropriate answer or select all that apply.

1. Match the problem for patients with cystocele and rectocele in the numbered column with the appropriate nursing intervention in the lettered column. Some interventions may be used more than once for one problem statement.

    1. _____ Stress incontinence
    2. _____ Constipation
    3. _____ Risk for infection
    4. _____ Acute pain

    A. Initial application of cold to reduce pain and swelling
    B. Teaching the patient Kegel exercises
    C. Emphasizing the need for a high-fiber diet
    D. Sitz baths and heat lamps
    E. Instructing the patient to report signs of urinary frequency, burning, or foul odor
    F. Use of indwelling or suprapubic catheter

2. Which of the following influence a person's chance for getting breast cancer? Select all that apply.
    1. Female
    2. Increased chance if mother or aunt has had breast cancer
    3. Increases markedly from the age of 35 on
    4. Early menarche
    5. Late menopause
    6. Mutation of the BRCA genes

3. What are ways the nurse can intervene to prevent or minimize lymphedema in the patient with a mastectomy? Select all that apply.
    1. Keep affected arm below heart level.
    2. Take blood pressure on the unaffected arm.
    3. No venipuncture or IV fluid administration in the affected arm.
    4. Deodorant may be applied in small amounts 3 days after surgery.
    5. Exercise arm on affected side frequently.

4. Internal radiation as a treatment for patients with ovarian cancer poses a nursing challenge. What are conditions related to internal radiation that make nursing interventions a challenge? Select all that apply.
    1. Radiation therapy may cause nausea, vomiting, and diarrhea.
    2. Movement of the patient is restricted.
    3. Total time for nursing care is restricted because nurses should not be exposed to radiation for more than 2 hours in a 24-hour period.

5. What types of medications may be prescribed for cancer patients receiving internal radiation to moderate radiation side effects and facilitate patient comfort? Select all that apply.
   1. Opioids
   2. Antiemetics
   3. Tranquilizers
   4. Diuretics
   5. Antidiarrheal medications

6. Which are contraindications for estrogen replacement therapy? Select all that apply.
   1. Certain types of cancer (such as estrogen receptor breast cancer)
   2. Hot flashes
   3. Undiagnosed uterine bleeding
   4. Thromboembolism

7. Which are problems related to patients with cancer of the cervix, ovaries, vulva, or vagina? Select all that apply.
   1. Altered sexuality patterns related to physical and emotional effects of cancer of the reproductive system
   2. Risk for injury related to trauma of the exposed uterus
   3. Acute pain related to inflammation
   4. Risk for injury (to patient and others) related to effects of radiotherapy, chemotherapy
   5. Stress incontinence related to pelvic muscle weakness

8. When a patient comes to a clinic with a female reproductive system problem, the opening question the nurse should ask is:
   1. "What is wrong with you today?"
   2. "What is the problem that made you come in?"
   3. "Why did you come to the clinic today?"
   4. "What is the reason for your visit?"

9. Which are common problems for a patient who has had a hysterectomy? Select all that apply.
   1. Deficient knowledge of information or misinterpretation of effects of hormone replacement therapy (HRT)
   2. Risk for fluid volume deficit related to postoperative bleeding
   3. Urinary retention related to surgical manipulation, local tissue edema, temporary sensory or motor impairment
   4. Self-esteem disturbance related to perceived potential changes in femininity, effect on sexual relationship
   5. Risk for injury related to trauma of the exposed uterus
   6. Constipation related to weakening of abdominal musculature, abdominal pain, decreased physical activity, dietary changes, environmental changes

Nursing Care Plan.
Refer to Nursing Care Plan, The Patient with a Hysterectomy, p. 1104 in the textbook, and answer questions 10-11.

10. What is the priority postoperative nursing diagnosis for this patient?

11. What are data collected from the health history and physical examination that indicate a need for hysterectomy?

Male Reproductive Disorders

 Go to http://evolve.elsevier.com/Linton/medsurg/ for additional activities and exercises.

NCLEX CATEGORIES:

Safe and Effective Care Environment:
Coordinated Care, Safety and Infection Control

Health Promotion and Maintenance

Psychosocial Integrity

Physiological Integrity: Basic Care and Comfort, Pharmacological Therapies, Reduction of Risk Potential, Physiological Adaptation

OBJECTIVES

1. Describe the major structures and functions of the normal male reproductive system.
2. Identify data to be collected when assessing a male patient with a reproductive system disorder.
3. Discuss commonly performed diagnostic tests and procedures and the nursing implications of each.
4. Identify common therapeutic measures used to treat disorders of the male reproductive system and the nursing implications of each.
5. For selected disorders of the male reproductive system, explain the pathophysiology, signs and symptoms, complications, medical diagnosis, and medical treatment.
6. Assist in developing a nursing care plan for a male patient with a reproductive system disorder.

PART I: MASTERING THE BASICS

A. Anatomy and Physiology.

Match the description or definition in the numbered column with the most appropriate term in the lettered column. Some terms may be used more than once.

1. _____ Male reproductive organs
2. _____ Extends from the bladder to the urinary meatus at the end of the penis
3. _____ The production of sperm
4. _____ Produces alkaline liquid that enhances motility and fertility of sperm
5. _____ A hormone necessary for the development of male reproductive organs, descent of the testicles, and production of sperm
6. _____ Provides outflow for semen during ejaculation
7. _____ The condition when the testes are located outside a dependent scrotal position
8. _____ The surgical removal of a portion of the vas deferens

A. Testosterone
B. Cryptorchidism
C. Urethra
D. Prostate
E. Vasectomy
F. Spermatogenesis
G. Testes

B. Erectile Dysfunction.

Complete the statement in the numbered column with the most appropriate term in the lettered column. Some terms may be used more than once, and some may not be used.

1. In erectile dysfunction, arteriosclerosis compromises the ability to fill with blood because of _____.

2. Two conditions in patients with diabetes mellitus that may contribute to erectile dysfunction are autonomic neuropathy and _____.

3. The type of erectile dysfunction likely to be caused by high blood pressure and its treatment is _____.

4. Two treatments that may be recommended for treating erectile dysfunction in the diabetic patient are papaverine self-injection and _____.

5. Spinal cord injuries that are more complete and more likely to cause erectile dysfunction are those injuries that are _____.

6. The most likely drugs to cause erectile dysfunction are _____.

A. Failure to store
B. Low
C. Antihypertensives
D. Failure to initiate
E. Atherosclerosis
F. Penile implant
G. Vascular surgery
H. High
I. Failure to fill
J. Antibiotics
K. Reduced blood flow
L. Neurologic disorders

C. Cancer.

What are the three most common parts of the male reproductive system that may be affected by cancer? Select all that apply.

1. Epididymis
2. Penis
3. Testicles
4. Scrotum
5. Prostate gland

D. Drug Therapy.

Match characteristics of drugs used to treat disorders of the male reproductive system in the numbered column with the drugs in the lettered column. Some terms may be used more than once.

1. _____ Prescribed for failure to fill or store

2. _____ Replacement for low hormone levels in men

3. _____ Decreases testosterone level; used to treat prostate cancer

4. _____ Examples are Viagra (sildenafil), Levitra (vardenafil), and Cialis (tadalafil)

5. _____ Relaxes smooth muscle in corpus cavernosum, increasing blood flow

6. _____ Used with luteinizing-hormone–releasing hormone (LHRH) to treat prostate cancer, decreasing testosterone level

A. Testosterone
B. Agents used to treat erectile dysfunction
C. Estrogen products (Tace)
D. Testosterone inhibitors

E. Male Reproductive System.

Using the figure below, label the parts of the male reproductive system (A–Q) from the terms (1–17) below.

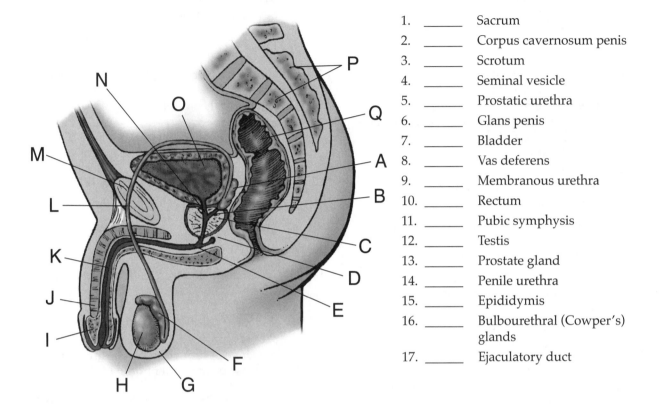

1. _____ Sacrum
2. _____ Corpus cavernosum penis
3. _____ Scrotum
4. _____ Seminal vesicle
5. _____ Prostatic urethra
6. _____ Glans penis
7. _____ Bladder
8. _____ Vas deferens
9. _____ Membranous urethra
10. _____ Rectum
11. _____ Pubic symphysis
12. _____ Testis
13. _____ Prostate gland
14. _____ Penile urethra
15. _____ Epididymis
16. _____ Bulbourethral (Cowper's) glands
17. _____ Ejaculatory duct

PART II: PUTTING IT ALL TOGETHER

F. Multiple Choice/Multiple Response.

Choose the most appropriate answer or select all that apply.

1. Three normal changes that may occur in the male reproductive system due to aging are decreased testosterone, a longer refractory period between erections, and:
   1. penile discharge.
   2. pain with urination.
   3. slower arousal.
   4. descent of testicles.

2. Erectile dysfunction related to diabetes mellitus may be caused by:
   1. spinal cord injury.
   2. atherosclerosis.
   3. low hormone levels.
   4. medication side effects.

3. Autonomic neuropathy inhibits muscle relaxation of lacunar spaces of the erectile chambers, which may make:
   1. the patient anxious about performance.
   2. adequate filling of the penis with blood for an erection impossible.
   3. testosterone levels abnormally low.
   4. the patient sterile.

4. Which factors may make assessment of the male reproductive system difficult for some patients? Select all that apply.
   1. Chronic disease
   2. Advanced age
   3. Defensiveness about sexual behavior
   4. Lack of sexual experience
   5. Health beliefs
   6. Need for privacy

5. Which test is done to document sterilization after a vasectomy?
   1. Ultrasonography
   2. Radiography
   3. Analysis of semen
   4. CBC

6. Past medical history helps link the current male reproductive problem of a patient with previous problems and should include information about injuries, diseases, surgeries, allergies, medications, and:
   1. marital status.
   2. treatments.
   3. age and health of siblings.
   4. age and health of parents.

7. The health history should include information about medications the patient is taking because they may:
   1. impair his cognitive abilities.
   2. make him too tired to participate in the assessment.
   3. impair sexual function.
   4. impair gastrointestinal function.

8. Physical examination of the male reproductive system can be accomplished by inspection and:
   1. palpation.
   2. auscultation.
   3. percussion.
   4. radiography.

9. Which drug may cause hypotension and cardiovascular collapse in patients who are taking nitrate vasodilators?
   1. Alprostadil
   2. Sildenafil
   3. Papaverine
   4. Testosterone

10. Transurethral prostatectomy is the most common surgical procedure for benign prostatic hypertrophy (BPH). In this procedure:
    1. the prostate is approached through the bladder by way of a low abdominal incision.
    2. portions of the prostate are cut away through a resectoscope inserted into the urethra.
    3. access to the prostate is gained through an incision between the scrotum and the anus.
    4. the surgeon reaches the prostate through a low abdominal incision and opens the front of the prostate.

11. Which is the most common problem for the patient with BPH?
    1. Risk for infection
    2. Sexual dysfunction
    3. Pain
    4. Impaired urinary elimination

12. Men with low sperm counts should be evaluated for:
    1. congestive heart failure.
    2. anemia.
    3. thyroid function.
    4. renal disease.

13. A common obstructive symptom of BPH is:
    1. urine retention.
    2. nocturia.
    3. frequency.
    4. hematuria.

14. The reason for bladder irrigation following a transurethral prostatectomy (TURP) procedure is to:
    1. decrease postoperative infection.
    2. prevent constriction of the urethra.
    3. prevent clot formation and obstruction.
    4. decrease urinary retention.

15. If postvoid dribbling occurs in a postoperative TURP patient after removal of the catheter, the nurse should:
    1. suggest perineal exercises.
    2. recommend biofeedback.
    3. use isotonic fluid for irrigation.
    4. monitor for signs of infection.

16. Drugs most likely to interfere with erection are:
    1. antihistamines.
    2. decongestants.
    3. analgesics.
    4. antihypertensives.

17. Which herb is thought to increase penile blood flow?
    1. Ginkgo biloba
    2. Kava kava
    3. Garlic
    4. Oil of jasmine

18. Which is an established risk factor for testicular cancer?
    1. Multiple sex partners
    2. African-American
    3. Caucasian
    4. High-fat diet

19. A cancer that occurs much more frequently among African-American men than Caucasians is:
    1. prostatic cancer.
    2. testicular cancer.
    3. penile cancer.
    4. bladder cancer.

20. Which intervention is appropriate for a patient with BPH?
    1. Place a rolled towel across the patient's thighs to elevate the scrotum and reduce pain.
    2. Provide bedrest, scrotal support, and local heat to the scrotum.
    3. Drink at least eight glasses of fluids throughout the day.
    4. Eat a high-protein diet.

21. Which is an irritative symptom of BPH?
    1. Nocturia
    2. Urine retention
    3. Postvoid dribbling
    4. Decreased force of urinary stream

22. Which drugs may cause urinary retention in patients with BPH?
    1. Smooth muscle relaxants
    2. Cold remedies
    3. Analgesics
    4. Antacids

23. Which drug is given to a postprostatectomy patient to relieve bladder spasms?
    1. Propantheline bromide (Pro-Banthine)
    2. Tansudosin (Flomax)
    3. Phenoxybenzamine HCl (Dibenzyline)
    4. Finasteride (Proscar)

24. Which herb can give a false negative result in patients with prostate cancer?
    1. Garlic
    2. Ginkgo biloba
    3. Siberian ginseng
    4. Saw palmetto

25. Which are treatment methods for a patient with epididymitis? Select all that apply.
    1. Bedrest
    2. Local heat
    3. Ice packs
    4. Sitz baths
    5. Analgesics
    6. Scrotal support

26. Which are factors that may trigger urinary retention in a patient with BPH? Select all that apply.
    1. Infections
    2. Delayed voiding
    3. Bedrest
    4. Antiinflammatory agents
    5. Antihistamines
    6. Chilling

27. Which drug actions are related to tamsulosin (Flomax) and Cardura (alpha-adrenergic blocking agents)? Select all that apply.
    1. Relax smooth muscle in the bladder neck and prostate
    2. Decrease testosterone levels
    3. Suppress prostatic tissue growth
    4. Reduce obstruction to urinary flow

PART III: CHALLENGE YOURSELF!

G. Getting Ready for NCLEX.

Choose the most appropriate answer or select all that apply.

1. Which are problems for the patient with testicular cancer? Select all that apply.
    1. Anxiety
    2. Acute pain
    3. Impaired urinary elimination
    4. Risk for injury
    5. Constipation
    6. Situational low self-esteem
    7. Risk for deficient fluid volume

2. Which are nursing interventions for a patient with a prostatectomy who is experiencing acute pain related to urinary obstruction and bladder spasms? Select all that apply.
    1. Reposition tubing
    2. Inspect urine, dressing, and wound drainage for excess bleeding
    3. Watch for water intoxication
    4. Monitor for signs of infection (temperature above 101° F [38.3° C])
    5. Give antispasmodics and analgesics

3. Which are nursing interventions for a patient with a prostatectomy who is experiencing risk for infection related to invasive procedures of the urinary tract or catheterization? Select all that apply.
    1. Maintain urine flow
    2. Use strict aseptic technique
    3. Keep closed urinary drainage systems intact
    4. Monitor for signs of infection (temperature above 101° F [38.3° C]; purulent wound drainage, and confusion)
    5. Monitor output

4. Which is a problem for a patient with BPH?
    1. Risk for deficient fluid volume related to hemorrhage
    2. Risk for infection related to invasive procedures of the urinary tract and surgical incision
    3. Acute pain related to tissue trauma and bladder spasms
    4. Impaired urinary elimination related to obstruction

Nursing Care Plan.

Refer to Nursing Care Plan, The Patient with a Prostatectomy, p. 1139 in the textbook, and answer question 5.

5. What is the priority problem for this patient?

Sexually Transmitted Infections

chapter
49

 Go to http://evolve.elsevier.com/Linton/medsurg/ for additional activities and exercises.

NCLEX CATEGORIES:

Safe and Effective Care Environment:
Coordinated Care, Safety and Infection Control

Health Promotion and Maintenance

Psychosocial Integrity

Physiological Integrity: Basic Care and Comfort, Pharmacological Therapies, Reduction of Risk Potential, Physiological Adaptation

OBJECTIVES

1. List infectious diseases classified as *sexually transmitted infections*.
2. Explain the importance of the nurse's approach when dealing with patients who have sexually transmitted infections.
3. Discuss tests used to diagnose sexually transmitted infections and the nursing considerations associated with each.
4. Explain why sexually transmitted infections must be reported to the health department.
5. Describe the pathophysiology, signs and symptoms, complications, and medical treatment for selected sexually transmitted infections.
6. Design a teaching plan on the prevention of sexually transmitted infections.
7. List nursing considerations when a patient is on drug therapy for a sexually transmitted infection.
8. Identify data to be collected when assessing a patient with a sexually transmitted infection.
9. Assist in developing a nursing care plan for a patient with a sexually transmitted infection.

PART I: MASTERING THE BASICS

A. Key Terms.
Match the definition in the numbered column with the most appropriate term in the lettered column.

1. _____ A papule that breaks down into a painless ulcer at the site of entry of the organism that causes syphilis

2. _____ Most common sexually transmitted infection (STI) in the U.S.; often has no symptoms

3. _____ An infection of the ovaries, fallopian tubes, and pelvic area

4. _____ Dormant; during this period of a disease, there are no signs or symptoms of the disease

5. _____ Burning of tissue

6. _____ A disease that can be transmitted by intimate genital, oral, or rectal contact

A. Latent
B. Cautery
C. Chlamydial infection
D. Sexually transmitted infection
E. Pelvic inflammatory disease
F. Chancre

B. Drug Therapy.

1. Which drugs are used to treat gonorrhea? Select all that apply.
   1. Cipro
   2. Bactrim
   3. Penicillin G
   4. Erythromycin
   5. Rocephin
   6. Achromycin
   7. Flagyl
   8. Acyclovir

2. Which group of drugs is used to treat genital herpes infections?
   1. Antibacterials
   2. Tetracyclines
   3. Sulfonamides
   4. Antivirals

C. Diagnostic Tests.

Which of the following STIs involve a vaginal or penile discharge for which smears and cultures are taken for diagnosis? Select all that apply.
   1. Chlamydial infection
   2. Herpes simplex virus (HSV)
   3. Trichomoniasis
   4. Syphilis
   5. Venereal warts
   6. HIV infection

D. Reporting.

Which STIs (confirmed cases) must be reported to the local health department? Select all that apply.
   1. HIV
   2. HSV
   3. Gonorrhea
   4. Syphilis
   5. Trichomonas infections
   6. Chlamydia

PART II: PUTTING IT ALL TOGETHER

E. Multiple Choice/Multiple Response.

Choose the most appropriate answer or select all that apply.

1. What percentage of all cases of STIs involve people between the ages of 15 and 24?
   1. 50%
   2. 65%
   3. 75%
   4. 85%

2. Serologic tests for STIs are designed to detect infectious diseases by measuring:
   1. white blood cells.
   2. red blood cells.
   3. clotting factors.
   4. antigens or antibodies.

3. Patients with gonococcal, chlamydial, HSV, trichomonal, or yeast infections often have:
   1. vaginal or penile discharge.
   2. increased temperature or tachycardia.
   3. generalized infection and rash.
   4. mouth sores and pharyngitis.

4. If males have a whitish- or greenish-colored discharge from the penis and complain of a burning sensation during urination, this is suggestive of:
   1. HSV infection.
   2. chlamydia.
   3. gonorrhea.
   4. syphilis.

5. Female patients with gonorrhea are likely to have vaginal discharge, a burning sensation during urination, abnormal menstruation, and:
   1. dyspnea.
   2. abdominal pain.
   3. hypotension.
   4. edema.

6. Paralysis, mental illness, blindness, and heart disease may occur as complications of:
   1. HSV infection.
   2. cervicitis.
   3. syphilis.
   4. gonorrhea.

7. Two screening tests for syphilis include the rapid plasma reagin (RPR) and the:
   1. VDRL.
   2. RBC.
   3. WBC.
   4. BUN.

8. The treatment of choice for syphilis is:
   1. doxycycline calcium (Vibramycin).
   2. erythromycin.
   3. tetracycline.
   4. penicillin.

9. After completing treatment for primary or secondary syphilis, the patient is advised not to engage in sexual activity for:
   1. 5 days.
   2. 2 weeks.
   3. 1 month.
   4. 6 months.

10. If untreated, sterility, prostatitis in males, and pelvic inflammatory disease in females may result from:
    1. syphilis.
    2. gonorrhea.
    3. HSV infection.
    4. venereal warts.

11. Which STI can be transmitted through the placenta, causing an infant to be born with the disease?
    1. HSV infection
    2. gonorrhea
    3. syphilis
    4. chlamydia

12. With an STI, common reasons that patients give for seeking medical care include pain, fever, lesions, or genital:
    1. itching.
    2. edema.
    3. bleeding.
    4. discharge.

13. Specimens collected during a pelvic exam are handled as:
    1. infective material.
    2. clean specimens.
    3. sterile specimens.
    4. chemically unstable material.

14. Untreated STIs can lead to serious complications such as pelvic inflammatory disease and:
    1. edema.
    2. sterility.
    3. shock.
    4. kidney failure.

15. Which emergency drugs for possible hypersensitivity reactions need to be kept on hand when administering drug therapy to patients with STIs? Select all that apply.
    1. Acyclovir (Zovirax)
    2. Diphenhydramine hydrochloride (Benadryl)
    3. Didanosine (Videx)
    4. Pentamidine isethionate (Pentam)
    5. Epinephrine
    6. Corticosteroids

16. Related to altered sexuality patterns in patients with STIs, the nurse explains that sexual dysfunction may be overcome by dealing with:
    1. the adverse drug effects of prescribed medications.
    2. the need for more exercise.
    3. emotional reactions to the disease.
    4. conflict resolution.

17. Females with HSV infections are advised to have annual Papanicolaou smears because they are at increased risk of:
    1. pyelonephritis.
    2. cervical cancer.
    3. kidney failure.
    4. AIDS.

18. How is HSV transmitted? Select all that apply.
    1. Air droplets
    2. Mouth-to-nose contact
    3. Fecal contamination
    4. Hand contact
    5. Sexual contact

19. Which is the drug of choice from treating HSV?
    1. Penicillin G
    2. Tetracycline hydrochloride (Achromycin)
    3. Acyclovir (Zovirax)
    4. Metronidazole (Flagyl)

20. Which STI has symptoms similar to those of gonorrhea?
    1. Syphilis
    2. Herpes simplex
    3. Chlamydia
    4. HIV

21. Gonorrhea can be found in the pharynx, urethra, uterus, and:
    1. kidney.
    2. rectum.
    3. heart.
    4. lungs.

22. Gonorrhea is transmitted most often by:
    1. infected mothers to newborn infants.
    2. direct sexual contact.
    3. skin lacerations of medical personnel.
    4. toilet seats and doorknobs.

23. The heart, joints, skin, and meninges may become involved with which systemic infection?
    1. Gonorrhea
    2. Syphilis
    3. Chlamydia
    4. Genital warts

24. The treatment for gonorrhea is a single dose of IM ceftriaxone sodium (Rocephin), followed by 7 days of oral:
    1. erythromycin.
    2. Vibramycin.
    3. penicillin.
    4. tetracycline.

25. What is the correct treatment for a patient who has trichomoniasis?
    1. Penicillin
    2. Metronidazole (Flagyl)
    3. Acyclovir
    4. Tetracycline

26. Which of the following is the cause of venereal warts?
    1. Human papilloma virus (HPV)
    2. HSV
    3. *Chlamydia trachomatis*
    4. *Neisseria gonorrhoeae*

27. What do Papanicolaou smears detect?
    1. Syphilis
    2. Gonorrhea
    3. Cancer of the cervix
    4. HSV infection

28. Which STI is the most common bacterial STI because people have no symptoms?
    1. Syphilis
    2. Gonorrhea
    3. Venereal warts
    4. Chlamydia

29. Some STIs are painless, but patients may have pain associated with oral lesions, rectal lesions, or:
    1. vaginal bleeding.
    2. genital edema.
    3. nerve irritation.
    4. pelvic infection.

30. Which statements are related to syphilis? Select all that apply.
    1. Characterized by a papule that becomes a painless red ulcer within a week.
    2. Patients are cured when the chancre disappears.
    3. The first sign of this disease is a chancre.
    4. During the secondary stage, pustules, fever, sore throat and aching are symptoms that occur.

31. Which statements are related to *Chlamydia trachomatis*? Select all that apply.
    1. An infection that is transmitted by contact with the mucous membranes in the mouth, eyes, urethra, vagina, or rectum
    2. Characterized by genital irritation; a thin, gray discharge, and a fish odor
    3. Treatment consists of antiviral drugs
    4. Characterized by a cauliflower-like mass
    5. Symptoms include a penile discharge that is initially thin and then creamy, accompanied by painful urination
    6. The most common STI in the United States

32. A patient with gonorrhea is being treated with Rocephin. Which side effects would the nurse expect to see? Select all that apply.
    1. Discoloration of teeth
    2. Allergic reactions in patients allergic to cephalosporins or penicillin
    3. Nephrotoxicity
    4. Superinfections

33. Which STIs can be cured with drug therapy? Select all that apply.
    1. Herpes simplex (HSV-2)
    2. Chlamydia
    3. Venereal warts
    4. Gonorrhea
    5. Syphilis

34. Which are signs and symptoms of chlamydia infection? Select all that apply.
    1. Greenish yellow urethral discharge
    2. May be no signs or symptoms
    3. Painful, frequent urination in males
    4. Lower abdominal pain in females
    5. Enlarged lymph nodes

35. Which are signs and symptoms of syphilis? Select all that apply.
    1. Round ulcer with well-defined margin (chancre) is present
    2. Sore throat
    3. Regional lymphadenopathy
    4. Profuse, watery vaginal discharge

PART III: CHALLENGE YOURSELF!

F. Getting Ready for NCLEX.

Choose the most appropriate answer or select all that apply.

1. The nurse is taking care of a patient with syphilis who is being treated with penicillin G. Which of the following manifestations may occur during the first 24 hours in patients with syphilis who are treated with penicillin? Select all that apply.
    1. Numbness of the extremities
    2. Sore throat
    3. Headache
    4. Fever
    5. Muscle aches

2. The nurse is taking care a patient with genital warts. Which treatments would the nurse expect to be used for a patient with genital warts? Select all that apply.
    1. Administration of penicillin
    2. Cryotherapy
    3. Surgical removal
    4. Injection of interferon into the lesions

3. The nurse is taking care of a patient with gonorrhea and is implementing a discharge teaching plan. Which of the following are ways to reduce the risk of gonorrhea that the nurse would explain to this patient? Select all that apply.
    1. Have all sexual partners treated.
    2. Take complete prescription of Cipro or tetracycline, even if symptoms disappear.
    3. Avoid unprotected sex until patient and sexual partners have been treated.
    4. Ensure that VDRL blood studies are done.

4. The nurse is presenting an education program to a school district advisory council meeting about prevention of STIs. Which are considered unsafe sexual practices in preventing transmission of infection that the nurse would include in the presentation? Select all that apply.
    1. Oral sex without condom
    2. Mutual masturbation
    3. Vaginal or anal intercourse with properly used condom
    4. Ingestion of urine or semen
    5. Open-mouthed kissing

5. Which of the following are common problems for a patient with an STI? Select all that apply.
    1. Deficient fluid volume related to anorexia
    2. Imbalanced nutrition: less than body requirements related to vomiting
    3. Sexual dysfunction related to fear of transmission
    4. Situational low self-esteem related to diagnosis
    5. Risk for injury related to disease process
    6. Acute pain related to lesions and inflammation
    7. Activity intolerance related to prescribed bedrest
    8. Excess fluid volume related to renal dysfunction

6. When collecting a sample of vaginal discharge for culture and sensitivity tests, the nurse or person collecting the sample always wears:
   1. goggles.
   2. a mask.
   3. gloves.
   4. a gown.

7. A discussion of sexual behavior can be awkward for the nurse and the patient. Before nurses can deal with patients' sexuality, they must:
   1. present the patient with written information.
   2. be aware of their own values.
   3. ask the patient to demonstrate understanding of the material presented by stating information in his/her own words.
   4. check the patient's chart to see whether he/she has an STI.

8. What is the priority patient problem related to lesions or inflammation for patients with STIs?
   1. Anxiety
   2. Acute pain
   3. Situational low self-esteem
   4. Ineffective management of therapeutic regimen: noncompliance

9. A patient problem related to possible effects of STI or partner reaction to the STI is:
   1. Pain.
   2. Risk for injury.
   3. Anxiety.
   4. Impaired tissue integrity.

10. What is the most important problem related to the stigma associated with STIs, shame, and anger?
    1. Sexual dysfunction
    2. Pain
    3. Ineffective coping
    4. Risk for infection

11. In order to identify and treat infected individuals so that transmission of the STI can be slowed, the nurse recognizes that partners may be notified and confirmed cases of certain STIs must be reported to the:
    1. United States Department of Health.
    2. hospital administrator.
    3. Department of Public Safety.
    4. local public health department.

Nursing Care Plan.

Refer to Nursing Care Plan, The Patient with Gonorrhea, p. 1167 in the textbook, and answer questions 12-15.

12. What is the priority nursing diagnosis?

13. What are risk factors for this patient who has gonorrhea?

14. What data collected in the health history and physical examination indicate the presence of a gonococcal infection?

15. What are five complications this patient with gonorrhea may face if not treated?

Skin Disorders

 Go to http://evolve.elsevier.com/Linton/medsurg/ for additional activities and exercises.

NCLEX CATEGORIES:

Safe and Effective Care Environment:
Coordinated Care, Safety and Infection Control

Health Promotion and Maintenance

Psychosocial Integrity

Physiological Integrity: Basic Care and Comfort, Pharmacological Therapies, Reduction of Risk Potential, Physiological Adaptation

OBJECTIVES

1. Describe the structure and functions of the skin.
2. List the components of the nursing assessment of the skin.
3. Define terms used to describe the skin and skin lesions.
4. Explain the tests and procedures used to diagnose skin disorders.
5. Explain the nurse's responsibilities regarding the tests and procedures for diagnosing skin disorders.
6. Explain the therapeutic benefits and nursing considerations for patients who receive dressings, soaks and wet wraps, phototherapy, and drug therapy for skin problems.
7. Describe the pathophysiology, signs and symptoms, diagnostic tests, and medical treatment for selected skin disorders.
8. Assist in developing a nursing care plan for the patient with a skin disorder.

PART I: MASTERING THE BASICS

A. Diagnostic Tests.

1. Match the description or definition in the numbered column with the most appropriate term in the lettered column. Some terms may be used more than once, and some terms may not be used.

   1. _____ A test used to diagnose viral skin infections
   2. _____ Used to diagnose fungal infections by studying a skin specimen
   3. _____ An examination in which the patient's skin is inspected under a black light in a darkened room
   4. _____ A test used to identify allergens in which common irritants are applied to the skin
   5. _____ The removal of skin for microscopic examination
   6. _____ A specimen no deeper than the dermis is obtained with a scalpel
   7. _____ The type of biopsy in which a circular tool cuts around the lesion, which is then lifted and severed
   8. _____ The type of biopsy indicated for deep specimens in which sutures are required to close the site
   9. _____ Used to detect mites

   A. Biopsy
   B. Punch biopsy
   C. Wood's light
   D. Shave biopsy
   E. Surgical excision
   F. Tzanck's smear
   G. Patch testing
   H. Scabies scraping
   I. KOH examination

2. Skin Biopsy. Answer the numbered questions below using the letters in Figure 50-5 (p. 1179) below. Answers may be used more than once.

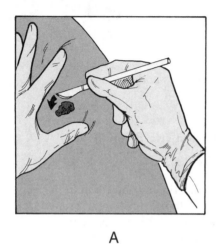

A

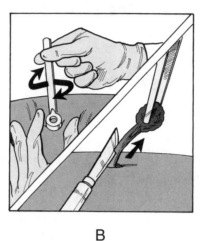

B

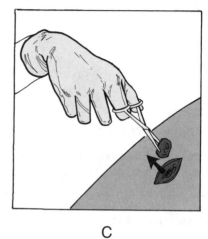

C

1. What do these pictures show?

2. _____ Which figure shows a punch biopsy?

3. _____ Which figure shows surgical excision?

4. _____ Which figure is a relatively shallow excision in which pressure or chemicals usually control bleeding?

5. _____ Which figure requires sutures?

6. _____ Which procedure involves minimal bleeding that is controlled with pressure, cautery, or chemicals?

B. Skin Cancers.

Match the statement in the numbered column with the most appropriate term in the lettered column. Answers may be used more than once.

1. _____ Type of carcinomas, unlike basal cell carcinomas, that grow rapidly and metastasize.

2. _____ A chronic autoimmune condition in which bullae (blisters) develop on the face, back, chest, groin, and umbilicus.

3. _____ A condition with painless, nodular lesions that have a pearly appearance

4. _____ Disorder that arises from the pigment-producing cells in the skin

5. _____ Characterized by scaly ulcers or raised lesions

6. _____ Carcinomas that grow slowly and rarely metastasize, but they should be removed because they can cause local tissue destruction.

7. _____ Usually caused by overuse of alcohol and tobacco.

8. _____ Treatment used is Mohs' surgery to determine margins of malignancy.

A. Melanoma
B. Squamous cell carcinoma
C. Pemphigus
D. Basal cell carcinoma

C. Burns.

Match the description in the numbered column with the type of burn in the lettered column. Answers may be used more than once.

1. _____ Pink to red and painful, like a sunburn

2. _____ Large, thick-walled blisters or edema

3. _____ Burned tissue lacking sensation

4. _____ Burn affecting only the epidermis

5. _____ Burn involving the epidermis, dermis, and underlying tissues, including fat, muscle, and bone

6. _____ Burned tissue is painful and sensitive to cold air

7. _____ Blistered, weepy, and pale to red or pink

8. _____ Dry, leathery, and sometimes red, white, brown, or black

9. _____ Weeping, cherry-red, exposed dermis

10. _____ A severe sunburn

A. Superficial burn
B. Superficial partial-thickness burn
C. Deep partial-thickness burn
D. Full-thickness burn

D. Skin Lesions.

1. Match the characteristics and examples of common skin lesions in the numbered column with the letters in Figure 50-3 (p. 1177) below. Some answers are used more than one time and some are not used.

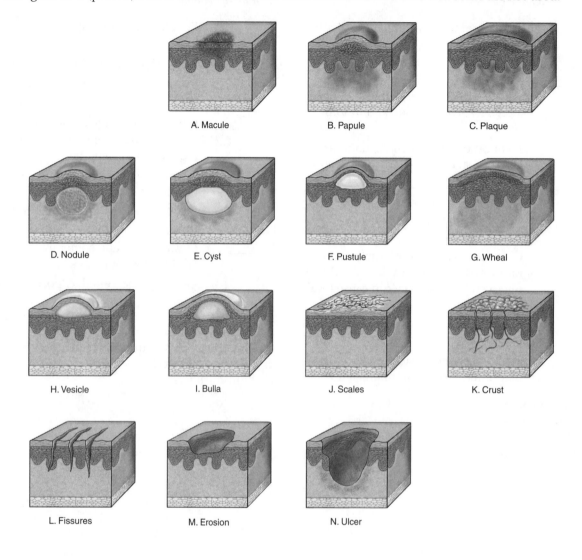

A. Macule   B. Papule   C. Plaque

D. Nodule   E. Cyst   F. Pustule   G. Wheal

H. Vesicle   I. Bulla   J. Scales   K. Crust

L. Fissures   M. Erosion   N. Ulcer

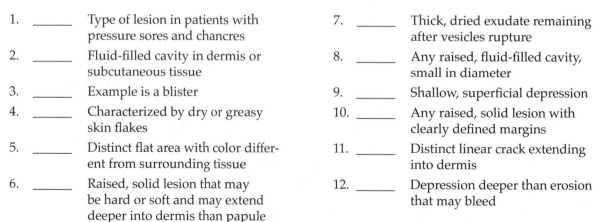

1. _____ Type of lesion in patients with pressure sores and chancres
2. _____ Fluid-filled cavity in dermis or subcutaneous tissue
3. _____ Example is a blister
4. _____ Characterized by dry or greasy skin flakes
5. _____ Distinct flat area with color different from surrounding tissue
6. _____ Raised, solid lesion that may be hard or soft and may extend deeper into dermis than papule

7. _____ Thick, dried exudate remaining after vesicles rupture
8. _____ Any raised, fluid-filled cavity, small in diameter
9. _____ Shallow, superficial depression
10. _____ Any raised, solid lesion with clearly defined margins
11. _____ Distinct linear crack extending into dermis
12. _____ Depression deeper than erosion that may bleed

2. Match the example or description in the numbered column with the appropriate type of lesion in the lettered column.

   1. _____ Freckle, petechia, hypopigmentation
   2. _____ Mole, wart
   3. _____ Herpes simplex, herpes zoster
   4. _____ Acne, impetigo
   5. _____ Vitiligo
   6. _____ Psoriasis
   7. _____ Fibroma
   8. _____ Allergic response, insect bite, hives

   A. Plaque
   B. Wheal
   C. Papule
   D. Patch
   E. Pustule
   F. Vesicle
   G. Nodule
   H. Macule

E. Drug Therapy.

Match the actions and uses in the numbered column with the appropriate drug classification in the lettered column.

1. _____ Interfere with viral replication
2. _____ Decrease proliferation of epidermal cells in psoriasis
3. _____ Reduce inflammation in various skin disorders
4. _____ Kill parasites and their eggs; used to treat pediculosis (lice) and scabies (mite) infestations
5. _____ Dissolve keratin and slow bacterial growth; used to treat acne and psoriasis
6. _____ Effective against fungi; used to treat fungal infections
7. _____ Used to treat psoriasis
8. _____ Destroy microorganisms; used to treat skin infections
9. _____ Reduce formation of comedones; increase mitosis of epithelial cells; used to treat acne

A. Keratolytics (for example, coal tar)
B. Topical antibacterials (for example, bacitracin)
C. Antiviral agents (for example, acyclovir)
D. Photosensitivity drugs (for example, methoxsalen)
E. Topical antifungal agents (for example, nystatin)
F. Topical antiinflammatories (for example, hydrocortisone)
G. Vitamin A derivatives (for example, tretinoin [Retin-A])
H. Pediculicides and scabicides (for example, lindane [Kwell])
I. Antipsoriatics (for example, anthralin)

F. Skin Infections.

1. Which are true statements about impetigo? Select all that apply.
   1. Vesicle or pustule that ruptures, leaving a thick crust
   2. Inflamed hair follicles with white pustules
   3. Inflamed skin and subcutaneous tissue with deep, inflamed nodules
   4. Treated with antibiotic therapy: erythromycin or dicloxacillin

2. Which are true statements about cellulitis? Select all that apply.
   1. Local tenderness and redness at first, then malaise, chills, and fever
   2. At first, small shiny lesions; then they enlarge and become rough
   3. Treated with electrical current to destroy lesion followed by removal with curette, cryotherapy (freezing), topical medications
   4. Site becomes more erythematous; nodules and vesicles may form; vesicles may rupture, releasing purulent material

G. Burns.

Match the appearance characteristics in the numbered column with the sensations experienced (in the same depth of burn) in the lettered column.

1. _____ Large, thick-walled blisters covering extensive areas (vesiculation); edema; mottled red base; broken epidermis; wet, shiny, weeping surface

2. _____ Variable—for example, deep red, black, white, brown; dry surface; edema; fat exposed; tissue disrupted

3. _____ Mild to severe erythema; skin blanches with pressure

A. Little pain, insensate
B. Painful, sensitive to cold air
C. Painful, hyperesthetic, tingling, pain eased by cooling

H. Treatment of Burns.

Match the definition or description in the numbered column with the most appropriate term in the lettered column. Some terms may be used more than once.

1. _____ Removal of necrotic tissue from a wound

2. _____ Covering a wound with skin

3. _____ Can be reduced by use of pressure dressings in early stages of care

4. _____ May be accomplished by mechanical means, surgical excision, or enzymes

5. _____ Can be reduced by use of custom-fitted garments that apply continuous pressure 24 hours a day

A. Skin grafting
B. Scarring
C. Débridement

I. Plastic Surgery.

Match the conditions treated with plastic surgery in the numbered column with the type of surgery used in the lettered column. Answers may be used more than once.

1. _____ Birthmarks
2. _____ Excess tissue around the eyes
3. _____ Developmental defects
4. _____ Disfiguring scars
5. _____ Receding chin
6. _____ Facial wrinkles

A. Aesthetic surgery
B. Reconstructive surgery

J. Skin Infestations.

Match the signs and symptoms of skin infestations in the numbered column with infestation in the lettered column.

1. _____ Thin, red lines on skin; itching

2. _____ Itching of hairy areas of body (head, pubis); nits (eggs) seen as tiny white particles attached to hair shafts

A. Lice
B. Scabies

K. Parts of the Skin.

Using Figure 50-1 (p. 1174) below, label the parts of the skin (A–L) from the terms provided (1–12).

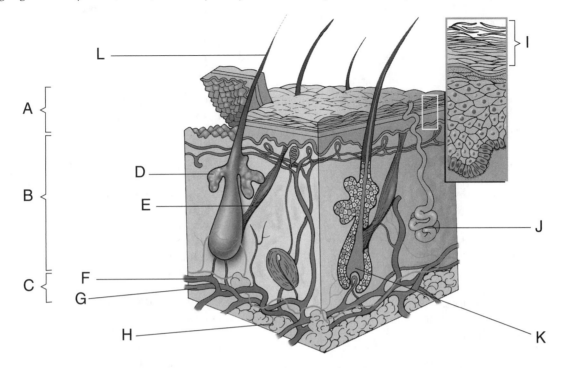

1. _____	Sebaceous gland	7. _____ Vein
2. _____	Hair follicle	8. _____ Epidermis
3. _____	Dermis	9. _____ Arrector pili muscle
4. _____	Hair shaft	10. _____ Sweat gland
5. _____	Stratum corneum	11. _____ Adipose tissue
6. _____	Artery	12. _____ Subcutaneous tissue

PART II: PUTTING IT ALL TOGETHER

L. Multiple Choice/Multiple Response.

Choose the most appropriate answer or select all that apply.

1. Which are changes that occur in older men and women? Select all that apply.
   1. Increased elastic tissue
   2. Increased facial hair
   3. Increased subcutaneous tissue
   4. Thickening of capillaries
   5. Thinning of scalp hair

2. Nevi (moles) are carefully inspected for pigmentation, ulcerations, changes in surrounding skin, and:
   1. vascular irregularities.
   2. amount of edema.
   3. amount of pus.
   4. irregularities in shape.

3. When assessing capillary refill, after applying pressure to cause blanching and then releasing the pressure, the nurse should observe that the color returns to normal within:
   1. 1–2 minutes.
   2. 3–5 seconds.
   3. 30–40 seconds.
   4. 50–60 seconds.

4. The potassium hydroxide (KOH) examination is used in combination with a culture to diagnose infections of the skin, hair, or nails that are:
   1. viral.
   2. bacterial.
   3. caused by parasites.
   4. fungal.

5. Which are assessments of the fingernails and toenails that nurses monitor? Select all that apply.
   1. Capillary refill
   2. Edema
   3. Hemorrhage
   4. Mobility
   5. Color of nail bed

6. The most common problem for patients with pruritus is Risk for impaired skin integrity related to:
   1. excessive dryness.
   2. intense itching.
   3. moist environment.
   4. inadequate circulation.

7. Nursing diagnoses for the patient with atopic dermatitis may include Impaired skin integrity related to:
   1. decreased resistance to infection.
   2. self-care practices.
   3. poor peripheral circulation.
   4. excessive dryness.

8. The assessment of patients with seborrheic dermatitis includes inspecting affected areas for:
   1. bleeding and exudate.
   2. edema and redness.
   3. scales and crusts.
   4. yellow skin and ascites.

9. A common risk factor for developing candidiasis is:
   1. hypertension.
   2. antibiotic therapy.
   3. emotional stress.
   4. tachycardia.

10. A primary problem for patients with candidiasis is:
    1. Activity intolerance.
    2. Altered oral mucous membranes.
    3. Decreased cardiac output.
    4. Self-care deficit.

11. Acne is caused by:
    1. eating too much chocolate.
    2. fatty foods.
    3. poor hygiene.
    4. blocked hair follicles.

12. The nurse advises the patient with shingles that the condition is communicable to people who have never been exposed to:
    1. measles.
    2. pertussis.
    3. chickenpox.
    4. mumps.

13. The most serious form of skin cancer is:
    1. basal cell carcinoma.
    2. melanoma.
    3. squamous cell carcinoma.
    4. cutaneous T-cell lymphoma.

14. Following a burn injury, plasma leaks into the tissue due to increased capillary:
    1. constriction.
    2. dilation.
    3. production.
    4. permeability.

15. After a burn injury, shifts in fluids and electrolytes cause local edema and a decrease in:
    1. respiratory rate.
    2. CNS stimulation.
    3. cardiac output.
    4. red blood cell production.

16. A patient with a burn experiences a shift of plasma proteins from the capillaries. This is likely to result in:
    1. hypoproteinemia.
    2. increased blood volume.
    3. dehydration.
    4. increased urine output.

17. Which is a complication of untreated fluid shifts in burn patients?
    1. Hypovolemic shock
    2. Kidney failure
    3. Pneumonia
    4. Convulsions

18. A type of therapy used in the treatment of psoriasis, vitiligo, and chronic eczema is:
    1. phototherapy.
    2. soaks.
    3. wet wraps.
    4. débridement.

19. Vitamin A is essential for:
    1. blood clotting.
    2. bone formation.
    3. wound healing.
    4. healthy skin.

20. Food allergies can cause:
    1. scabies.
    2. basal cell carcinoma.
    3. psoriasis.
    4. atopic dermatitis.

21. Which is a topical herbal preparation used as an emollient?
    1. Aloe
    2. Angelica
    3. Balm of Gilead
    4. Ginseng

22. What should be included in the teaching plan for a patient with atopic dermatitis? Select all that apply.
    1. Avoid constrictive clothing.
    2. Use sunscreens and moisturizers.
    3. Topical corticosteroids provide the best control of inflammation.
    4. It is helpful to take nystatin for itching.

23. Acne lesions develop when there is:
    1. increased fatty food intake.
    2. increased sebum production.
    3. increased chocolate intake.
    4. poor hygiene.

24. Which drug used to remove heavy scales in patients with psoriasis can stain normal skin and hair?
    1. Tazarotene (Tazorac)
    2. Glucocorticoids
    3. Methotrexate sodium
    4. Anthralin (Anthra-Derm)

25. Which skin disorder characterized by irritation and redness in body folds is fairly common among patients in long-term care facilities?
    1. Intertrigo
    2. Impetigo
    3. Candidiasis
    4. Pemphigus

26. Which should *not* be used in patients with intertrigo because it supports the growth of *C. albicans*?
    1. Topical corticosteroid
    2. Cornstarch
    3. Anthralin (Anthra-Derm)
    4. Moisturizer

27. Who is at greatest risk for skin cancer?
    1. Caucasians
    2. African-Americans
    3. Native Americans
    4. Hispanics

28. A prominent symptom of psoriasis, dermatitis, eczema, and insect bites is:
    1. fever.
    2. pain.
    3. pruritus.
    4. edema.

29. If one arm and one leg are burned, what is the estimated burn size, according to the rule of nines?
    1. 18%
    2. 27%
    3. 36%
    4. 54%

30. The burn patient is at great risk for:
    1. hyperthermia.
    2. paralysis.
    3. edema.
    4. infection.

31. A patient has just been prescribed isotretinoin (Accutane) for resistant acne. Which are teaching points for this patient? Select all that apply.
    1. A serious adverse effect of isotretinoin (Accutane) is fetal deformities.
    2. Isotretinoin (Accutane) can cause mental depression, possibly leading to suicidal ideation.
    3. Do not apply to eyes, mouth, or angles of the nose.
    4. Avoid sun exposure and use sunscreen.

32. Which are true statements about acne skin dis-
    orders? Select all that apply.
    1. Mild cases of acne respond well to
       Acyclovir (Zovirax).
    2. Comedones (whiteheads and blackheads),
       pustules, and cysts are characteristics of
       acne.
    3. Two oral antibiotics that are frequently
       given for acne are tetracycline and erythro-
       mycin.
    4. A drug prescribed for patients if acne is
       severe and unresponsive to antibiotics is
       isotretinoin (Accutane).
    5. Acne is a condition in which androgenic
       hormones cause increased sebum produc-
       tion and bacteria proliferation, causing hair
       follicles to block and become inflamed.

33. Which are true statements about herpes zoster
    virus? Select all that apply.
    1. Older adults are especially susceptible to
       complications, including ophthalmic in-
       volvement, from herpes zoster virus.
    2. Patients with herpes zoster virus exhibit
       early symptoms of heightened sensitivity
       along a nerve pathway, pain, and itching.
    3. Cold sores or fever blisters are oral lesions
       caused by herpes zoster virus.
    4. The sites most often infected by herpes
       zoster virus are the nose, lips, cheeks, ears,
       and genitalia.
    5. Wet dressings soaked in Burow's solution
       may be used to treat lesions associated
       with herpes zoster virus.
    6. Herpes zoster infection is commonly called
       shingles.

34. Which are true statements about candidiasis?
    Select all that apply.
    1. Candidiasis infections, which are mani-
       fested as red lesions with white plaques,
       are found on the mucous membranes.
    2. Three common sites for candidiasis include
       the mouth, skin, and vagina.
    3. Candidiasis is a bacterial infection caused
       by herpes simplex.
    4. Oral candidiasis is treated with nystatin.
    5. One area that is susceptible to candidia-
       sis, owing to the constant moisture found
       there, is the ostomy site.

35. Which are skin changes related to malnutri-
    tion? Select all that apply.
    1. Hives
    2. Pruritus
    3. Cracked skin
    4. Dermatitis
    5. Dry skin (xerosis)

PART III: CHALLENGE YOURSELF!

M. Getting Ready for NCLEX.
*Choose the most appropriate answer or select all that
apply.*

1. Which types of skin lesions require contact precautions? Select all that apply.
   1. Wart lesions
   2. Infected lesions
   3. Plaque lesions
   4. Draining lesions
   5. Weeping lesions
   6. Scaly lesions

2. Which problems are most likely to occur in the
   emergent stage of patients with burns? Select
   all that apply.
   1. Risk for infection
   2. Risk for imbalanced nutrition
   3. Decreased cardiac output
   4. Excess fluid volume

3. Which of the following problems are related to
   patients with burns? Select all that apply.
   1. Acute pain related to tissue trauma
   2. Risk for infection related to loss of protec-
      tive skin barrier
   3. Impaired skin integrity related to scratch-
      ing
   4. Hypothermia related to impaired heat-
      regulating ability of injured skin
   5. Impaired physical mobility related to con-
      tractures, pain
   6. Impaired skin integrity related to inflam-
      mation

4. Which is a problem for the patient with shingles?
   1. Impaired skin integrity related to excessive dryness, scratching
   2. Risk for infection related to moist environment, broken skin
   3. Disturbed body image related to comedones, pustules, and cysts
   4. Acute pain related to lesions or postherpetic neuralgia

5. Which are problems for the patient with psoriasis? Select all that apply.
   1. Risk for injury related to improper nail trimming, poor peripheral circulation
   2. Decreased cardiac output related to hypovolemia secondary to shift of fluid from vascular to extracellular compartment
   3. Disturbed body image related to lesions and scales on skin
   4. Excess fluid volume related to changes in capillary permeability and accumulation of fluid in body tissues
   5. Social isolation related to embarrassment about flaky skin lesions

6. When a skin biopsy is scheduled, the physician may advise the patient to avoid which drug before the procedure to reduce bleeding?
   1. Diphenhydramine
   2. Tetracycline
   3. Aminophylline
   4. Aspirin

7. Which foods are vital for healthy skin? Select all that apply.
   1. Liver
   2. Sweet potato
   3. Grapefruit
   4. Bananas
   5. Cantaloupe
   6. Spinach
   7. Carrots

Nursing Care Plan.
Refer to Nursing Care Plan, The Patient with Psoriasis, p. 1188 in the textbook, and answer questions 8-9.

8. What is the priority problem for this patient?

9. What data collected in the health history and physical examination are indicative of a patient with psoriasis?

Eye and Vision Disorders

 Go to http://evolve.elsevier.com/Linton/medsurg/ for additional activities and exercises.

NCLEX CATEGORIES:

Safe and Effective Care Environment:
Coordinated Care, Safety and Infection Control

Health Promotion and Maintenance

Psychosocial Integrity

Physiological Integrity: Basic Care and Comfort, Pharmacological Therapies, Reduction of Risk Potential, Physiological Adaptation

OBJECTIVES

1. Identify the data to be collected in the nursing assessment of the eye and vision.
2. Identify the nursing responsibilities for patients having diagnostic tests or procedures to diagnose eye disorders.
3. List measures to reduce the risk of eye injuries.
4. Describe the nursing care of patients who require common therapeutic measures for eye disorders: irrigation, application of ophthalmic drugs, and surgery.
5. Describe the pathophysiology, signs and symptoms, diagnosis, and treatment of selected eye conditions.
6. Assist in developing a nursing care plan for the patient with an eye disorder.

PART I: MASTERING THE BASICS

A. Eye Disorders.

Match the definition in the numbered column with the most appropriate term in the lettered column. Some terms may be used more than once, and some terms may not be used.

1. _____ Measurement of pressure, such as intraocular pressure

2. _____ Agent that causes the pupil to constrict

3. _____ Error of refraction caused by uneven curvature of the cornea or lens; causes visual distortion

4. _____ Inflammation of the cornea

5. _____ Inflammation of the membrane lining the eyelids and the eyeball

6. _____ Clouding or opacity of the normally transparent lens within the eye; causes blurred vision and objects to take on a yellowish hue

7. _____ Agent that paralyzes the ciliary muscle so that the eye does not accommodate

8. _____ Bending of light rays

9. _____ Farsightedness

10. _____ Agent that causes the pupil to dilate

11. _____ Visual impairment associated with older age

12. _____ Nearsightedness

A. Keratitis
B. Myopia
C. Tonometry
D. Cycloplegic
E. Conjunctivitis
F. Refraction
G. Presbyopia
H. Miotic
I. Mydriatic
J. Cataract
K. Astigmatism
L. Hyperopia

B. Glaucoma.

1. Which are true statements about glaucoma? Select all that apply.
    1. Tunnel vision occurring in patients with glaucoma
    2. A condition in which intraocular pressure is decreased below normal
    3. Excess pressure impairs blood flow to the optic nerve, resulting in vision impairment
    4. The type of vision that is lost first in glaucoma

2. Which are true statements about drugs used to treat glaucoma? Select all that apply.
    1. Timolol maleate (Timoptic), used in glaucoma to lower intraocular pressure, is classified as a beta blocker.
    2. Acetazolamide (Diamox) is used to reduce intraocular pressure by increasing the production of aqueous humor.
    3. Chronic glaucoma, open-angle glaucoma, is usually treated first with drug therapy, which includes miotics.
    4. Adrenergics are used to decrease intraocular pressure, by decreasing the formation of aqueous humor and increasing its outflow.

C. Drug Therapy.

Match the actions and uses in the numbered column with the most appropriate drug classification in the lettered column.

1. _____   Used to treat or prevent eye infections
2. _____   Used to treat herpes simplex keratitis
3. _____   Dilate pupil; used in open-angle glaucoma; decrease corneal congestion; controls hemorrhage
4. _____   Prevent redness and swelling caused by inflammation due to causes other than bacterial infection
5. _____   Used primarily to treat glaucoma
6. _____   Block sensation in external eye for tonometry; used in removal of sutures or foreign bodies and in some surgical procedures
7. _____   Are effective against some fungal infections of eye
8. _____   Dilate pupil; used before eye exams and for uveitis; decrease lacrimal gland secretion

A. Antibacterials
B. Antiinflammatory agents
C. Miotics
D. Antifungals
E. Topical anesthetics
F. Anticholinergics
G. Antivirals
H. Adrenergics

D. Drug Therapy for Glaucoma.

1. Which medications are used in the treatment of glaucoma? Select all that apply.
    1. Anticholinergics
    2. Beta-adrenergic blockers
    3. Adrenergics
    4. Cholinergics
    5. Carbonic anhydrase inhibitors
    6. Antihistamines
    7. Hyperosmotic agents

2. Match the actions and uses in the numbered column with the classification of drugs used to treat glaucoma in the lettered column. Some classifications may be used more than once.

1. _____   Treatment of acute glaucoma
2. _____   Initial treatment of acute and chronic glaucoma
3. _____   Preoperative preparation for glaucoma surgery
4. _____   Treatment of chronic glaucoma
5. _____   Action of these topical drugs is to lower intraocular pressure by decreasing the production of aqueous humor
6. _____   Action of drugs is to constrict the pupil, facilitating the outflow of aqueous humor
7. _____   Action of drugs is to decrease intraocular pressure by decreasing the formation of aqueous humor and increasing its outflow

A. Cholinergic miotics
B. Osmotic diuretics
C. Beta-adrenergic blockers
D. Adrenergics

E. Diseases of the Eye.

Match the disease in the numbered column with the effect on the eyes in the lettered column.

1. _____ Elevated blood glucose in patients with diabetes

2. _____ Changes in retina due to diabetes

3. _____ Vision problem in neurologic disorders (brain tumors, head injuries, and strokes)

4. _____ Problem with movement of the eyes in neurologic disorders (brain tumors, head injuries, and strokes)

5. _____ Hyperthyroidism

6. _____ Changes in blood vessels of the eye in patients with hypertension

A. May cause bulging eyes (exophthalmos)
B. Causes temporary blurring of vision
C. May cause blindness
D. Inability to move eyes
E. May be impaired, blurred, diplopia, and loss of part of visual fields
F. May lead to vision loss

F. Eye Structures.

Using Figure 51-2 (p. 1211) below, label the internal structures of the eye (A–O) by using the terms (1–15) below.

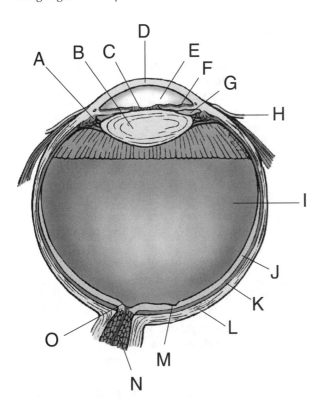

1. _____ Anterior chamber
2. _____ Choroid
3. _____ Ciliary muscle
4. _____ Conjunctiva
5. _____ Cornea
6. _____ Fovea
7. _____ Iris
8. _____ Lens
9. _____ Optic disk
10. _____ Vitreous body
11. _____ Optic nerve
12. _____ Posterior chamber
13. _____ Pupil
14. _____ Retina
15. _____ Sclera

PART II: PUTTING IT ALL TOGETHER

G. Multiple Choice/Multiple Response.

Choose the most appropriate answer or select all that apply.

1. As light enters the eye, it passes through the transparent cornea, aqueous humor, lens, and:
   1. conjunctiva.
   2. sclera.
   3. vitreous humor.
   4. lacrimal glands.

2. Dark spots that are actually bits of debris in the vitreous are called:
   1. flashes.
   2. floaters.
   3. blind spots.
   4. cataracts.

3. If a patient has sensitivity to light, the nurse would document this as:
   1. photophobia.
   2. presbyopia.
   3. myopia.
   4. hyperopia.

4. When the nurse is performing a physical assessment of the eyes, the lids should cover the eyeball completely when closed; when the eyes are open, the lower lid should be at the level of the:
   1. conjunctiva.
   2. retina.
   3. iris.
   4. lacrimal gland.

5. The eyeball is inspected for color and moisture; the sclera should be clear:
   1. yellow.
   2. white.
   3. gray.
   4. black.

6. The pupils are assessed for size, equality, and reaction to light; pupils that are unequal, dilated, or do not respond to light suggest:
   1. diabetes.
   2. liver dysfunction.
   3. inflammation.
   4. neurologic problems.

7. When the nurse asks the patient to focus on the nurse's finger as it is moved slowly toward the patient's nose, the nurse is assessing:
   1. presbyopia.
   2. astigmatism.
   3. accommodation.
   4. refraction.

8. Visual acuity is commonly tested using:
   1. the Snellen chart.
   2. the accommodation test.
   3. tonometry.
   4. fluorescein angiography.

9. Eye surgery may involve surgical incisions, the application of cold probes (cryotherapy), or the use of:
   1. tonometry.
   2. lasers.
   3. fluorescein angiography.
   4. topical dyes.

10. Following eye surgery, the patient is usually positioned:
    1. flat in bed.
    2. prone.
    3. side-lying on affected side.
    4. with the head of bed elevated.

11. An important aspect of the care of postoperative eye patients is to prevent increased:
    1. blood pressure.
    2. cardiac output.
    3. intraocular pressure.
    4. ocular movement.

12. Medications prescribed after cataract surgery usually include antibiotics and:
    1. miotics.
    2. antihistamines.
    3. anticholinergics.
    4. corticosteroids.

13. One of the leading causes of blindness in the United States is:
    1. conjunctivitis.
    2. retinal detachment.
    3. glaucoma.
    4. cataracts.

14. Which drug has a side effect of vision disturbances?
    1. Digitalis
    2. Lasix
    3. Aspirin
    4. Synthroid

15. A vision of 20/30 on the Snellen chart means that the person can:
    1. read at 20 feet from the left eye and 30 feet from the right eye what a normal person reads at these distances.
    2. read at 20 feet what a normal person reads at 50 feet.
    3. read at 30 feet what a person with normal vision reads at 20 feet.
    4. read at 20 feet what a person with normal vision reads at 30 feet.

16. The measurement of pressure in the anterior chamber of the eye is:
    1. refraction.
    2. electroretinopathy.
    3. tonometry.
    4. angiography.

17. Which is an inflammation of hair follicles along the eyelid?
    1. Hordeolum (stye)
    2. Conjunctivitis
    3. Blepharitis
    4. Keratitis

18. Corticosteroids are contraindicated in patients with conjunctivitis caused by:
    1. herpes.
    2. bacteria.
    3. fungi.
    4. chlamydia.

19. Which drug is ordered before surgery for a patient with cataracts?
    1. An analgesic
    2. A mydriatic
    3. A miotic
    4. An anticholinergic

20. Which herb should not be taken by patients with glaucoma because it increases intraocular pressure?
    1. Kava kava
    2. Garlic
    3. Ginkgo
    4. Ephedra

21. A patient sees floaters and states: "It is like a curtain has come down across my vision." This is a symptom of:
    1. cataracts.
    2. macular degeneration.
    3. retinal detachment.
    4. glaucoma.

22. Which antioxidant is believed to slow the progression of age-related macular degeneration?
    1. Vitamin A
    2. Vitamin B
    3. Vitamin E
    4. Vitamin K

23. Which are signs and symptoms of cataracts? Select all that apply.
    1. Tunnel vision
    2. Loss of peripheral vision
    3. Cloudy vision
    4. Seeing spots
    5. Floaters in eyes

PART III: CHALLENGE YOURSELF!

H. Getting Ready for NCLEX.

Choose the most appropriate answer or select all that apply.

1. Match the most appropriate nursing diagnosis for patients following eye surgery in the numbered column with the "related to" statement in the lettered column.

    1. _____ Acute pain
    2. _____ Anxiety
    3. _____ Risk for injury
    4. _____ Disturbed sensory perception (visual)

    A. Tissue trauma
    B. Temporary vision impairment
    C. Disease process, trauma to the eye, patching
    D. Pressure or trauma

2. Which are interventions that relate to lighting for patients who are partially sighted? Select all that apply.
    1. Reduce glare because it interferes with vision.
    2. Make sure the furniture is a different color from the floors and walls.
    3. Use dishes and cups with a solid, single color to facilitate self-feeding and reduce spills.

3. Which are the most common problems for patients with impaired vision? Select all that apply.
    1. Disturbed sensory perception related to inflammation, rejection of transplanted tissue
    2. Ineffective coping related to decreased independence
    3. Disturbed sensory perception related to altered reception, transmission, and interpretation of visual stimuli
    4. Self-care deficit (feeding, hygiene, grooming) related to visual impairment

4. Which are problems for patients with glaucoma? Select all that apply.
   1. Disturbed sensory perception related to vision changes caused by rejection of transplanted tissue
   2. Fear related to actual or potential loss of vision
   3. Acute pain related to acute increased intraocular pressure

5. What are the goals/patient outcomes related to risk for injury for a patient who is postoperative eye surgery? Select all that apply.
   1. Patient states pain is relieved.
   2. Patient avoids rubbing eyes.
   3. Patient is careful not to bend forward.
   4. Patient demonstrates self-care activities.

6. If more than one eye medication is being given, the nurse must wait how long between each medication?
   1. 60 seconds
   2. 5 minutes
   3. 30 minutes
   4. 60 minutes

7. Nurses can teach people how to care for their eyes in order to protect their vision; it is important to tell people that:
   1. burning sensations in the eyes should be reported to the physician.
   2. watching too much television or sitting too close to the television injures the eyes.
   3. eating foods with high vitamin A content will improve vision.
   4. eyes need to be rinsed regularly to protect vision.

8. The nurse should treat nausea promptly in the postoperative eye surgery patient in order to prevent:
   1. infection.
   2. hemorrhage.
   3. pain.
   4. increased intraocular drainage.

9. Which is correct patient teaching regarding protection of health of the eyes?
   1. "Watching too much TV or sitting too close to the TV can injure your eyes."
   2. "Gently cleanse your eyelids each time you wash your face."
   3. "Eating foods that contain large amounts of vitamin A improves vision."
   4. "Eyes need to be rinsed on a daily basis."

10. A primary consideration of the patient with visual impairment is:
    1. safety.
    2. infection.
    3. hemorrhage.
    4. nutrition.

11. Following cataract surgery, the nurse should:
    1. advise the patient to sleep on the affected side.
    2. have the patient cough and deep-breathe.
    3. administer mydriatic agents.
    4. keep the bed low.

Nursing Care Plan.
Refer to Nursing Care Plan, The Patient Having Cataract Surgery, p. 1231 in the textbook, and answer questions 12-13.

12. What is the priority problem for this patient?

13. Which nursing interventions for the patient are planned to prevent increased intraocular pressure? Select all that apply.
    1. Keep the bed in low position.
    2. Keep head of bed elevated.
    3. Instruct the patient not to rub the operative eye, strain, or lean forward.
    4. Instruct the patient to lie on the affected side.
    5. Administer antiemetics immediately as ordered for nausea and vomiting.
    6. Encourage patient to take stool softeners as ordered to prevent constipation.
    7. Acknowledge fear of vision loss common with eye surgery.

Ear and Hearing Disorders

chapter
52

 Go to http://evolve.elsevier.com/Linton/medsurg/ for additional activities and exercises.

NCLEX CATEGORIES:

Safe and Effective Care Environment:
Coordinated Care, Safety and Infection Control

Health Promotion and Maintenance

Psychosocial Integrity

Physiological Integrity: Basic Care and Comfort, Pharmacological Therapies, Reduction of Risk Potential, Physiological Adaptation

OBJECTIVES

1. Identify the data to be collected for the assessment of a patient with a disorder affecting the ear, hearing, or balance.
2. Describe the tests and procedures used to diagnose disorders of the ear, hearing, or balance.
3. Explain the nursing considerations for each of the tests and procedures.
4. Explain the nursing involvement for patients receiving common therapeutic measures for disorders of the ear, hearing, or balance.
5. Describe the pathophysiology, signs and symptoms, complications, and medical or surgical treatment for selected disorders.
6. Assist in the development of a nursing care plan for a patient with a disorder of the ear, hearing, or balance.
7. Identify measures the nurse can take to reduce the risk of hearing impairment and to detect problems early.

PART I: MASTERING THE BASICS

A. Key Terms.
Match the definition in the numbered column with the most appropriate term in the lettered column.

1. _____ Eardrum; the structure that separates the external and middle portions of the ear
2. _____ Waxy secretion in the external auditory canal; earwax
3. _____ Ringing, buzzing, or roaring noise in the ears
4. _____ State of balance needed for walking, standing, and sitting
5. _____ Feeling of unsteadiness
6. _____ Sensation that one's body or one's surroundings are rotating
7. _____ Capable of injuring the eighth cranial nerve (acoustic) of hearing and balance structures in the ear
8. _____ Pain in the ear
9. _____ Hearing loss associated with age

A. Tinnitus
B. Cerumen
C. Tympanic membrane
D. Otalgia
E. Equilibrium
F. Vertigo
G. Dizziness
H. Ototoxic
I. Presbycusis

B. Hearing Loss.

1. Which statements are related to sensorineural hearing loss? Select all that apply.
   1. Patients who hear better in noisy settings than in quiet settings have sensorineural hearing loss.
   2. Causes include congenital problems, noise trauma, aging, Meniere's syndrome, ototoxicity, diabetes, and syphilis.
   3. A condition in which the stapes in the middle ear does not vibrate.
   4. A disturbance of the neural structures in the inner ear or the nerve pathways to the brain.
   5. Sometimes called *nerve deafness*.
   6. Patients can hear sounds but have difficulty understanding speech.

2. Which statements are related to conductive hearing loss? Select all that apply.
   1. Patients who either cannot perceive or cannot interpret sounds that are heard
   2. A hearing loss that results from interference with the transmission of sound waves from the external or middle ear to the inner ear
   3. People with conductive hearing losses are usually helped to hear by hearing aids
   4. May be caused by otosclerosis or obstruction of the external canal or eustachian tube
   5. Patients either cannot perceive or cannot interpret sounds that are heard

C. External Ear Infections.

Which are true statements about otitis externa? Select all that apply.
   1. It is also called *swimmer's ear*.
   2. Treatment of otitis externa includes topical corticosteroids and diuretics.
   3. Drainage in otitis externa may be blood-tinged or purulent.
   4. May be caused by scratching or cleaning the ear with sharp objects.
   5. The most characteristic symptom of otitis externa is itching.

D. Ototoxic Drugs.

Match the ototoxic drugs in the numbered column with their most appropriate classification in the lettered column. Some classifications may be used more than once, and some classifications may not be used.

1. _____ Aspirin
2. _____ Erythromycin estolate (Ilosone)
3. _____ Furosemide (Lasix)
4. _____ Cisplatin (Platinol-AQ)
5. _____ Indomethacin (Indocin)
6. _____ Streptomycin sulfate
7. _____ Ethacrynic acid (Edecrin)
8. _____ Quinidine
9. _____ Tetracycline
10. _____ Bleomycin (Blenoxane)

A. Antiarrhythmics
B. Antibiotics/aminoglycosides
C. Antineoplastics/chemotherapy drugs
D. Antihistamines
E. Salicylates
F. Diuretics

E. Ear.
Using Figure 52-1 (p. 1241) below, label all parts of the ear (A–L) from the terms (1–12) below.

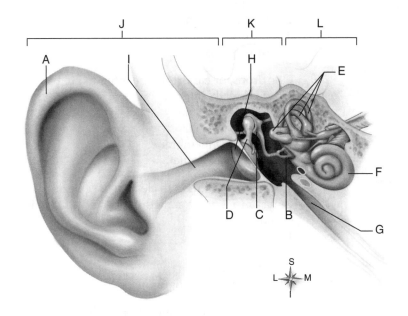

1. _____	Auricle (pinna)
2. _____	External ear
3. _____	Stapes
4. _____	Malleus
5. _____	Inner ear
6. _____	Semicircular canals
7. _____	Auditory (eustachian) tube
8. _____	Incus
9. _____	Middle ear
10. _____	Tympanic membrane
11. _____	Cochlea
12. _____	External acoustic meatus (ear canal)

F. Hearing.
Trace the sound waves from the external ear to the brain in Figure 52-3 (p. 1242) below. Label each step (A–F) from the terms (1–6) below.

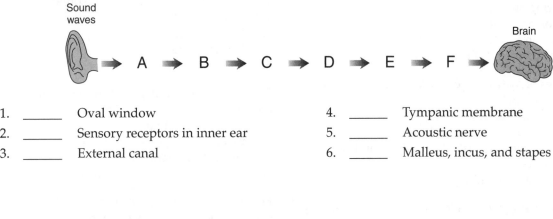

1. _____	Oval window	4. _____	Tympanic membrane
2. _____	Sensory receptors in inner ear	5. _____	Acoustic nerve
3. _____	External canal	6. _____	Malleus, incus, and stapes

G. Diagnostic Procedures.
Match the description in the numbered column with diagnostic test in lettered column. Answers may be used more than once.

1. _____ Detects hearing impairment by assessing the patient's ability to hear a range of sounds.

2. _____ Measures the ability to hear spoken words.

3. _____ Test is conducted in a sound-isolated room.

4. _____ Patient listens to simple words through earphones and repeats them.

5. _____ Test is conducted in a sound-isolated room. A tuning fork is used to measure when vibrating sounds are heard.

6. _____ Examples are the Rinne's test and the Weber's test.

A. Speech audiometry
B. Pure tone audiometry test
C. Tuning fork tests

PART II: PUTTING IT ALL TOGETHER

H. Multiple Choice/Multiple Response.

Choose the most appropriate answer or select all that apply.

1. Age-related changes in the inner ear affect sensitivity to sound, understanding of speech, and:
   1. balance.
   2. infection.
   3. cerumen production.
   4. blood pressure.

2. The type of hearing loss usually associated with aging is:
   1. otitis media.
   2. cholesteatoma.
   3. otosclerosis.
   4. presbycusis.

3. Pain in the ear is called:
   1. otosclerosis.
   2. otitis.
   3. ototoxicity.
   4. otalgia.

4. Ototoxicity means that a drug can damage the eighth cranial nerve or the organs of:
   1. hearing and balance.
   2. vision and sight.
   3. smell and taste.
   4. movement and coordination.

5. Examples of drugs that can have ototoxic effects are:
   1. aspirin and antibiotics.
   2. anticoagulants and corticosteroids.
   3. central nervous system stimulants and adrenergics.
   4. diuretics and antihypertensives.

6. When assessing the position of the auricles, the nurse should observe that the top of the auricle normally will be at about the level of the:
   1. nostrils.
   2. forehead.
   3. eye.
   4. mouth.

7. The external auditory canal is inspected for obvious obstructions or:
   1. edema.
   2. cyanosis.
   3. drainage.
   4. jaundice.

8. Which is the only normal secretion in the external auditory canal?
   1. Sebum
   2. Purulent drainage
   3. Cerumen
   4. Mucus

9. Otic drops, or ear drops, are intended to be placed directly into the:
   1. middle ear canal.
   2. inner ear canal.
   3. tympanic membrane.
   4. external ear canal.

10. The use of a solution to cleanse the external ear canal or to remove something from the canal is called:
    1. audiometry.
    2. irrigation.
    3. débridement.
    4. electronystagmography.

11. Which is a common indication for irrigation?
    1. Clot formation
    2. Impacted cerumen
    3. Purulent drainage
    4. Bleeding

12. Which is a device that amplifies sound?
    1. An audiometer
    2. A tuning fork
    3. A hearing aid
    4. An otoscope

13. People who benefit the most from hearing aids are those with:
    1. sensorineural loss.
    2. mixed hearing loss.
    3. conductive hearing loss.
    4. hearing loss due to Meniere's disease.

14. Postoperative dizziness or vertigo following ear surgery may put the patient at risk for:
    1. injury.
    2. impaired skin integrity.
    3. infection.
    4. pain.

15. Patients who have had ear surgery may have altered auditory sensory perception as a result of:
    1. dizziness or vertigo.
    2. knowledge deficit.
    3. self-care deficit.
    4. packing and edema in affected ear.

16. Following ear surgery, patients often complain of the sensation that the room is spinning or that their bodies are spinning. This is documented as:
    1. dizziness.
    2. otalgia.
    3. edema.
    4. vertigo.

17. After ear surgery, patients are advised to move slowly and carefully and to avoid sudden movement, which may cause:
    1. hemorrhage.
    2. vertigo.
    3. infection.
    4. edema.

18. Of all patients with sensory disorders, people who probably suffer the most severe social isolation are those with:
    1. hearing impairment.
    2. sight impairment.
    3. smell impairment.
    4. taste impairment.

19. To prevent one form of congenital hearing impairment, all women of childbearing age should be immunized for:
    1. pertussis.
    2. influenza.
    3. rubella.
    4. hepatitis B.

20. One of the most common causes of obstruction of the external ear canal is:
    1. hemorrhage.
    2. infection.
    3. impacted cerumen.
    4. blood clots.

21. Patients with impacted cerumen may complain of hearing loss or:
    1. sharp pain.
    2. tinnitus.
    3. bloody discharge.
    4. headache.

22. A very common problem after mastoidectomy or middle ear surgery is:
    1. nausea.
    2. constipation.
    3. oliguria.
    4. seizures.

23. Because the fixed stapes cannot vibrate in patients with otosclerosis, sound waves cannot be transmitted to the:
    1. middle ear.
    2. tympanic membrane.
    3. inner ear.
    4. external auditory canal.

24. Slow progressive hearing loss in the absence of infection is the primary symptom of:
    1. acute otitis media.
    2. labyrinthitis.
    3. perforated eardrum.
    4. otosclerosis.

25. The most common treatment for otosclerosis is a surgical procedure called:
    1. myringotomy.
    2. stapedectomy.
    3. mastoidectomy.
    4. incision and drainage.

26. A hereditary condition in which an abnormal growth causes the footplate of the stapes to become fixed is:
    1. cholesteatoma.
    2. otosclerosis.
    3. labyrinthitis.
    4. conductive hearing loss.

27. An inner ear infection that usually follows an upper respiratory infection and that may lead to Meniere's disease is:
    1. otitis media.
    2. otosclerosis.
    3. mastoiditis.
    4. labyrinthitis.

28. The treatment for labyrinthitis is:
    1. antiemetics.
    2. analgesics.
    3. corticosteroids.
    4. beta blockers.

29. Which is a major concern for a patient with vertigo?
    1. Infection
    2. Safety
    3. Nutrition
    4. Edema

30. Which is the primary symptom of ototoxicity with salicylates?
    1. Vertigo
    2. Tinnitus
    3. Dizziness
    4. Anorexia

31. A low buzzing sound that sometimes becomes a roar and that is a symptom of Meniere's disease is documented as:
    1. vertigo.
    2. tinnitus.
    3. dizziness.
    4. otitis.

32. When the caloric test or electronystagmography is done in patients with Meniere's disease, they will experience severe:
    1. vertigo.
    2. seizures.
    3. headache.
    4. flushing.

33. Following surgery for Meniere's disease, the nurse needs to assess the patient for:
    1. facial nerve damage.
    2. fluid volume excess.
    3. decreased cardiac output.
    4. urinary retention.

34. Presbycusis is the result of changes in one or more parts of the:
    1. middle ear.
    2. external auditory canal.
    3. eustachian tube.
    4. cochlea.

35. A labyrinth disorder in which there is an accumulation of fluid in the inner ear is:
    1. otosclerosis.
    2. otitis media.
    3. Meniere's disease.
    4. presbycusis.

36. Drugs that can cause permanent hearing loss are:
    1. antihypertensives.
    2. aminoglycosides (antibiotics).
    3. anticholinergics.
    4. diuretics.

37. Patients who are at special risk of developing ototoxicity because their bodies excrete drugs more slowly are those with:
    1. renal failure.
    2. pneumonia.
    3. myocardial infarction.
    4. liver disease.

38. Rinne's and Weber's tests use a tuning fork to assess the:
    1. ability to hear whispers.
    2. presence of lesions in the vestibule.
    3. conduction of sound by air and bone.
    4. function of the eighth cranial nerve.

39. Which diet may be recommended for patients with Meniere's disease?
    1. Increased calcium
    2. Increased vitamin K
    3. Increased potassium
    4. Low sodium

40. Which are potential complications of surgery for Meniere's disease? Select all that apply.
    1. Tinnitus
    2. Infection
    3. Hearing loss
    4. Ataxia
    5. Loss of cerebral spinal fluid
    6. Damage to cranial nerve VII (facial nerve)

41. Which is true about drying agents used as drug therapy for patients with ear infections? Select all that apply.
    1. Decrease risk of infection by drying the external canal after swimming or bathing.
    2. Prevent or treat nausea, vomiting, motion sickness.
    3. They soften ear wax.
    4. An example is boric acid.
    5. Contraindicated with perforated tympanic membrane
    6. Used with ear surgery.

42. Which are true statements about the use of topical corticosteroids for patients with ear infections? Select all that apply.
    1. Prevent or treat nausea, vomiting, and motion sickness.
    2. Treat inflammation, pruritus, and allergic response.
    3. Side effects include sedation, drowsiness, and dry mouth.
    4. Side effects include hypersensitivity: redness, rash, burning.
    5. Otocort, neomycin, colistin (Coly-Mycin S Otic), and polymyxin B are examples.

PART III: CHALLENGE YOURSELF!

I. Getting Ready for NCLEX.

Choose the most appropriate answer or select all that apply.

1. A patient with rheumatoid arthritis is taking aspirin. The nurse will monitor the patient for which signs and symptoms of toxicity? Select all that apply.
    1. Hearing loss
    2. Ataxia
    3. Infection
    4. Tinnitus
    5. Dizziness
    6. Drainage

2. The nurse is taking care of a patient with Meniere's disease. Which of the following is the priority problem for this patient?
    1. Impaired verbal communication related to inability to hear
    2. Risk for deficient fluid volume related to vomiting
    3. Social isolation related to inability to communicate verbally
    4. Ineffective coping related to change in social interaction

3. Which is the correct postoperative intervention for a patient who has had ear surgery?
    1. Position patient on the unaffected side to promote drainage.
    2. Instruct patient to keep his mouth closed if he needs to cough or sneeze.
    3. Increase vitamin K and protein intake in the diet.
    4. Avoid shampooing for 2 weeks.

4. Which is the priority intervention for patients with impaired verbal communication?
    1. Provide adequate lighting away from the patient's face.
    2. Raise the tone your voice.
    3. If the patient has a good ear, speak to that side.
    4. Explain the use of the call button and bedside intercom.

Nursing Care Plan.
Refer to Nursing Care Plan, The Patient with Meniere's Disease, p. 1258 in the textbook, and answer questions 5-7.

5. What is the priority nursing diagnosis?

6. What data collected during the health history and physical examination indicate the presence of Meniere's disease?
    1. _____
    2. _____
    3. _____
    4. _____
    5. _____

7. Which tasks may be assigned to unlicensed assistive personnel?
    1. _____
    2. _____
    3. _____
    4. _____
    5. _____
    6. _____

Nose, Sinus, and Throat Disorders

 Go to http://evolve.elsevier.com/Linton/medsurg/ for additional activities and exercises.

NCLEX CATEGORIES:

Safe and Effective Care Environment:
Coordinated Care, Safety and Infection Control

Health Promotion and Maintenance

Psychosocial Integrity

Physiological Integrity: Basic Care and Comfort, Pharmacological Therapies, Reduction of Risk Potential, Physiological Adaptation

OBJECTIVES

1. Describe the nursing assessment of the nose, sinuses, and throat.
2. Identify nursing responsibilities for patients undergoing tests or procedures to diagnose disorders of the nose, sinuses, or throat.
3. Describe the nurse's role when the following common therapeutic measures are instituted: administration of topical medications, irrigations, humidification, suctioning, tracheostomy care, and surgery.
4. Explain the pathophysiology, signs and symptoms, complications, and medical or surgical treatment of selected disorders of the nose, sinuses, and throat.
5. Assist in developing nursing care plans for patients with disorders of the nose, sinuses, or throat.

PART I: MASTERING THE BASICS

A. Key Terms.
Complete the statement in the numbered column with the most appropriate term in the lettered column. Some terms may be used more than once.

1. The terms *maxillary, frontal, ethmoid,* and *sphenoid* refer to _____.

2. Projections that increase the surface area where inspired air moves are called _____.

3. The procedure by which the nurse shines a special light into the patient's mouth to see whether the sinus cavities are filled with air is _____.

4. Spaces in the bones of the skull are called _____.

5. The sinuses are lined with _____.

6. Particles that are trapped in the mucus are swept toward the throat by _____.

7. Type of cells that line the roof of the nasal cavity are _____.

8. Specialized sensory cells detect odors and relay information about odors to the brain by way of the _____.

9. The sinuses produce mucus that drains into the _____.

10. Air spaces that act as sound chambers for the voice and reduce the weight of the skull are called _____.

A. Cilia
B. Nasal cavity
C. Olfactory nerve
D. Turbinates
E. Mucous membrane
F. Sinuses
G. Transillumination
H. Olfactory

B. Obstructive Sleep Apnea (OSA).

Refer to Figure 53-6 (p. 1279) below.

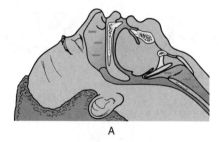

A

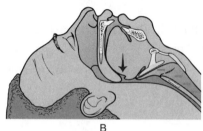

B

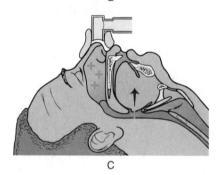

C

1. _____ Which figure shows the nasal CPAP in place?

2. _____ Which figure shows a patient predisposed to obstructive sleep apnea (OSA) with a small pharyngeal airway?

3. _____ Which figure shows the relaxation of the pharyngeal muscles, allowing the airway to close, resulting in repeated apneic episodes?

4. Which of the following are symptoms of OSA? Select all that apply.
   1. Sore throat
   2. Epistaxis
   3. Irritable and sleepy during the day
   4. Impaired concentration and memory
   5. Muscle aches
   6. Loud snoring
   7. Hypotension
   8. Cardiac dysrhythmias

5. Which diagnostic test is done to confirm OSA?
   1. Laryngoscopy
   2. Bronchoscopy
   3. Polysomnography
   4. Blood gases

C. Laryngectomy Key Terms.

Complete the statement in the numbered column with the most appropriate term in the lettered column.

1. Following laryngectomy, many patients are able to learn to control and use air to produce sounds, which is called _____.

2. Following laryngectomy, some patients use an electronic device to produce sound, which is called a(n) _____.

3. A procedure used for small tumors of the larynx is _____.

4. Surgery in which the voice is preserved is _____.

A. Laser surgery
B. Artificial larynx
C. Esophageal speech
D. Hemilaryngectomy

D. Drug Therapy.

Match the actions and uses of the drugs in the numbered column with the classification of drugs in the lettered column.

1. _____ Anesthetic effect on skin and mucous membranes
2. _____ Reduce body temperature, treat fever
3. _____ Decongestion, vasoconstriction
4. _____ Treat allergic reactions, prevent motion sickness
5. _____ Reduce pain
6. _____ Kill or suppress growth of microorganisms
7. _____ Decrease salivary and respiratory secretions

A. Sympathomimetics
B. Anticholinergics
C. Antihistamines
D. Antipyretics
E. Analgesics
F. Topical anesthetics
G. Antiinfectives

E. Bacterial Pharyngitis.

Indicate for each characteristic below whether it refers to (A) viral or (B) bacterial pharyngitis.

1. _____ Positive culture
2. _____ Dysphagia
3. _____ Normal CBC
4. _____ Rhinorrhea
5. _____ Abrupt onset of symptoms
6. _____ Malaise
7. _____ Mild elevation of temperature
8. _____ Gradual onset of symptoms
9. _____ Joint and muscle pain
10. _____ Rare complications

F. Age-Related Changes.

Which are age-related changes of the nose, throat, and sinuses? Select all that apply.

1. Decreased nasal obstruction
2. Cartilage of the external nose hardens
3. Increased, more serious side effects of nasal decongestants
4. Production of mucus increases
5. Mucous membrane becomes thinner
6. Sense of smell declines
7. Occurrence of epistaxis (nosebleed) increases
8. Esophageal sphincter may weaken, causing gastric content to flow back into the throat when patients lie down
9. Tissues of the larynx become drier and less elastic

G. Nose and Throat.

Using Figure 53-2 (p. 1263) below, label the structures of the nose and throat (A–J) by using the terms (1–10) below.

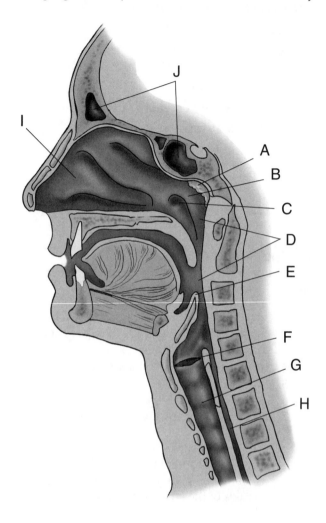

1. _____ Nasal cavity
2. _____ Sinuses
3. _____ Area of pharynx
4. _____ Orifice of auditory tube
5. _____ Vocal cord
6. _____ Esophagus
7. _____ Pharyngeal tonsils (adenoids)
8. _____ Epiglottis
9. _____ Area of nasopharynx
10. _____ Larynx

PART II: PUTTING IT ALL TOGETHER

H. Multiple Choice/Multiple Response.

Choose the most appropriate answer or select all that apply.

1. For patients with throat disorders, for what does the nurse inspect the mucous membranes and tonsils of the throat? Select all that apply.
   1. Cyanosis
   2. Lesions
   3. Pallor
   4. Redness
   5. Drainage
   6. Swelling

2. Inspection and palpation of the neck may reveal enlarged:
   1. lymph nodes.
   2. tonsils.
   3. adenoids.
   4. vocal cords.

3. Epistaxis (nosebleed) is more common in older people, especially in those taking:
   1. antibiotics.
   2. analgesics.
   3. anticoagulants.
   4. diuretics.

4. A patient has a weakened esophageal sphincter that allows gastric contents to flow back into the throat when the patient lies down. Where does this patient experience a burning sensation?
   1. Larynx
   2. Nares
   3. Trachea
   4. Stomach

5. Following laryngoscopy, the patient takes nothing by mouth until:
   1. respirations are normal.
   2. vomiting has stopped.
   3. the gag reflex returns.
   4. 24 hours after surgery.

6. Before suctioning a patient, it is important to:
   1. administer antiemetics as ordered.
   2. ambulate the patient.
   3. oxygenate the patient.
   4. administer antibiotics as ordered.

7. Which is a key point to remember when suctioning a patient?
   1. Keep the vent closed when inserting the catheter.
   2. Apply suction continuously as the catheter is withdrawn.
   3. Suction for no longer than 30 seconds.
   4. Use sterile procedure.

8. When providing tracheostomy care to a patient, which is the appropriate intervention?
   1. Use Standard Precautions.
   2. Suction the tracheostomy after removing the old dressings.
   3. Use a sterile solution of iodine to clean the inner cannula.
   4. Cut a new pad to fit around the tracheostomy site.

9. Which are common problems the nurse monitors in a patient who has had nasal surgery? Select all that apply.
   1. Tachycardia
   2. Dyspnea
   3. Pain
   4. Pressure
   5. Anxiety
   6. Hypotension
   7. Pallor

10. After nasal surgery, the patient's vital signs are monitored to detect signs of which of the following?
    1. Hypokalemia
    2. Hypernatremia
    3. Hypovolemia
    4. Inadequate circulation

11. The patient who has had nasal surgery may be at risk for decreased cardiac output because of:
    1. blood loss from nasal passageways.
    2. nasal packing.
    3. airway obstruction.
    4. facial bruising.

12. Following nasal surgery, what is the priority problem for this patient?
    1. Hemorrhage
    2. Infection
    3. Hypertension
    4. Confusion

13. Laxatives or stool softeners may be ordered for patients after nasal surgery in order to prevent which of the following?
    1. Diarrhea
    2. Vomiting
    3. Hypertension
    4. Straining

14. Which is the best position for patients after nasal surgery to help control swelling?
    1. Lying flat in bed
    2. Lying with the head of bed elevated
    3. Side-lying
    4. Supine

15. When the nasal cavity is packed following surgery, the patient is breathing through the mouth. Which is the best measure that helps decrease dryness of the mucous membranes?
    1. Frequent oral hygiene
    2. Humidifiers
    3. Oral fluids high in vitamin C
    4. Ice packs

16. Patients may experience disturbed body image following nasal surgery due to:
    1. airway obstruction.
    2. blood loss.
    3. hypovolemia.
    4. facial bruises.

17. Serious neurologic complications should be suspected in patients with sinusitis if the patient develops which of the following?
    1. Tachycardia and restlessness
    2. High fever and seizures
    3. Confusion and cyanosis
    4. Dyspnea and anxiety

18. Which is the type of surgery performed for chronic maxillary sinusitis?
    1. Laryngoscopy
    2. Tonsillectomy and adenoidectomy
    3. The Caldwell-Luc operation
    4. Nasal septoplasty

19. Desensitizing injections, or "allergy shots," are composed of dilute solutions of which of the following?
    1. Allergens
    2. Histamines
    3. Antihistamines
    4. Plasma

20. A deviated septum may obstruct the nasal passage and block which of the following?
    1. Sinus drainage
    2. Eustachian tube drainage
    3. Pharyngeal drainage
    4. Jugular vein drainage

21. Patients with a deviated septum may complain of epistaxis, sinusitis, and:
    1. palpitations.
    2. headaches.
    3. insomnia.
    4. sweating.

22. When epistaxis occurs, the patient should sit down and lean forward and direct pressure should be applied for:
    1. 1–2 minutes.
    2. 3–5 minutes.
    3. 7–10 minutes.
    4. 15–20 minutes.

23. Suctioning is limited to 10 seconds because prolonged suctioning may lead to which of the following?
    1. Hypoxia
    2. Hypertension
    3. Increased intracranial pressure
    4. Bradycardia

24. Patients with severe epistaxis may be at high risk for infection due to:
    1. possible airway obstruction.
    2. nasal packing.
    3. hypotension.
    4. hypovolemia.

25. The two major problems that may develop in the postoperative phase of tonsillectomy are respiratory distress and:
    1. infection.
    2. hemorrhage.
    3. hypersensitivity reaction.
    4. cardiac dysrhythmia.

26. Following a tonsillectomy, a treatment that may be applied to the neck to decrease swelling and pain is:
    1. a heating pad.
    2. a TENS unit.
    3. antibiotic ointment.
    4. an ice collar.

27. A postoperative tonsillectomy patient is ready to be discharged. Which symptoms should be reported to the physician if the nurse observes them?
    1. Bleeding
    2. Earache
    3. White patches in the throat (surgical site)
    4. Sore throat

28. Which treatment is usually prescribed to reduce irritation of the larynx in patients with laryngitis?
    1. Surgery
    2. Voice rest
    3. Intravenous fluids
    4. Application of heat

29. A primary nursing diagnosis for patients with laryngitis due to aphonia is:
    1. Risk for infection.
    2. Risk for injury.
    3. Impaired verbal communication.
    4. Altered tissue perfusion.

30. What is the correct term for benign masses of fibrous tissue that result primarily from overuse of the voice or that follow infections?
    1. Nodules
    2. Myomas
    3. Fibromas
    4. Tumors

31. The only symptom of laryngeal nodules is:
    1. pain.
    2. fever.
    3. dysphagia.
    4. hoarseness.

32. Which is the term for a swollen mass of mucous membrane attached to the vocal cord?
    1. Nodule
    2. Tumor
    3. Cancer
    4. Polyp

33. Individuals who both smoke and use alcohol are at particularly high risk for:
    1. tonsillitis.
    2. pneumonia.
    3. cancer of the larynx.
    4. nasal polyps.

34. What is the most common site of metastasis in a patient with laryngeal cancer?
    1. Liver
    2. Colon
    3. Lung
    4. Brain

35. Total laryngectomy causes permanent loss of the:
    1. voice.
    2. cough.
    3. sternocleidomastoid muscle movement.
    4. swallow reflex.

36. A total laryngectomy involves removal of the entire larynx, vocal cords, and which of the following?
    1. Pharynx
    2. Epiglottis
    3. Tonsils
    4. Esophagus

37. Gently closing one naris at a time and instructing the patient to breathe through the other naris is a way to assess:
    1. lung sounds.
    2. aphonia.
    3. sense of smell.
    4. patency of the nostrils.

38. Normally, the frontal and maxillary sinuses are filled with which of the following?
    1. Fluid
    2. Air
    3. Polyps
    4. Cysts

39. In the immediate postoperative period after total laryngectomy, the nurse's assessment focuses on comfort, circulation, and:
    1. fluid balance.
    2. oxygenation.
    3. infection.
    4. hypovolemia.

40. Which position promotes maximal lung expansion in the patient with a laryngectomy?
    1. Semi-prone
    2. Flat
    3. Semi-Fowler's
    4. Side-lying

41. To prevent pooling of secretions in the lungs of patients with laryngectomies, which should the nurse encourage?
    1. Coughing and deep-breathing
    2. Increased fluid intake
    3. Early ambulation
    4. Avoidance of dusty places

42. Which herb is used to boost the immune system and is taken by some to decrease the severity of a cold?
    1. Ginseng
    2. Ephedra
    3. Echinacea
    4. St. John's wort

43. To decrease the patient's reaction to offending allergens, the allergist may recommend injections for what purpose?
    1. Prevent inflammation
    2. Treat tissue injury
    3. Increase immunity
    4. Provide desensitization

44. Which are true statements about sinusitis? Select all that apply.
    1. Pain or a feeling of heaviness over the frontal or maxillary area is a common symptom.
    2. Toothache-like pain is a common symptom of sinusitis that involves the frontal sinus.
    3. Complications of sinusitis include brain abscess and meningitis.
    4. Most sinus infections are caused by a virus.

45. Which are true statements about acute viral coryza? Select all that apply.
    1. Acute viral coryza is contagious and spread by droplet infection.
    2. Complications of acute viral coryza are more common in people with increased resistance.
    3. Complications of acute viral coryza include otitis media, sinusitis, bronchitis, and pneumonia.
    4. Antibiotics are effective against acute viral coryza.
    5. Decongestants and antihistamines are used to treat acute viral coryza.

46. Which are true statements about pharyngitis? Select all that apply.
    1. Pharyngitis is treated with rest, fluids, analgesics, and throat gargles.
    2. A soft or liquid diet may be ordered because of nausea.
    3. A treatment that may be ordered is humidification.
    4. The recommended daily fluid intake for patients with pharyngitis is 1000–1500 ml.

47. Which are complications of bacterial pharyngitis that may occur 1–5 weeks after the throat infection? Select all that apply.
    1. Acute glomerulonephritis
    2. Meningitis
    3. Sinusitis
    4. Brain abscess
    5. Rheumatic fever

PART III: CHALLENGE YOURSELF!

I. Getting Ready for NCLEX.

Choose the most appropriate answer or select all that apply.

1. Which are true statements about patients with tonsillitis? Select all that apply.
    1. Tonsillitis is a contagious infection spread by food or airborne routes.
    2. A patient with tonsillitis usually reports a sore throat, difficulty swallowing, fever, chills, and muscle aches.
    3. If swollen tissue blocks the eustachian tubes in patients with tonsillitis, there may also be pain in the lungs.
    4. An elevated white blood cell count in patients with tonsillitis suggests a viral infection.
    5. The medical treatment of tonsillitis usually includes the use of antibiotics.

2. Which are common problems for a patient with epistaxis? Select all that apply.
    1. Ineffective airway clearance related to increased pulmonary secretions or weak cough
    2. Decreased cardiac output related to hypovolemia secondary to hemorrhage
    3. Risk for injury related to pressure (of packing, balloon) and possible airway obstruction
    4. Risk for infection related to presence of nasal packing
    5. Disturbed body image related to facial bruising

3. With facial trauma or nasal fracture, the recommended treatment initially is application of:
    1. an ice pack.
    2. a warm compress.
    3. direct pressure.
    4. heat.

4. Which are early signs of inadequate oxygenation in the postoperative tonsillectomy patient? Select all that apply.
   1. Cyanosis
   2. Pallor
   3. Numbness
   4. Confusion
   5. Restlessness
   6. Increased pulse rate

5. Which foods should be avoided in patients after a tonsillectomy?
   1. Frozen liquids
   2. Ice cream
   3. Applesauce
   4. Citrus juices

6. In the patient with a laryngectomy, the nurse monitors the need for suctioning by observing which of the following? Select all that apply.
   1. Increased pulse
   2. Swelling
   3. Pain
   4. Restlessness
   5. audible or visible mucus

7. The nurse is taking care of a patient who has had a laryngectomy. Which of the following are factors that affect the respiratory status of this patient? Select all that apply.
   1. Nutrition
   2. Verbal communication
   3. Humidification
   4. Personal hygiene
   5. Positioning
   6. fluids

8. An older adult has pharyngitis. Why must fluids be increased slowly in older adults?
   1. They do not adjust well to sudden changes in blood volume.
   2. They have decreased kidney function.
   3. They may develop cardiac edema if the fluids are given too rapidly.
   4. The esophagus is more narrow.

Nursing Care Plan.
Refer to Nursing Care Plan, The Patient Having Tonsillectomy, p. 1278 in the textbook, and answer questions 9-14.

9. What is the priority nursing diagnosis?

10. What were this patient's signs and symptoms listed in the health history that indicate a need for a tonsillectomy?
    1. _____
    2. _____
    3. _____
    4. _____
    5. _____

11. Which three nursing interventions will the nurse perform first?
    1. _____
    2. _____
    3. _____

12. Which data in the physical examination indicate the need to watch for excessive bleeding in this patient?
    1. _____
    2. _____

13. In what position should this patient be placed?

14. Which of the following should be included in this patient's discharge teaching? Select all that apply.
    1. Consume soft, high-calorie, high-protein diet for 10 days.
    2. Drink 6–8 8-ounce glasses of fluids daily.
    3. Avoid strenuous activity or straining for 2 weeks.
    4. Do not take aspirin.
    5. Headaches are common following surgery.

Psychological Responses to Illness

ⓔ Go to http://evolve.elsevier.com/Linton/medsurg/ for additional activities and exercises.

NCLEX CATEGORIES:

Safe and Effective Care Environment:
Coordinated Care, Safety and Infection Control

Health Promotion and Maintenance

Psychosocial Integrity

Physiological Integrity: Basic Care and Comfort, Pharmacological Therapies, Reduction of Risk Potential, Physiological Adaptation

OBJECTIVES

1. Define mental health.
2. Discuss the concepts of stress, anxiety, adaptation, and homeostasis.
3. Discuss how age and cultural and spiritual beliefs affect an individual's ability to cope with illness.
4. Identify some basic coping strategies (defense mechanisms).
5. Discuss the concepts of anxiety, fear, stress, loss, grief, hopelessness, and powerlessness in relation to illness.
6. Describe several factors that may precipitate adaptive or maladaptive coping behaviors in response to illness.
7. Discuss implementation of the nursing process to enhance a patient's mental health as the patient deals with the stresses of illness.

PART I: MASTERING THE BASICS

A. Key Terms. Defense Mechanisms.
Match or complete the statement in the numbered column with the most appropriate term in the lettered column.

1. _____ Refusal to acknowledge a real situation

2. _____ An attempt to make up for real or imagined weakness

3. _____ Use of logic, reasoning, and analysis to avoid unacceptable feelings

4. _____ Transferring unacceptable feelings or impulses to another

5. _____ Avoidance of unacceptable thoughts and behaviors by expressing opposing thoughts or behaviors

6. _____ Withdrawing to an earlier level of development to benefit from the associated comfort levels

7. _____ Transfer of painful feelings to body parts; the person's feelings are expressed in the form of a physical symptom

8. _____ An emotional conflict is turned into a physical symptom, that provides the individual with some sort of benefit (secondary gain)

A. Compensation
B. Rationalization or intellectualization
C. Somatization
D. Denial
E. Conversion
F. Projection
G. Reaction formation
H. Regression

B. Coping Strategies.

Which of the following are relaxation strategies? Select all that apply.

1. Biofeedback
2. Role-playing
3. Meditation
4. Discussion with clients about a higher power or their beliefs
5. Yoga
6. Deep-breathing exercises

C. Mental Health Definition.

1. Which are characteristics of healthy individuals, according to Maslow? Select all that apply.
   1. Positive self-esteem
   2. Accurate perception of reality
   3. Sense of spirituality
   4. Ability to accept oneself and others
   5. Ability to be spontaneous
   6. Need for privacy
   7. Need for isolation
   8. Independence or autonomy
   9. Frequent "peak experiences"
   10. Sense of ethics
   11. Sense of conformity
   12. Identification with humankind

2. Match the descriptions in the numbered column with the dimensions of a complete person in the lettered column.

   1. _____ Ability to experience and express feelings and emotions
   2. _____ Skills in living as a member of a family and a community
   3. _____ Ability to formulate thoughts, process information, and solve problems
   4. _____ Person's internal environment
   5. _____ Reflects a person's individuality

   A. Physical dimension
   B. Cognitive dimension
   C. Affective dimension
   D. Behavioral dimension
   E. Social dimension

D. Powerlessness.

Which of the following are characteristics of powerlessness? Select all that apply.

1. Loss of motivation
2. Passivity
3. Nonparticipation in self-care and decision-making
4. Dependence on others, which may lead to anger, resentment, or guilt

E. Nursing Diagnoses.

Which of the following are patient problems that are often identified in persons or families with inadequate coping? Select all that apply.

1. Activity intolerance
2. Interrupted family processes
3. Ineffective role performance
4. Acute confusion
5. Disturbed body image
6. Fear
7. Low self-esteem
8. Deficient fluid volume
9. Disturbed sleep pattern
10. Sedentary lifestyle
11. Complicated grieving

PART II: PUTTING IT ALL TOGETHER

F. Multiple-Choice Questions.

Choose the most appropriate answer.

1. Defense mechanisms are adopted by the individual as protective measures to allow the ego relief from:
   1. rationalization.
   2. denial.
   3. anxiety.
   4. repression.

2. A factor that is basic to helping the patient cope with illness is the nurse's:
   1. caring attitude.
   2. educational background.
   3. professionalism.
   4. organization.

3. Effective nursing interventions can be made only after patients have been assessed as:
   1. members of a particular culture.
   2. members of a particular sex.
   3. members of a certain race.
   4. unique individuals.

4. A group's affiliation because of a shared language, race, and values is:
   1. culture.
   2. behavior.
   3. morality.
   4. ethnicity.

5. People subjected to prolonged stressors eventually become:
   1. defensive.
   2. exhausted.
   3. cognitive.
   4. emotional.

6. What is often an early response to illness?
   1. Grief
   2. Depression
   3. Anxiety
   4. Loss

7. What is the process called when a person with a severe illness is forced to relinquish original hopes?
   1. Mourning
   2. Grief
   3. Anxiety
   4. Fear

8. The experience of loss is related to the individual's:
   1. self-concept.
   2. sense of belonging.
   3. anxiety.
   4. depression.

9. Any change in a person's life creates:
   1. fear.
   2. anxiety.
   3. stress.
   4. mourning.

10. Unconscious coping mechanisms are referred to as:
    1. stressors.
    2. defense mechanisms.
    3. self-concepts.
    4. illusions.

11. Passivity and verbal expression of loss of control over situations are characteristics of:
    1. gratification.
    2. denial.
    3. intellectualization.
    4. powerlessness.

12. Denial of obvious problems and weaknesses is related to the nursing diagnosis of:
    1. Ineffective individual coping.
    2. Activity intolerance.
    3. Altered growth and development.
    4. Ineffective self health care management.

13. Passivity and dependence on others are characteristics of:
    1. helplessness.
    2. powerlessness.
    3. denial.
    4. displacement.

14. Minimizing the severity of an illness by a patient is an example of:
    1. denial.
    2. repression.
    3. compensation.
    4. regression.

15. Ineffective coping mechanisms may evolve from a sense of:
    1. isolation.
    2. projection.
    3. powerlessness.
    4. reaction formation.

16. Which is an example of conversion?
    1. A woman finds a suspicious lump in her breast and does not keep appointments for a breast biopsy.
    2. An individual witnesses a murder and then experiences sudden blindness without an organic cause.
    3. A child starts sucking her thumb when her new baby brother comes home from the hospital.
    4. A man who is angry at his boss comes home and yells at his dog.

PART III: CHALLENGE YOURSELF!

G. Getting Ready for NCLEX.

Choose the most appropriate answer or select all that apply.

Patient Teaching Plan.

Refer to Patient Teaching Plan, Helping Patients and Their Families Cope with a Serious Diagnosis, p. 1292 in the textbook, and answer question 1.

1. A patient has just been admitted with heart failure, and the nurse is teaching the patient steps to help him deal effectively with his initial diagnosis, and steps to make the best possible decisions for himself and his family. Arrange the following actions in the appropriate order for teaching the patient about dealing with his illness.

   A. _____ The patient should talk with members of the health team, as good communication will increase satisfaction with the care received.

   B. _____ The patient should decide on a treatment plan with the health care team so that he is involved in a plan that best meets his needs.

   C. _____ The patient should take the time he needs and not rush important decisions about his health.

   D. _____ The patient should seek out information that is based on scientific evidence.

   E. _____ The patient should get the support he needs from family, friends, and people who are going through the same problem.

Nursing Care Plan.

Refer to Nursing Care Plan, Patient Ineffectively Coping with Illness, Box 54-1, p. 1297 in the textbook, and answer question 2.

2. Which are nursing interventions for this patient? Select all that apply.

   1. Use confrontational techniques to help the patient accept the problem of coping.
   2. Give the patient an opportunity to verbalize feelings of powerlessness by approaching patient care in an unhurried manner.
   3. Establish a no-harm contract with the patient.
   4. Collect data about the patient's and family's current coping strategies and behaviors.
   5. Involve the dietitian in planning an adequate diet.
   6. Implement stress-reduction strategies, such as music therapy, to help the patient deal with stressful moments.

Psychiatric Disorders

chapter
55

 Go to http://evolve.elsevier.com/Linton/medsurg/ for additional activities and exercises.

NCLEX CATEGORIES:

Safe and Effective Care Environment:
Coordinated Care, Safety and Infection Control

Health Promotion and Maintenance

Psychosocial Integrity

Physiological Integrity: Basic Care and Comfort, Pharmacological Therapies, Reduction of Risk Potential, Physiological Adaptation

OBJECTIVES

1. Describe the differences between social relationships and therapeutic relationships.
2. Describe key strategies in communicating therapeutically.
3. Describe the components of the mental status examination.
4. Identify target symptoms, behaviors, and potential side effects for the following types of medications: antianxiety (anxiolytic), antipsychotic, and antidepressant drugs.
5. Summarize current thinking about the etiology of schizophrenia and mood disorders.
6. Identify key features of the mental status examination and their relevance in anxiety disorders, schizophrenia, mood disorders, cognitive disorders, and personality disorders.
7. Identify common nursing diagnoses, goals, and interventions for people with anxiety disorders, schizophrenia, mood disorders, cognitive disorders, and personality disorders.

PART I: MASTERING THE BASICS

A. Key Terms.
Match the definition or description in the numbered column with the most appropriate term in the lettered column.

1. _____ Frequently irreversible side effect of antipsychotic medication that develops after years of use; symptoms include involuntary movements of face, jaw, and tongue, leading to grimacing; jerky movements of upper extremities; and tonic contractions of neck and back

2. _____ A state in which a person's perception of reality is impaired, thereby interfering with the capacity to function and to relate to others

3. _____ Assumes that mental disorders are related to physiologic changes within the central nervous system

4. _____ Level of consciousness and orientation to time, place, person, and self

5. _____ Based on the theory that people function at different levels of awareness (conscious to unconscious) and that ego defense mechanisms, such as denial and repression, are used to prevent anxiety

6. _____ A defense mechanism in which particular feelings or specific aspects of reality are excluded from awareness

7. _____ A defense mechanism in which one sees others as a source of one's own unacceptable thoughts, feelings, or impulses

8. _____ Side effects of antipsychotic drugs on the portion of the central nervous system controlling involuntary movements

9. _____ Refers to behaviors and symptoms of masklike face, rigid posture, shuffling gait, and resting tremors

10. _____ A state of feeling outside of oneself; that is, watching what is happening as if it were happening to someone else

11. _____ The patient learns new ways to behave in a therapeutic relationship built on trust

A. Sensorium
B. Depersonalization
C. Projection
D. Psychosis
E. Parkinsonian syndrome
F. Psychoanalytic approach
G. Tardive dyskinesia
H. Extrapyramidal effects
I. Interpersonal approach
J. Biologic approach
K. Denial

B. Mental Health Disorders.
Match the definition or description in the numbered column with the most appropriate term in the lettered column.

1. _____ Involves deficits in orientation, memory, language comprehension, and judgment

2. _____ A very serious group of usually chronic thought disorders in which patients' ability to interpret the world around them is severely impaired

3. _____ A mental disorder that involves a change in identity, memory, or consciousness that enables patients to remove themselves from anxiety-provoking situations

4. _____ Periods of elevated mood (manic episodes) and depression

5. _____ Fear of situations outside the home

6. _____ A mental state that is characterized by cognitive and intellectual deficits severe enough to impair social or occupational functioning (memory, abstract thinking, and judgment)

7. _____ Patient experiences a marked, persistent fear that is excessive and works hard to avoid the feared object or situation

8. _____ Patient experiences intense episodes of apprehension to the point of terror

9. _____ Patient exhibits unstable relationships, unstable self-image, and unstable mood

A. Dissociative disorder
B. Dementia
C. Organic mental disorder
D. Borderline personality disorder
E. Bipolar disorder
F. Panic disorder
G. Agoraphobia
H. Schizophrenia
I. Specific phobia disorder

C. Mental Health Disorders.
Match the definition or description in the numbered column with the most appropriate term in the lettered column.

1. _____ Person exhibits two or more distinct personalities

2. _____ Loss of body function (e.g., paralysis) without physiologic cause

3. _____ A disorder that is characterized by vague, multiple, recurring physical complaints that are not caused by real physical illness

4. _____ Pervasive, chronic, and maladaptive personality characteristics that interfere with normal functioning

5. _____ A psychological disorder experienced following a traumatic event that is characterized by flashbacks, detachment, and sleeping and eating difficulties

6. _____ Recurrent obsessions or compulsions, or both, that produce distress and interfere with daily functioning

7. _____ Belief that a serious medical condition exists when medical findings are absent

8. _____ Persistent depressed mood

9. _____ Disorder that occurs after exposure to a recent distressing event that is characterized by detachment, derealization, depersonalization, and dissociative amnesia

A. Post-traumatic stress disorder
B. Major depression
C. Dissociative identity disorder
D. Hypochondriasis
E. Somatoform disorder
F. Personality disorder
G. Obsessive-compulsive disorder
H. Conversion disorder
I. Acute stress disorder

D. Mental Status Examination.
Which features are assessed during the mental status examination? Select all that apply.
1. Heart rate
2. Blood pressure
3. Appearance
4. Mood and affect
5. Speech and language
6. Thought content
7. Respirations
8. Perceptual disturbances
9. Insight and judgment
10. Sensorium
11. Emotional responses
12. Memory and attention

E. Therapeutic Relationship.
Match the description in the numbered column with (A) therapeutic or (B) social relationship.

1. _____ May or may not have clear boundaries and a clear ending.

2. _____ Focus is on personal and emotional needs of patient.

3. _____ Purpose is to benefit both participants in the relationship.

4. _____ Participants are not formally responsible for evaluating their interaction.

5. _____ Helper has responsibility for evaluating the interaction and the changing behavior.

6. _____ Relationship has some boundaries (purpose, place, time) and clear ending.

7. _____ Relationship develops spontaneously.

F. Therapeutic Relationship.
Which are interpersonal strategies of a therapeutic relationship? Select all that apply.
1. Sharing observations
2. Responsibility
3. Accepting silence
4. Listening
5. Professionalism
6. Clarifying
7. Being available
8. Giving advice

G. Schizophrenia.
Which are correct interventions for a patient who is experiencing disturbed thought processes? Select all that apply.
1. Encourage involvement in activities.
2. Focus on reality.
3. Make brief, frequent contacts with the patient to interrupt hallucinatory experiences.
4. Let the patient know that the nurse does not share the delusion.
5. Connect delusions with anxiety-provoking situations.
6. Encourage the patient to pay attention to what is occurring in the environment (instead of internal stimuli).
7. Inform the patient that hallucinations are part of the disease process.
8. Encourage the patient to express feelings and anxiety.

H. Drug Therapy.

Refer to Table 55-5, p. 1312 in the textbook. Match the descriptions in the numbered column with the drug classification in the lettered column. Answers may be used more than once.

1. _____ Antidepressant drug that affects serotonin and epinephrine/norepinephrine; may cause cardiac complications

2. _____ Used in the treatment of bipolar disorders with narrow therapeutic range; may cause toxicity signs, including tremors

3. _____ Antipsychotic agent that is helpful in the treatment of schizophrenia; may cause drowsiness, hypotension, dry mouth, extrapyramidal symptoms (EPS), and tardive dyskinesia

4. _____ Antidepressants that can be taken once a day without being cardiotoxic; useful in treatment of panic disorder and obsessive-compulsive disorder

5. _____ Antipsychotic agents that treat both positive and negative symptoms of schizophrenia; examples are Clozaril, Zyprexa, and Seroquel

6. _____ Important to maintain hydration, and monitor renal function and serum blood levels of drug

7. _____ Antidepressant drugs that require strict diet restriction to avoid hypertensive crisis

8. _____ Mood-stabilizer used in the treatment of bipolar disorders

A. Typical neuroleptics
B. Atypical neuroleptics
C. SSRIs
D. Tricyclics
E. MAOIs
F. Lithium
G. Valproic acid (Depakote)

PART II: PUTTING IT ALL TOGETHER

I. Multiple Choice/Multiple Response.

Choose the most appropriate answer or select all that apply.

1. Repeated checking to see whether the door is locked is an example of:
   1. obsession.
   2. hallucination.
   3. delusion.
   4. compulsion.

2. Many people with obsessive-compulsive disorders have become symptom-free once therapeutic levels of which drug have been reached?
   1. Analgesics
   2. Antihistamines
   3. Antidepressants
   4. Anticonvulsants

3. Conversion disorders and hypochondriasis are examples of:
   1. mood disorders.
   2. somatoform disorders.
   3. panic disorders.
   4. obsessive-compulsive disorders.

4. Amnesia and multiple personality disorder are examples of:
   1. somatoform disorders.
   2. dissociative disorders.
   3. panic disorders.
   4. post-traumatic stress disorders.

5. A symptom of dissociative disorders is:
   1. depersonalization.
   2. hypochondriasis.
   3. agitation.
   4. hallucinations.

6. Most patients with dissociative identity disorder report severe:
   1. agoraphobia.
   2. hallucinations.
   3. delusions.
   4. childhood abuse.

7. The primary antianxiety medications are the:
   1. benzodiazepines.
   2. antihistamines.
   3. thiazides.
   4. salicylates.

8. Withdrawal from antianxiety medications should be medically supervised because of the effect(s) of:
   1. amnesia and confusion.
   2. negative feedback.
   3. hormones and histamines.
   4. physical and psychological dependence.

9. Which is a key problem for patients with anxiety disorders?
   1. Disturbed body image
   2. Powerlessness
   3. Spiritual distress
   4. Ineffective coping

10. One of the most common psychiatric disorders is:
    1. bipolar disorder.
    2. major depression.
    3. post-traumatic stress disorder.
    4. conversion disorder.

11. As patients respond to antidepressant medications and their energy level increases, what risk may increase?
    1. Mutism
    2. Panic
    3. Suicide
    4. Hypertension

12. A type of therapy that may be used for patients with severe depression when other forms of therapy have failed is:
    1. antidepressants.
    2. electroconvulsive therapy.
    3. psychotherapy.
    4. isolation therapy.

13. Possible side effects of electroconvulsive therapy are temporary memory loss and:
    1. orthostatic hypotension.
    2. confusion.
    3. tardive dyskinesia.
    4. parkinsonian syndrome.

14. Which are signs of major depression in a patient? Select all that apply.
    1. Psychomotor retardation
    2. Agoraphobia
    3. No spontaneous movements
    4. Post-traumatic stress syndrome
    5. Downcast gaze
    6. Agitated movements of hand wringing

15. Frequently assessing a patient's suicidal potential and maintaining continuous one-to-one contact, if indicated, are interventions for depressed patients who are at risk for:
    1. sleep pattern disturbance.
    2. anxiety.
    3. self-directed violence.
    4. self-esteem disturbance.

16. Learning to limit self-criticism and to give and receive compliments are interventions for patients who are experiencing:
    1. Risk for self-directed violence.
    2. Chronic low self-esteem.
    3. Anxiety.
    4. Dysfunctional grieving.

17. Offering small snacks and warm baths and teaching relaxation exercises to be used before retiring for the evening are interventions for patients with:
    1. Chronic low self-esteem.
    2. Risk for self-directed violence.
    3. Hopelessness.
    4. Disturbed sleep pattern.

18. The key medication for patients with manic episodes is:
    1. alprazolam (Xanax).
    2. fluoxetine hydrochloride (Prozac).
    3. lithium.
    4. benztropine mesylate (Cogentin).

19. The key problems for people with organic mental disorders stem from:
    1. speech and language impairments.
    2. anxiety disorders.
    3. conversion disorders.
    4. cognitive impairments.

20. Which herbal preparation is used by many people to relieve depression?
    1. Ephedra
    2. Ginkgo
    3. Ginseng
    4. St. John's wort

21. Which of the following are common physical signs and symptoms of anxiety? Select all that apply.
    1. Decreased heart rate
    2. Elevated blood pressure
    3. Sweaty palms
    4. Drowsiness
    5. Urinary frequency
    6. Diarrhea
    7. Ataxia
    8. A tight sensation in the chest
    9. Difficulty breathing
    10. Confusion

22. What are side effects of antianxiety medications that are associated with sedation? Select all that apply.
    1. Nausea
    2. Drowsiness
    3. Fatigue
    4. Dizziness
    5. Confusion
    6. Fever

23. Which of the following are typical symptoms of schizophrenia? Select all that apply.
    1. Feelings of panic
    2. Disturbed thought processes
    3. Delusions
    4. Hallucinations
    5. Bizarre behavior
    6. Disturbed emotional responses

24. Which of the following are side effects of drug therapy (antipsychotic and antiparkinsonian medications) used for patients with schizophrenia? Select all that apply.
    1. Agitation
    2. Akathisia (restlessness and inability to sit still)
    3. Orthostatic hypotension
    4. Extrapyramidal effects
    5. Neuroleptic syndrome
    6. Hypertensive crisis
    7. Agranulocytosis

25. Which are probable etiologic factors of mood disorders? Select all that apply.
    1. Childhood trauma
    2. Neuroendocrine dysfunction
    3. Genetic factors
    4. Learned helplessness
    5. Loss of significant others

26. Which are types of antidepressant medications used for mood disorders? Select all that apply.
    1. Benzodiazepines
    2. Tricyclic antidepressants
    3. Second-generation antidepressants
    4. Monoamine oxidase (MAO) inhibitors

27. Which are four levels of consciousness? Select all that apply.
    1. Sluggish
    2. Comatose
    3. Drowsy
    4. Alert
    5. Stuporous

28. The nurse asks the patient, "What do you mean when you say, 'The world is falling apart'?" Which strategy in a therapeutic relationship does this represent?
    1. Sharing observations
    2. Listening
    3. Clarifying
    4. Being available

29. The nurse says, "You are saying that your life is falling apart, and you are also smiling." This is an example of which therapeutic communication intervention?
    1. Sharing observations
    2. Listening
    3. Clarifying
    4. Being available

30. Which are the main elements of suicide risk assessment that are part of data collection in the mental status examination? Select all that apply.
    1. Suicidal ideation (thoughts)
    2. General intellectual level
    3. Plans for committing suicide
    4. Intention to carry out suicide

31. Why are benzodiazepines typically used at the initial phase of treatment for a patient with anxiety?
    1. They are the fastest-acting drugs.
    2. They reduce symptoms until other medications can take effect.
    3. They work well with patients who have depression as well as anxiety.
    4. They depress the central nervous system.

PART III: CHALLENGE YOURSELF!

J. Getting Ready for NCLEX.

Choose the most appropriate answer or select all that apply.

1. In addition to counseling the patient, what are ways to prevent and manage increasing anxiety? Select all that apply.
   1. Rise slowly from sitting position
   2. Relaxation techniques
   3. Warm baths
   4. Positive self-talk
   5. Physical exercise

2. The nurse is caring for a patient with manic episodes. Which patient problems would the nurse expect to see in this patient? Select all that apply.
   1. Altered thought processes related to delusions
   2. Altered nutrition: less than body requirements related to hyperactivity
   3. Ineffective coping related to dissociation
   4. Risk for violence directed at others related to low frustration tolerance

3. The nurse is taking care of a patient with depression. Which problems would the nurse expect to see in this patient? Select all that apply.
   1. Risk for self-directed violence related to episodes of anger and impaired judgment
   2. Risk for self-directed violence related to hopelessness
   3. Disturbed personal identity related to splitting
   4. Chronic low self-esteem related to negative feelings about self
   5. Anxiety related to severe stress

4. A patient with depression tells the nurse that he is thinking about killing himself. Which is the best therapeutic response of the nurse? Select all that apply.
   1. "Have you had any past suicide attempts?"
   2. "How do you plan to kill yourself?"
   3. "What has happened to you to make you want to kill yourself?"
   4. "Do you intend to carry out your plan to kill yourself?"
   5. "Have you told your family about your thoughts of killing yourself?"

Nursing Care Plan.

Refer to Nursing Care Plan, The Patient with Major Depression, p. 1316 in the textbook, and answer questions 5-7.

5. What is the priority nursing diagnosis?

6. Which data collected in the health history and physical examination indicate the presence of major depression?

   1. _____
   2. _____
   3. _____
   4. _____
   5. _____
   6. _____

7. Which are nursing interventions related to the nursing diagnosis Risk for self-violence related to suicidal feelings? Select all that apply.
   1. Encourage patient to improve hygiene.
   2. Provide sleep-producing measures such as small snacks, warm baths, and relaxation exercises before going to bed.
   3. Establish a no-harm contract.
   4. Take necessary suicide precautions.
   5. Remove dangerous objects from the environment.
   6. Maintain continuous one-to-one contact.
   7. Assist in identifying symbols of hope in this patient's life.
   8. Involve dietitian in planning an adequate diet.

Substance-Related Disorders

chapter

56

Go to http://evolve.elsevier.com/Linton/medsurg/ for additional activities and exercises.

NCLEX CATEGORIES:

Safe and Effective Care Environment:
Coordinated Care, Safety and Infection Control

Health Promotion and Maintenance

Psychosocial Integrity

Physiological Integrity: Basic Care and Comfort, Pharmacological Therapies, Reduction of Risk Potential, Physiological Adaptation

OBJECTIVES

1. Discuss the biologic, sociocultural, behavioral, and interpersonal theories of the cause of substance abuse or dependence.
2. Describe the data to be collected for the nursing assessment of a patient with substance abuse or dependence.
3. Describe alcohol dependence, alcohol withdrawal syndrome, medical complications of alcohol dependence, and treatment of alcohol abuse and dependence.
4. Discuss the pathophysiologic effects of frequently abused drugs.
5. Describe disorders associated with substance abuse and dependence.
6. Differentiate between drug abuse treatment and alcohol abuse treatment.
7. Describe the nursing diagnoses and interventions associated with substance abuse and dependence.
8. Discuss populations that present special problems in relation to drug abuse and dependency.

PART I: MASTERING THE BASICS

A. Key Terms.
Match the definition in the numbered column with the most appropriate term in the lettered column.

1. _____ Maladaptive pattern of substance use that differs from generally accepted cultural norms; sometimes referred to as *chemical abuse* or *drug abuse*

2. _____ Self-help support process outlining 12 steps to overcoming a physical or psychological dependence on something outside oneself that has a destructive impact on one's life

3. _____ Intense cravings for the substance on which one is dependent without physical withdrawal symptoms

4. _____ Effect of habitual ingestion of a substance to the point of physical dependence; used interchangeably with the term *dependence*

5. _____ Occurs when body cells are dependent on alcohol to carry out metabolic processes

6. _____ Ingestion of substances in gradually increasing amounts due to a physical need; used interchangeably with the terms *chemical dependence* and *drug dependence*

7. _____ Unpleasant and sometimes life-threatening physical substance-specific syndrome occurring after stopping or reducing the habitual dose or frequency of an abused drug

8. _____ Simultaneous existence of a major psychiatric condition and a medical condition

9. _____ Lifelong process of maintaining abstinence from the substance to which one is addicted; a return to moderate substance use is never the end result

10. _____ Exaggerated dependent pattern of self-defeating behaviors, beliefs, and feelings learned as a result of pathologic relationship to a chemically dependent, or otherwise dysfunctional, person

11. _____ Need for increasing amounts of a substance to achieve the same effect brought about by the original amount

A. Substance dependence
B. Substance abuse
C. Tolerance
D. Physical dependence
E. Dual diagnosis
F. Codependence
G. Psychological dependence
H. Withdrawal
I. Twelve-step program
J. Recovery
K. Addiction

B. Substance Abuse Complications.

Complete the statement in the numbered column with the most appropriate term in the lettered column. Some terms may be used more than once, and some terms may not be used.

1. A recent addition to the methods for the detection of abused substances is _____.

2. A complication of chronic alcoholism that is due to thiamine and niacin deficiencies, which contribute to the degeneration of the cerebrum and the peripheral nervous system, is _____.

3. The preferred way of screening for the recent use of an unknown drug is _____.

4. Occurs when alcohol becomes integrated into physiologic processes at the cellular level _____.

5. Legal intoxication in most states occurs when a person's blood alcohol level is _____.

6. Requires sensitive technology and can detect drugs for up to 1 year after use _____.

7. Bugs, snakes, and rats are commonly described by patients with _____.

8. A critical sign of withdrawal in substance abusers is _____.

9. A medical complication that may cause low birth weight and heart defects in newborn babies is _____.

10. The presence of amphetamines, barbiturates, marijuana, narcotics, and benzodiazepines can be identified with _____.

11. The most accurate type of test available to measure the degree of intoxication on initiation of treatment for alcohol abuse is _____.

A. Urine drug screening
B. Hypertension
C. 0.1%
D. Withdrawal
E. Hair analysis
F. Fetal alcohol syndrome
G. Hallucinations
H. Physical addiction
I. 0.05%
J. Korsakoff's psychosis
K. Blood alcohol
L. 1.0%

C. Defense Mechanisms.

Which descriptions of substance abusers are related to the patient's use of denial? Select all that apply.

1. Drug abusers insist that they became addicted to alcohol as a result of pressure to drink socially with colleagues so that colleagues would not think they were prudes

2. Abusers attempt to justify their abuse of substances, making an excuse for their addiction

3. Abusers focus only on objective facts as a way of avoiding dealing with unconscious conflicts and the emotions they evoke

4. Patients state that they do not have a problem with drug abuse despite evidence to the contrary

5. Patients state that they must use heroin because the drugs their doctor gave them for their back injuries were not working

6. People shift blame for their behavior on someone else

7. Individuals may minimize their substance abuse problems by maintaining that they can stay sober by themselves

D. Withdrawal.

A few patients may not experience any physical withdrawal symptoms despite a history of prolonged, frequent, and heavy substance abuse. Which factors may affect the incidence of withdrawal effects? Select all that apply.

1. Weight of the patient
2. Stage of addiction
3. Baseline physical status of the patient
4. Type of drugs being misused
5. Defense mechanisms used

E. Signs of Abuse.

Which of the following are physical characteristics of the appearance of the average substance abuser? Select all that apply.

1. Obese
2. Malnourished
3. Poorly cared for
4. Evidence of physical trauma
5. Peripheral neuropathy

F. Drug Therapy.

Match the description in the numbered column with the drug in the lettered column. Answers may be used more than once.

1. _____ Synthetic opioid analgesic that is sometimes prescribed for chronic severe pain

2. _____ Used for opioid detoxification

3. _____ Opioid antagonist

4. _____ Counteracts respiratory depressant effects of heroin and other opioid overdose

5. _____ Controversial substance as it constitutes substituting another addictive drug for the one misused by the patient

6. _____ Side effects include constipation and sweating

A. Methadone
B. Naloxone (Narcan)

PART II: PUTTING IT ALL TOGETHER

G. Multiple Choice/Multiple Response.

Choose the most appropriate answer or select all that apply.

1. The least likely way to alienate an already defensive patient is to use a manner that is matter-of-fact and:
   1. nonjudgmental.
   2. assertive.
   3. reassuring.
   4. positive.

2. It is believed that the cause of hangover symptoms is related to the buildup of acetaldehyde and lactic acid in the blood and to:
   1. hyperkalemia.
   2. hyponatremia.
   3. hypoglycemia.
   4. hyperthyroidism.

3. Substance abusers who are overly sensitive and use critical self-talk may be experiencing:
   1. Ineffective coping.
   2. Risk for injury.
   3. Knowledge deficit.
   4. Chronic low self-esteem.

4. The biggest issue for a substance abuser to be addressed at first during rehabilitation is:
   1. rationalization.
   2. sublimation.
   3. denial.
   4. compensation.

5. Which are behaviors that often lead to relapse for a substance abuser? Select all that apply.
   1. Overtiredness
   2. Detoxification
   3. Withdrawal
   4. Argumentativeness
   5. Depression
   6. Self-pity
   7. Decreased participation in AA meetings

6. Older individuals who abuse substances over an extended period of time may experience significant medical problems as a result of decreased ability to:
   1. circulate and absorb drugs.
   2. utilize and react to drugs.
   3. metabolize and excrete drugs.
   4. transport and detoxify drugs.

7. Patients taking antianxiety or antidepressant agents with alcohol may risk accidental overdose due to:
   1. antagonist effects.
   2. idiosyncratic effects.
   3. stimulant effects.
   4. additive effects.

8. Programs designed to offer a supportive alternative to health professionals addicted to a substance so that they do not have their licenses revoked are called:
   1. Alcoholics Anonymous.
   2. peer assistance programs.
   3. Codependents Anonymous.
   4. Al-Anon.

9. Which are characteristics that substance abusers frequently have? Select all that apply.
   1. Damaged relationships
   2. Poor circulation
   3. Dysfunctional grieving
   4. Erratic and unprovoked mood swings
   5. Blackouts
   6. Significant problems at work
   7. Decreased activity levels

10. Individuals with chronic alcoholism may require supplements of vitamin:
    1. C.
    2. K.
    3. B_6.
    4. E.

11. Which findings should be reported to the physician because they may indicate physical withdrawal from alcohol abuse?
    1. Mental status changes
    2. High blood pressure
    3. Tachycardia
    4. Nausea and vomiting

12. A patient who has abused alcohol or a benzodiazepine must be monitored for signs of physical withdrawal, because the patient may be at risk for:
    1. paranoia.
    2. seizures.
    3. violence.
    4. euphoria.

13. Which drug is not identified in urine drug screening?
    1. Methadone
    2. Amphetamines
    3. Benzodiazepines
    4. Cocaine

14. Which supplements may be given to individuals with chronic alcoholism?
    1. Beta carotene and vitamin E
    2. Iron and vitamin C
    3. Folate and vitamin B_6
    4. Calcium and vitamin D

15. Which are symptoms of patients with an overdose of depressants? Select all that apply.
    1. Irritability
    2. Oversedation
    3. Respiratory depression
    4. Impaired coordination
    5. Hyperactivity
    6. Brain damage

16. Which of the following are stimulants? Select all that apply.
    1. Amphetamines
    2. Cocaine
    3. Barbiturates
    4. Hypnotics

17. A patient is dependent on barbiturates. What may happen if the patient abruptly stops taking these drugs?
    1. Rebound sedation
    2. Oversedation
    3. Psychosis
    4. Depression

18. Which are signs and symptoms of chronic inhalation of cocaine? Select all that apply.
    1. Runny nose
    2. Weight gain
    3. Hyperactivitiy
    4. Hypotension

19. Hyperactivity, irritability, combativeness, and paranoia are symptoms of the use of:
    1. opioids.
    2. depressants.
    3. anxiolytics.
    4. amphetamines.

20. Which are effects of opioids on substance abusers? Select all that apply.
    1. Stimulation
    2. Dilated pupils
    3. Analgesia
    4. Euphoria
    5. Restlessness
    6. Paranoia
    7. Sedation

21. Which is a common effect of xanthines (caffeine) and nicotine?
    1. Euphoria
    2. Poor judgment
    3. Stimulation
    4. Relaxation

22. Which substance produces euphoria?
    1. Alcohol
    2. Caffeine
    3. Nicotine
    4. Amphetamine

23. Which signs are related to a patient who abuses alcohol? Select all that apply.
    1. Incoordination
    2. Constipation
    3. Constricted pupils
    4. Slurred speech
    5. Nausea and vomiting
    6. Dysrhythmias
    7. Damage to kidneys

PART III: CHALLENGE YOURSELF!

H. Getting Ready for NCLEX.

Choose the most appropriate answer or select all that apply.

1. Which are goals of an intervention for an impaired nurse? Select all that apply.
    1. Assist the impaired nurse to receive treatment.
    2. Protect the public from an untreated nurse.
    3. Terminate employment of the impaired nurse.
    4. Help the recovering nurse reenter nursing in a planned, safe way.
    5. Assist in monitoring the continued recovery of the nurse for a period of time.

2. Usually there is a 2-year time period after intervention for an impaired nurse to comply with the peer assistance process. Which are steps to be accomplished by the impaired nurse in this 2-year period? Select all that apply.
    1. The nurse is required to attend AA or NA groups regularly.
    2. The nurse participates in peer support groups.
    3. The nurse meets routinely with an identified support person representing the peer assistance program.
    4. The nurse must report how substance abuse impaired his/her practice to the state board of nursing.
    5. The nurse submits random urine drug screens to ensure that no relapse has occurred.

3. Which of the following problems of a substance abuser put him at risk for injury? Select all that apply.
    1. Ineffective problem-solving and series of self-perpetuating crises
    2. Refusal to acknowledge actual consequences of substance abuse
    3. Excessive use of the drug and risk for relapse
    4. Driving while under the influence
    5. Returning to places where one used drugs
    6. Using substances to deal with anxiety, emotional discomfort, and stress

4. When patients abusing alcohol state that they can quit easily and that they do not have a problem, they may be experiencing:
    1. Chronic low self-esteem.
    2. Ineffective denial.
    3. Risk for injury.
    4. Impaired verbal communication.

5. Substance abusers who have driven under the influence of drugs and who engage in excessive drug use are at risk for:
    1. infection.
    2. injury.
    3. aspiration.
    4. activity intolerance.

6. Which are significant neurologic signs that may be associated with nutritional deficits in the substance abuser? Select all that apply.
   1. Paranoia
   2. Euphoria
   3. Confusion
   4. Memory loss
   5. Tremors
   6. Lack of coordination

7. Which of the following are typical stressors of aging that may cause older adults to use or abuse alcohol for the first time? Select all that apply.
   1. Cognitive decline
   2. Retirement
   3. Losses of significant others
   4. Confusion
   5. Family conflict
   6. Health problems
   7. Social isolation
   8. Loss of self-worth

Nursing Care Plan.
Refer to Nursing Care Plan, The Patient Abusing Alcohol, p. 1329 in the textbook, and answer questions 8-11.

8. What is the priority nursing diagnosis for this patient?

9. Which data collected in the health history and the physical examination indicate a problem of alcohol abuse? Select all that apply.
   1. Blood pressure 128/72 mm Hg
   2. Found lying on the floor at home, passed out
   3. Long history of alcohol abuse, but claims he does not have a problem, because he only drinks beer
   4. Lost his job due to tardiness at work
   5. Children are afraid of him when he drinks
   6. Pulse 80 bpm
   7. Respirations 20/min
   8. Yellowish tinge to eyes and skin
   9. Appears thin and wasted
   10. Age 37 years old

10. Which physical characteristics of this patient show evidence of substance abuse? Select all that apply.
    1. Malnourished
    2. Poorly cared for
    3. Evidence of physical trauma
    4. Jaundice

11. Which of the following is evidence of ineffective denial in this patient?
    1. Found lying on the floor at home
    2. Long history of alcohol abuse
    3. States he does not have problem with alcohol because he drinks beer
    4. Recently lost his job for not reporting to work on time

Notes

Notes